Geriatric Psychiatry Review and Exam Preparation Guide

A CASE-BASED APPROACH

T0256138

Geriatric psychiatry is a relatively young discipline within the field of psychiatry in North America. And with an aging population, developing a workforce that is equipped to meet the mental health needs of older adults is an urgent priority.

Geriatric Psychiatry Review and Exam Preparation Guide offers geriatric psychiatrists, general psychiatrists, and other healthcare workers a detailed and up-to-date reference that can be used to prepare for ward rounds, in case discussions, in educational sessions with patients and families, or for exam preparation. Experts from across Canada have contributed chapters on dementia; mood, anxiety, and other disorders; and other issues and topics unique to working with older adults and their caregivers. Each chapter includes a case scenario, concise point-form summaries of diagnostic and treatment approaches, up-to-date evidence syntheses, discussions of controversies, a series of practical and thought-provoking questions and answers, and recommended resources for further reading. The result is a succinct and advanced review of geriatric psychiatry that will help clinicians improve the psychiatric care of an aging population.

MARK J. RAPOPORT is an associate professor in the geriatric psychiatry division of the Department of Psychiatry at the University of Toronto. He is also an associate scientist at Sunnybrook Health Sciences Centre and President of the Canadian Academy of Geriatric Psychiatry.

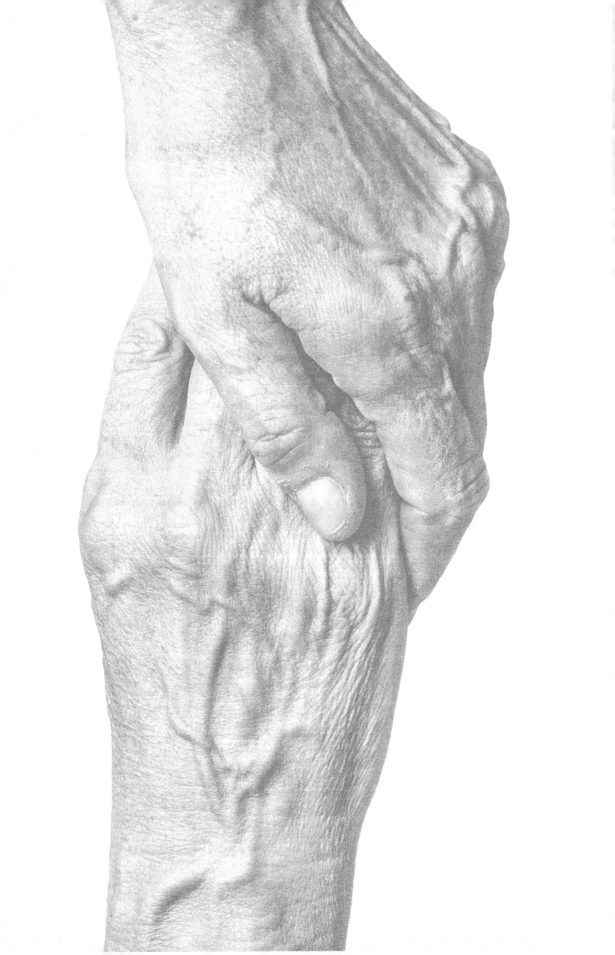

Geriatric Psychiatry Review and Exam Preparation Guide

A CASE-BASED APPROACH

EDITOR
Mark Rapoport

ASSOCIATE EDITORS
Dallas Seitz, Andrew Wiens, and Evan Lilly

UNIVERSITY OF TORONTO PRESS
Toronto Buffalo London

ISBN 978-1-4875-0088-7 (cloth)   ISBN 978-1-4426-2827-4 (paper)

Library and Archives Canada Cataloguing in Publication

Geriatric psychiatry review and exam preparation guide : a case-based approach /
editor, Mark Rapoport ; associate editors, Dallas Seitz, Andrew Wiens, and Evan Lilly.

Includes bibliographical references.
ISBN 978-1-4875-0088-7 (cloth).   ISBN 978-1-4426-2827-4 (paper)

1. Geriatric psychiatry – Examinations, questions, etc.   I. Rapoport, Mark, 1970–, editor

RC451.4.A5G47 2016   618.97'6890076   C2016-906500-6

University of Toronto Press acknowledges the financial assistance to its publishing program of the
Canada Council for the Arts and the Ontario Arts Council, an agency of the Government of Ontario.

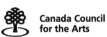

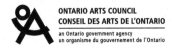

In recognition of their significant contributions to geriatric psychiatry in Canada, this book is dedicated to the past-presidents of the Canadian Academy of Geriatric Psychiatry, Drs Joel Sadavoy, Ken Le Clair, Marie-France Rivard, David Conn, Martha Donnelly, and Kiran Rabheru, in addition to Drs Melissa Andrew and Cathy Shea who ushered the profession through the crucial final stages culminating in the recognition of the subspecialty by the Royal College of Physicians and Surgeons of Canada.

A personal and heartfelt dedication to Dr Mark Rapoport's grandmother, Marjorie Detsky, who provided much love and inspiration in her devotion to successful aging for 93 years.

Contents

Foreword   ix

Acknowledgments   xi

Disclaimer   xiii

Introduction   3

SECTION 1: DEMENTIA

1.1 Neurobiology and Diagnosis of the Dementias   7

1.2 The Cognitive Examination in Geriatric Psychiatry   34

1.3 Neuropsychiatric Symptoms in Dementia   47

1.4 Nonpharmacological Management of Neuropsychiatric Symptoms of Dementia   64

1.5 Pharmacologic Treatment of Dementia: The Cognitive Enhancers   78

SECTION 2: MOOD AND ANXIETY DISORDERS

2.1 Recognition and Assessment of Depression in Older Adults   99

2.2 Bereavement in Older Adults   111

2.3 Pharmacotherapy of Depression in Older Adults   124

2.4 Bipolar Disorder in Older Adults   138

2.5 Anxiety Disorders in Older Adults   150

2.6 Electroconvulsive Therapy in Older Adults   164

2.7 Psychotherapy in Older Adults   181

2.8 Suicide among Older Adults   206

SECTION 3: OTHER DISORDERS

3.1 Primary Psychotic Disorders in Older Adults   231

3.2 Delirium in Older Adults   242

3.3 Sleep Difficulties and Disorders in Older Adults, and Their Management   261

3.4 Personality Disorders in Older Adults   289

3.5 Neuropsychiatric Disorders in Older Adults   300

SECTION 4: SPECIAL TOPICS

4.1 Epidemiology of Mental Illness in Older Adults   317

4.2 Aging and Psychopharmacology   332

4.3 Antipsychotics in Older Adults   342

4.4 Anticholinergic Drugs and Inappropriate Medications in Older Adults   356

4.5 Psychosocial Aspects of Care in Geriatric Psychiatry   364

4.6 Palliative Care in Geriatric Psychiatry   386

4.7 What Else?   396

Abbreviations   399

Authors and Affiliations   405

Disclosures   407

Foreword

In the relatively short period of time that has been the span of my career, I have seen the field of geriatric psychiatry grow rapidly into a subspecialty of psychiatry replete with its separate set of examinations both in the United States and most recently in Canada. Indeed, when I was a senior resident in psychiatry in the late 1970s, the few geriatric psychiatrists in Canada were imported from England. Canadian psychiatrists like Ken Shulman needed to travel there for their geriatric training because England was leading the field of geriatric psychiatry in the 1960s and 70s at the Maudsley Hospital with Felix Post and at the University of Nottingham with Tom Arie and many others. I was the beneficiary of this British connection by completing the first geriatric psychiatry fellowship in Canada in 1981 with Ken Shulman. Recalling my training, I was blessed with outstanding supervision from Ken but outside of the clinical experience, there was very little formal geriatric focused evidence-based literature to guide clinical practice.

When I look at this unique text book and study guide of almost 500 pages and the breadth and depth of available evidence today, it is absolutely staggering to see the difference in 34 years. This text and study guide is encyclopedic in scope. I am particularly struck by our increased understanding of the dementias and their classification, their behaviour and psychiatric sequelae, and the available bio/psycho/social approaches to treating these patients and supporting their caregivers. One quarter of the book is devoted to this topic.

In recent years, I have spent most of my time in the field of academic education exploring continuing professional development, and life-long and self-directed learning. Using my educator's lens, I would like to make a few comments on the utility of this textbook as a vehicle for teaching and learning.

Managing the knowledge explosion in medicine is one the biggest challenges for busy clinicians in practice. When a teacher/educator can synthesize a field of knowledge in point form, make complicated problems simpler, provide test questions with their answers, and contextualize the information with practical cases, frontline clinicians will cheer. I believe that is what this text succeeds in doing. It is on the one hand very comprehensive and on the other hand practical and practice-based.

There are multiple ways a learner or a teacher can use this text. A teacher can use the cases at the beginning of each chapter to lead small group discussions for medical students or residents. A family physician, psychiatrist, or geriatric psychiatrist can use the simple-to-read point form text and related tables as quick reference points to answer clinical questions "just-in-time" when the patient might still be in their office. A study group of residents, fellows, or psychiatrists preparing for their geriatric psychiatry examinations can use the entire text, especially the short-answer questions, their answers, and the references as a study guide.

Although written with physicians in mind, I think because of the bio-psycho-nature of the evidence presented and the related approaches to treatment, the text will also be of interest to the entire interprofessional geriatric psychiatry team – nurses, pharmacists, social workers, occupational therapists, physiotherapists, and recreational therapists. Indeed, the text would be an ideal reference and study guide for in-service teaching for the healthcare team. I also feel this text is international in scope. Learners and teachers will use this text for practice and study wherever geriatric psychiatry is practised.

The challenge for the editors going forward will be keeping the information updated. Knowing how rapidly new evidence for diagnosis and treatment is accumulating in the field and to maintain its prominence as *the* study guide for geriatric psychiatry, the editors will need to consider revising the text over time, or consider providing an e-text format that might make rapid revisions feasible. I think this text would also do very well in an app format, making it available on popular hand-held computers.

Congratulations to Editor Mark Rapoport and Associate Editors Dallas Seitz, Andrew Wiens, and Evan Lilly for their work planning and editing this outstanding teaching and learning resource. We are all learners and we are all teachers throughout our careers, working with the mentally ill who are elderly and their families. This text will facilitate our teaching and learning, and our patients and their families will be the beneficiaries.

Ivan Silver, MD, Med, FRCPC
Vice-President Education
Centre for Addiction and Mental Health
Professor, Department of Psychiatry
Faculty of Medicine
University of Toronto

Acknowledgments

The chapter authors would like to acknowledge the contributions of the following clinicians and researchers who provided ideas, suggestions, and peer-review for the content: Drs Rayan K. Al Jurdi, David Arciniegas, Nick Delva, Martha Donnelly, Alastair Flint, Caroline Gosselin, Adrian Grek, Zahinoor Ismail, Ron Keren, Marcus Law, Molyn Leszcz, Mario Masellis, Scott McCullagh, David Oslin, Kiran Rabheru, Ram Randhawa, Joel Sadavoy, David Streiner, Gayla Tennen, Lilian Thorpe, Zenovia Ursuliak, and Ari Zaretsky.

We are also grateful to the board members of the Canadian Academy of Geriatric Psychiatry from 2012 to the present, as well as the participants in our educational initiatives, to the Canadian Electroconvulsive Therapy Survey (CANECTS) group (www.canects.org), and to Eric Carlson, Stephen Shapiro, Lisa Jemison, Carolyn Zapf, and the staff of the University of Toronto Press.

The DSM-IV-TR and DSM-5 are summarized throughout the text but not reproduced.[1]

---

1 American Psychiatric Association. Diagnostic and statistical manual of mental disorders. 4th ed., text rev. (DSM-IV-TR). Washington, DC: APA; 2000; American Psychiatric Association. Diagnostic and statistical manual of mental disorders, 5th ed. (DSM-5). Washington, DC: APA; 2013.

Disclaimer

The case scenarios are anonymous conflations of the clinical experiences of the faculty and resemblance to actual patients, living or dead, events or settings are entirely coincidental. All efforts have been made to ensure that this book is as up-to-date as possible, but delays between writing and publishing should be taken into account by the reader. Any updates, should they be required, will be available at http://www.utppublishing.com/Geriatric-Psychiatry-Review-and-Exam-Preparation-Guide-A-Case-Based-Approach.html.

The assessment and treatment recommendations provided represent the views of the authors, and should not be taken to be an official position of the Canadian Academy of Geriatric Psychiatry or as a standard of practice. General readers are advised to seek medical advice, and not to rely on this book for self-diagnosis or treatment/prescription recommendations.

Geriatric Psychiatry Review and Exam Preparation Guide

A CASE-BASED APPROACH

Introduction

Geriatric psychiatry is a relatively young discipline within the field of North American psychiatry, with specialized organizations founded in the United States only since 1978, and in Canada since 1991. Ours is a discipline of complexity and uncertainty, and our colleagues in general psychiatry often lack the expertise and confidence in dealing with many of the mental health problems arising in older adulthood. After decades of lobbying the Royal College of Physicians and Surgeons of Canada to recognize geriatric psychiatry, official subspecialty status was granted to our discipline in 2011. In the United States, geriatric psychiatrists have had this designation for many years, and thus the bar is now set higher across North America for geriatric psychiatrists. For new trainees in Canada, a mandatory two years of training is required, as well as an examination. For geriatric psychiatrists already practising, the training has been "grandfathered," but not the examination. From 2012 to 2016, the Canadian Academy of Geriatric Psychiatry (CAGP) held five national review courses in three different provinces, both to help its members consolidate the vast array of knowledge in geriatric psychiatry and to help them feel prepared for an examination. Most of our members had not written examinations in decades! Expert faculty from across Canada who had no part in creating the examinations devoted much time to preparing concise, practical, clinically relevant, academic, and up-to-date summaries of the literature in their areas of interest, with little remuneration but with a considerable amount of gratitude from the membership. The CAGP also launched a popular asynchronous online study group and online course in which participants interacted with each other and the faculty on short-answer questions, practical clinical dilemmas, and broader areas of controversy.

The Institute of Medicine in the United States and the Mental Health Commission of Canada have emphasized the importance of developing a workforce to meet the mental health needs of older adults. Despite the advent of the cholinesterase inhibitors, a cure for Alzheimer's disease seems far off, with several recent disappointing clinical trials. Diagnostic categorization in psychiatry continues to be ever-shifting and somewhat out of touch with the clinical reality of our complex patients. There is an increasing appreciation for an expanding array of adverse effects of psychopharmacological agents, at the same time as novel approaches for treatment optimization are coming to light. New evidence-based psychotherapies are showing promise in the face of earlier pessimism about the ability of older adults to change thoughts and behaviour, although the literature in this regard is still in its infancy. Service delivery is increasingly taking centre stage, with recognition of the importance of specialized skills for management of behavioural disturbances in complex settings.

There is much for us to learn about the expert care of older adults. The geriatric psychiatrist must assess and treat patients today in face of the limitations of what we know, but also be armed with enthusiasm to create novel ways of impacting on the quality of life of patients with mental illness later in life that will help our patients and colleagues now and in the future. We are drawn to this work because of the richness of our patients' life histories, their complex medical and neurological comorbidities, and a desire to understand the meaning of older adult life and impact positively on its trajectory.

This book sprouted from the enthusiasm of faculty, participants, and residents who were eager for concise summaries of material. Physicians tend to be busy clinicians, administrators, and educators with little time for reading textbook material. The faculty involved with our educational initiatives readily agreed to summarize their material for this volume in order to help geriatric psychiatrists, general psychiatrists, other physicians, and trainees obtain a quick reference for up-to-date understanding of the knowledge base needed to meet the mental health needs of older adults.

A case scenario begins each chapter, emphasizing challenging aspects of topics in geriatric psychiatry. After brief introductions provided by the editors, the chapters include concise point-form summaries of diagnostic and treatment approaches, including up-to-date evidence and a brief discussion of controversies. A series of questions follows the point-form summary. These include short-answer questions and questions highlighting broader conceptual or controversial issues. Each chapter has a section titled "Recommended Resources for Review." Although these resources may not be specifically cited in the text, their approach informed the contents of the chapter, and they are recommended as useful further reading.

Our guide is intended for psychiatrists and other physicians and residents who are interested in a succinct, detailed, and up-to-date review of psychiatry at an advanced level. The book may be used to prepare for ward rounds, in case discussions with colleagues or supervisors, in educational sessions with patients and families, or for exam preparation.

Section one of the book is devoted to dementia. Chapters in this section discuss the neurobiology and diagnosis of dementia and mild cognitive impairment, the cognitive examination in geriatric psychiatry, neuropsychiatric symptoms in dementia, pharmacotherapy for the cognitive symptoms in dementia, and a nonpharmacological approach to the treatment of neuropsychiatric symptoms in dementia. Section two of the book focuses on mood and anxiety disorders. Chapters in this section focus on depression, bereavement, bipolar disorder, anxiety disorders, electroconvulsive therapy, psychotherapy, and suicide. Section three provides a review of other disorders including psychotic disorders, delirium, sleep disorders, personality disorders, and neuropsychiatric disorders. Special topics covered in the fourth section include epidemiology, psychopharmacology, antipsychotics, anticholinergic and other inappropriate drugs, consent and capacity, psychiatry in long-term care and community settings, caregiver burden, elder abuse and neglect, and palliative care. We have added a final chapter that includes helpful review references for topics not covered in the text.

I would finally like to acknowledge the contribution of Associate Editors Dallas Seitz and Andrew Wiens, who donated their time to edit many of the chapters in this text, and contributed countless hours of meetings for this book and for the educational initiatives from which the book originated. Special thanks to all faculty who contributed chapters for the book, as well as to the peer reviewers. The book would not exist without the support of the CAGP board and secretariat, as well as the attendees and participants in the CAGP educational initiatives who contributed creative ways of answering the difficult questions posed, and former medical student (now graduated) Evan Lilly, who meticulously assisted with the process of summarizing these and the final formatting.

Mark Rapoport, MD, FRCPC

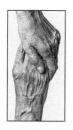

SECTION 1: DEMENTIA

1.1 Neurobiology and Diagnosis of the Dementias

Andrew Wiens, MD, FRCPC

INTRODUCTION

The dementias characterize a key difference between geriatric psychiatry and the rest of psychiatry. The aging population has also made these disorders more commonly seen by clinicians. Geriatric psychiatrists "share" these disorders with geriatric medicine, neurology, and family medicine, though we will focus on the behavioural effects of dementia more than other specialties do. In recent years, diagnostic systems have been updated to include current research findings that differentiate one disorder from another; these findings have also been included in the DSM-5. This chapter covers clinically relevant diagnostic features for the more common dementias that can help guide clinicians' assessment of these patients.

CASE SCENARIO

A 73-year-old man whom a geriatric psychiatrist had treated five years ago for depression was referred back to him. The patient was seen with his wife. She describes her husband as making embarrassing comments when out in public and having a heightened sex drive. She adds that he has been paranoid, thinking that items he had misplaced were stolen by other people, and has alienated some friends and family members because of this behaviour. He believes people on television speak to him, and is driven to eat when he sees food commercials. She notes he has been forgetful and has word-finding problems. Activities of daily living (ADLs) and instrumental activities of daily living (IADLs) are impaired. His Mini Mental State Examination (MMSE) was 26 a year earlier, losing points for attention and calculations, and his GP started him on donepezil, currently 10 mg QAM, but his wife has not noticed any change. A CT scan done six months ago showed perivascular patchiness, but no notable changes otherwise, and was read as being consistent with age.

1. What is the differential diagnosis?
2. What other information is needed to make the correct diagnosis?

OVERVIEW

1. Normal Cognitive Aging
(Harada, Natelson Love, & Triebel, 2013)

Declines with age
- Processing speed: yes
- Attention
  - Simple tasks: no
  - Complex tasks: yes
- Memory
  - Episodic (autobiographical): lifelong decline
  - Semantic (general knowledge): may improve in some; decline in late-life
  - Procedural: unchanged
- Language
  - In general: no
  - Visual confrontation naming, verbal fluency: yes
- Visuospatial function
  - Simple tasks: no
  - Complex tasks: yes
- Executive function
  - Concept formation, abstraction, and mental flexibility: yes, especially after age 70
  - Inductive reasoning: declines after age 45
  - Similarities, proverbs, reason about familiar material: stable

2. DSM-5 Neurocognitive Disorder (NCD)
(American Psychiatric Association, 2013; McKhann et al., 2011)

Decline in one or more of the following:
- Complex attention (sustained, divided, selective; processing speed)
- Executive function
- Learning and memory
- Language
- Perceptual-motor (includes visuoperceptive, visuoconstructive, perceptual-motor, praxis, and gnosis)
- Social cognition (recognition of emotions, theory of mind)

Decline must be:
- For mild NCD: "modest" [refers to 1–2 SD below norms (3rd to 16th percentile)]
- For major NCD: "significant" [refers to > 2 SD below norms (< 3rd percentile)]
- Not explained by a number of other factors capable of ↓ cognition
- Specify severity:
  - Mild NCD: independent; may need accommodation
  - Major NCD: ↓ independence – code severity
    - Mild: ↓ IADLs

- ▪ Moderate: ↓ basic ADLs
- ▪ Severe: fully dependent

3. Some Objective Assessments
(Albert et al., 2011)

- Memory: Rey Auditory Verbal Learning Test
- Executive function: Trail Making Test, Parts A and B
- Attention: digit span forward
- Language: Boston naming test, letter and category fluency
- Visuospatial abilities: figure copying
- Social cognition: recognition of emotions, theory of mind story cards

4. Clinical Screens That Test Multiple Cognitive Domains

See chapter 2.

5. Specifiers

5.1 Causal Specifiers

Specify whether due to:
- Alzheimer's disease (AD)
- Frontotemporal lobar degeneration (FTLD)
- Lewy body disease
- Vascular disease
- Traumatic brain injury
- Substance/medication use
- HIV infection
- Prion disease
- Parkinson's disease
- Huntington's disease
- Another medical condition
- Multiple etiologies
- Unspecified

If "major NCD," code medical etiology as well

5.2 Behavioural Specifiers

- Without behavioural disturbance
- With behavioural disturbance (specify disturbance):
  - Psychotic symptoms
  - Mood disturbance
  - Agitation
  - Apathy
  - Other behavioural symptoms

6. Mild Cognitive Impairment
(Loewenstein et al., 2009; Molano et al., 2010; Petersen et al., 2009; Petersen, 2011)

- Approximates mild NCD in DSM-5 (American Psychiatric Association, 2013)

6.1 Epidemiology of Mild Cognitive Impairment (MCI)

- A decline in cognitive function beyond normal
- Prevalence: 10–20% > 65 years
- Progression to dementia:
    - Community: 5–10%/year
    - Specialty clinic: 10–15%/year
- Reversion to normal: up to 25–30%/year

6.2 Neuropathology of MCI

- 60% have evidence of Alzheimer's
- Vascular disease is significant
- Non-amnestic form: less common and may be early form of non-Alzheimer's dementia, e.g., frontotemporal dementia (FTD) or Lewy body

6.3 Factors Predicting More Rapid Progression in MCI
(Petersen, 2011)

- Increased clinical severity: closer to dementia threshold
- Apo ε4 carrier status: however, routine testing not recommended
- Atrophy on MRI: 2–3x rate if hippocampus volume ≤ 25th vs ≥ 75th percentile
- Fluorodeoxyglucose (FDG) positron emission tomography (PET) pattern of AD: temporal and parietal hypometabolism
- Cerebrospinal fluid (CSF) markers compatible with AD: low $A\beta42$ and elevated tau
- Positive amyloid imaging: using Pittsburgh compound B

6.4 Neuropsychiatric Manifestations in MCI
(Apostolova & Cummings, 2008; Panza et al., 2010; Teng, Lu, & Cummings, 2007)

- Common: reported in 35–75%
- Similar to those seen in AD: depression, apathy, anxiety, and irritability
- May identify subgroup with prodromal AD, especially depression and apathy

7. Dementia in Canada
(Canadian Study of Health and Aging, 1994; Canadian Study of Health and Aging Working Group, 2000; Lindsay et al., 2004)

Prevalence:
- Doubles every ~5 years
- 8% > 65 years
    - Ages 65 to 74: 2.4%
    - Ages 75 to 84: 11.1%
    - Ages 85+: 34.5%
- Females > males

8. Neuropathology of Dementia
(Schneider et al., 2007)

Fifty autopsy cases of dementia from a sample set of 141

- 30% were found to have AD (atrophy, plaques, tangles) with no additional pathology
- 54% AD with additional pathology
  - 38% AD + infarcts
  - 12% AD + Parkinson's disease/Lewy body disease
  - 4% AD + infarcts + Parkinson's disease/Lewy body disease
- 16% No AD
  - 12% infarcts
  - 2% Parkinson's disease/Lewy body disease
  - 2% other (tumours, amyloid angiopathy, and hemorrhages)

9. Four Syndromes Encapsulate Most of Dementia

- AD: episodic memory, word/way finding
- Frontotemporal dementia (FTD): younger onset
- Parkinson's disease dementia (PDD)/dementia with Lewy bodies (DLB)
- Vascular dementia: vascular risk factors, focal signs, temporal relationship

10. Alzheimer's Disease (AD)
(Knopman et al., 2001; Mayeux, 2010)

- A progressive degenerative disease
- Average 7–10 years from onset of symptoms to death

Incidence (Canadian Study of Health and Aging, 1994):

- 5% of population over 65
- 1% between 60 and 70 years
- Doubles every 5 years
- 6–8% at 85 or older

10.1 Neurocognitive Disorder Due to AD
(American Psychiatric Association, 2013)

- Meets DSM-5 major or mild NCD
- Progressive ↓ in ≥ 1 domain for mild NCD, and ≥ 2 domains in major NCD
- Rank probability
  - Major NCD due to AD:
    - For probable, requires:
      - Known mutation, or
      - ↓ Memory and learning + 1 other domain (usually visuoconstructional/ perceptual-motor ability, and language), progressive decline without extended plateau, and not mixed etiology
    - If above not met: possible

- Mild NCD due to AD:
  - Probable: known mutation
  - Possible: requires ↓ memory and learning, progressive decline without extended plateau, and not mixed etiology
- Not better explained by other NCD

10.2 Variant AD Syndromes
(Alladi et al., 2007; Crutch et al., 2012; Snowden et al., 2007; Warren, Fletcher, & Golden, 2012)

- Non-amnestic focal cortical syndromes secondary to AD pathology
- Do not fit conventional AD criteria
- Epidemiology poorly defined: screens usually emphasize memory so can miss these variants
- Of AD with onset:
  - > 65: 5% are variant
  - < 65: 1/3 are variant
- Effect of current treatments unknown

10.2.1 Posterior Cortical Atrophy

- Also known as visual or bi-parietal variant of AD
- Progressive decline in visuospatial and/or visuoperceptive abilities, literacy, and praxic skills in various combinations
- Parieto-occipital atrophy with relative sparing of medial temporal lobes
- F > M, low incidence of family history, present in middle age
- Pathology: > 80% AD, some corticobasilar atrophy, DLB, prion diseases

10.2.2 Frontal AD

- Frontal > posterior deficits: more behavioural changes
- Frontal, anterior temporal atrophy
- Tend to be younger, M > F, strong family history
- More likely to have memory difficulty and delusions/hallucinations and agitation than FTD (Mendez et al., 2013)

10.2.3 Logopenic Variant Primary Progressive Aphasia (lvPPA)

- Prolonged word-finding pauses, impaired auditory verbal short-term memory → more difficulty in repeating and comprehending sentences than single words
- Temporoparietal and posterior temporal atrophy
- Pathology: > 60% AD, some FTD

10.2.4 Rapid Progressive AD

- > 3 point ↓MMSE/6 months
- 10% of AD

- Predictors
  - Demographics
    - High educational attainment
    - Younger age of onset
    - Male
  - Clinical characteristics
    - Severe cognitive impairment at onset
    - Medical problems: poor nutritional, diabetes mellitus (DM)
    - Neurologic: focal signs, seizures, signs of DLB
    - Psychotic symptoms: e.g., delusions, hallucinations (primarily visual)
    - Cortical signs: apraxia
    - Subcortical signs: e.g., apathy, deficits in executive function and attention
    - Behavioural: e.g., aggression, agitation, wandering
  - Genetic: *APOE4* positive, *PSEN1*, *BuChE*, and others
- Many potential causes, including Creutzfeldt-Jakob (reportable in Canada)
- If diagnosis remains uncertain: refer to specialty settings
- Known AD with faster-than-expected clinical decline should be reassessed for co-morbid conditions

10.2.5 *Other Variants*
(Gauthier et al., 2012; Warren, Fletcher, & Golden, 2012; Schmidt et al., 2011; Stopford et al., 2007; Gauthier et al., 2006)

- Younger onset
  - < 5% of AD
  - Usually more rapid progression
  - More severe visuospatial, attention, executive deficits
- Distinct memory profiles: working memory, visual recall, verbal recall, recognition, and personal memory can break down separately
- Markedly slow progression: more often pure amnestic

10.3 *If Prominent, These Features Suggest Something Other than Alzheimer's*
(Kawas, 2003)

- Abrupt onset, stepwise deterioration: vascular dementia (VaD)
- Prominent behaviour changes: FTD
- Profound apathy: FTD
- Prominent aphasia: FTD, VaD
- Progressive gait disorder: VaD, hydrocephalus
- Prominent fluctuations in levels of consciousness or cognitive abilities: delirium; DLB; seizures
- Hallucinations or delusions: delirium; DLB
- Extrapyramidal signs or gait: Parkinsonian syndromes, VaD
- Eye-movement abnormalities: progressive supranuclear palsy (PSP), Wernicke's encephalopathy

10.4 Alzheimer Dementia Risk Factors

10.4.1 Non-Modifiable Risk Factors
(Bertram & Tanzi, 2008; Farlow, 2007; Patterson et al., 2007)

MCI

Age

Female sex

Genetics

- 1° relative with AD ~4x risk
- Downs
- Early-onset AD: *APP, PSEN1, PSEN2*
  - Age of onset: 30 to 60
- Late-onset AD: *APOE4*
  - Gene on chromosome 19
    - 3 alleles: ε2, ε3, ε4
      - Allele ε4: 20% population
        - ε4/ε4: 50% risk AD in 60s
        - ε4 heterozygote: 50% risk in 70s
  - APOE screening *not recommended* due to low sensitivity/specificity and low +ve and −ve predictive values

Many others of little or unknown significance

10.4.2 Potentially Modifiable

Worldwide estimates of potentially attributable risk of developing Alzheimer's are shown in Figure 1.1.1 (last bar on graph adjusts for overlap between listed factors; Norton et al., 2014).

Figure 1.1.1: Worldwide Estimates of Potentially Attributable Risk of Developing Alzheimer's Disease

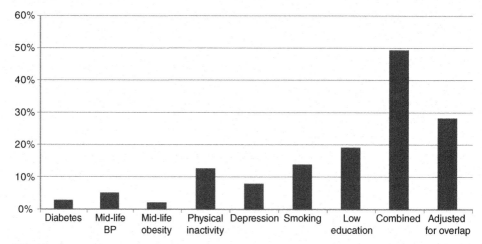

BP = blood pressure
Adapted from Norton et al., 2014.

10.5 Alzheimer's Dementia Protective Factors ~½ Risk
(Williams et al., 2010)

10.5.1 Lifestyle

- Cognitive engagement: multiple activities/socialization
- Head protection
- Mediterranean diet
- Moderate wine intake? There is no current consensus (Piazza-Gardner, Gaffud, & Barry, 2013)

10.5.2 Medications

- Avoid non-steroidal anti-inflammatory drugs (NSAIDs), acetylsalicylic acid (ASA), steroids (Jaturapatporn et al., 2012)
- Avoid estrogen with progesterone

10.6 Pathology of AD
(Dickson, 2009a)

- Senile plaques composed of:
  - Extra-cellular protein deposits
    - Amyloid:
      - α-secretase ➔ γ-secretase: aβ40
      - β-secretase ➔ γ-secretase: aβ42 ➔ toxic effect initiates pathophysiologic cascade
    - Non-amyloid: APOE, clusterin, complement
  - Dystrophic neurites
  - Reactive glia: astrocytes and microglia
- Neurofibrillary tangles display a gradually spreading distribution (Braak stage) that correlates with cognitive decline. Also seen in some normals, but confined to medial temporal lobe
- Amyloid angiopathy: can lead to lobar hemorrhages

10.7 Mixed Vascular/AD

- Mixed pathology of AD is common (Dickson, 2009a; Bugiani, 2004; Haan et al., 1999)
- Age associated with higher frequency of mixed pathology in AD

10.8 Major Neurochemical Changes in AD
(Perry et al., 1978; Rodríguez-Puertas et al., 1997; Whitehouse et al., 1982)

10.8.1 Acetylcholine

- Loss of cholinergic neurons in basal forebrain
- Decline in choline acetyltransferase (ChAT) activity
- Depletion of acetylcholine (especially mod-severe stage)
  - Reduced acetyl cholinesterase
  - Reduced butyryl cholinesterase

10.8.2 Glutamate

- Primary excitatory neurotransmitter
- Normal activity: role in pathways associated with learning and memory via long-term potentiation
- Hyperexcitation in Alzheimer's:
  - Neuronal toxicity
  - May impair learning

11. Frontotemporal Lobar Degeneration (FTLD)
(Feldman et al., 2003; Freedman, 2007; Neary, Snowden, & Mann, 2005; Pereira et al., 2009; Seelaar et al., 2011)

- FTLD refers to the neuropathologic findings; FTD refers to the clinical presentation
- Characterized by progressive behavioural changes and frontal executive deficits and/or selective language difficulties
- Clinical picture determined by location of atrophy
- Early onset: ages 45–65 (range 21–85)
  - Tends to affect people in prime of life = disproportionate impact on families and society
  - 10% of FTD have onset at > 70 years
- 5% of patients with dementia referred to Canadian dementia centres
  - 12% of those before age 70: 2nd most common after AD
  - 2% of those after age 70
- Lasts 6–8 years (3 in FTD with motor neuron disease [FTD-MND])

11.1 DSM-5 Possible Major or Mild Frontotemporal Neurocognitive Disorder
(American Psychiatric Association, 2013)

- Meets DSM-5 major or mild NCD
- Progressive decline
- Two types:
  - Behaviour variant:
    - ↓ social cognition and/or executive abilities, plus
    - 2 or more of the following:
      - Disinhibition
      - Apathy
      - Loss of empathy
      - Perseverative, stereotyped, or compulsive behaviour
      - Hyperorality
  - Language variant: prominent decline in language abilities
- Mostly spared learning and memory, and perceptual-motor
- Not explained by a number of other factors capable of ↓ cognition
- For "probable": add known mutation or imaging evidence, otherwise "possible"

11.2 FTLD: Clinical Neuropathology (Simplified)

(Chare et al., 2014; Loy et al., 2014; Masellis et al., 2013; Seelaar et al., 2011; Rascovsky et al., 2011)

11.2.1 Behavioural Variant FTD (bvFTD)

- Accounts for half of cases
- ~One-third familial
- Atrophy bilateral (or R) orbitofrontal

11.2.2 Language Variant; Primary Progressive Aphasia (PPA)

- Accounts for half of cases
- < 10%, predominantly left-sided pathology

11.2.2.1 NON-FLUENT/AGRAMMATIC VARIANT PPA (NFPPA)
- Atrophy: left posterior frontotemporal

11.2.2.2 SEMANTIC VARIANT PPA (SVPPA)
- Atrophy: bilateral anterior temporal (L > R)

11.3 FTD Is Frequently Misdiagnosed

(Mendez et al., 2007)

Initial diagnosis 2 years before formal diagnosis of FTD

- 47% FTD
- 27% Psychiatric
    - 11% Depression/bipolar
    - 5% Psychosis
    - 4% Anxiety
    - 4% Personality disorder
    - 3% Adjustment disorder
- 12% Alzheimer's
- 7% Neurological disorder
- 7% Unknown

11.4 Neurotransmitter Deficits in FTD

(Huey, Putnam, & Grafman, 2006; Kaye et al., 2010)

- Consistent: post-synaptic serotonin deficit
- Some evidence for dopaminergic deficit
- Cholinergic system is relatively spared
- Little research in noradrenaline, glutamate or γ-aminobutyric acid (GABA)

11.5 Other Illnesses Associated with FTD

(Mathew, Bak, & Hodges, 2012)

11.5.1 FTD-MND (Motor Neuron Disease)

- Degeneration of bulbar (brain-stem) neurons and anterior horn cells
- Associated with bvFTD and svPPA

11.5.2 Corticobasilar Degeneration Syndrome (CBS)

- Motor: akinetic rigidity +/− dystonia and myoclonus
- Sensorimotor: asymmetric apraxia +/− alien limb syndrome (in ~50%)
- Cognitive: aphasia +/− frontal deficits, and can overlap with…

11.5.3. Progressive Supranuclear Palsy (PSP)

- Symmetric with vertical gaze palsy
- Both CBS and PSP can be associated with bvFTD and nfPPA

12. Dementia with Lewy Bodies (DLB)

12.1 DSM-5 NCD with Lewy Bodies
(American Psychiatric Association, 2013; McKeith et al., 2005)

- Meets major or minor NCD
- Probability:
    - Probable: > 2 core or 1 core + > 1 suggestive
    - Possible: any one of core or suggestive
- Core features:
    - Fluctuating cognition: can be difficult to differentiate from delirium
    - Recurrent well-formed and detailed visual hallucinations
    - Spontaneous Parkinsonism with onset after cognitive ↓
- Suggestive features:
    - Rapid eye movement (REM) sleep behaviour disorder
    - Severe neuroleptic sensitivity: D2 blockers; in ~50%
- Exclusion: a number of other factors capable of ↓ cognition

12.2 Other Features of DLB
(Galasko, 2007; McKeith et al., 2005)

12.2.1 Neuropsychiatric

- Hallucinations in other modalities
- Systematized delusions: usually related to visual hallucinations
- Depression: can be very severe

12.2.2 Autonomic Impairment

- Orthostatic hypotension
- Repeated falls and syncope: due to carotid sinus sensitivity
- Transient unexplained loss of consciousness
- Abnormal metaiodobenzylguanidine scintigraphy: cardiac autonomic denervation

12.2.3 Diagnosis Less Likely

- Evidence of cerebrovascular disease: focal neurologic signs or on brain imaging

- Sufficient physical illness or brain disorder to account for the clinical picture
- Parkinsonism only appears for the first time at a stage of severe dementia

12.3 Parkinson's Disease Dementia
(Ballard, Kahn, & Corbett, 2011; McKeith et al., 2004; McKeith, 2007)

12.3.1 Dementia in Parkinson's

- In about 30–80%
- Mean of 10 years into Parkinson's
- One year rule: Parkinson's disease occurred one or more years before onset of cognitive decline

12.3.2 Differences between PDD and DLB

- Age of onset, temporal course, and possibly levodopa responsiveness
- More attention deficits in DLB
- More postural instability and gait difficulties in DLB
- Only 2/3 of DLB have Parkinsonian symptoms, and are more often symmetrical
- More severe reaction antipsychotics in DLB

12.3.3 DSM-5 Major or Mild NCD Due to Parkinson's Disease
(American Psychiatric Association, 2013)

- Meets DSM-5 major or mild NCD
- Gradual decline
- Established Parkinson's
- Probability:
    - Probable: both of…; Possible: one of…
        - No mixed etiology
        - Parkinson's came first
- Not explained by a number of other factors capable of ↓ cognition

12.4 Pathology of PDD and DLB
(Dickson, 2009b; Taipa, Pinho, & Melo-Pires, 2012; Tröster, 2008)

- Two clinical phenotypes of disorders due to alpha-synuclein accumulation in the form of:
    - Lewy bodies: large spherical cytoplasmic inclusions
    - Lewy neurites: smaller curvilinear or dot-shaped processes represent the bulk of alpha-synuclein
- Display a brain-stem to cortex progression:
    - PDD: greater nigral neuron loss (maybe due to disease severity and duration)
    - DLB: greater cortical amyloid deposition

13. Vascular Dementia/Vascular Cognitive Impairment (VaD/VCI)
(Pendlebury & Rothwell, 2009; Sahathevan, Brodtmann, & Donnan, 2012)

Cognitive disorder caused by vascular lesions
Clinical features depend on location and size of lesion

- Epidemiology:
  - Mixed (VaD and AD +/or other): 25 to > 50% of dementias
- Post-stroke dementia:
  - 10% had dementia before first stroke (2 × normal)
  - 10% of first stroke survivors (excludes pre-existing)
  - 1/3 of recurrent stroke survivors

13.1 DSM-5 Major or Mild Vascular NCD
(American Psychiatric Association, 2013)

1. Meets DSM-5 major or mild NCD
2. Sufficient cerebrovascular disease (Hx, exam, +/or imaging)
- Either of:
  - Temporal relationship between 1 and 2 above
  - Decreased complex attention and executive function
- Probability:
  - Probable: ≥ 1 of…; Possible: no imaging or none of….
    - a. Sufficient changes on imaging
    - b. Temporally related
    - c. Clinical and genetic evidence
- Exclusion: other brain disease or systemic disorder

13.1 Vascular Cognitive Impairment: Risk Factors
(Gorelick & Nyenhuis, 2013)

- Demographic factors
  - Advancing age
- Lifestyle factors
  - Low education
  - ? Diet (antioxidants, fish oil, vitamin D, B-vitamins, Mediterranean diet, and moderate alcohol)
  - Lack of physical activity/exercise
  - Obesity
  - Smoking
  - Lack of social support/networks
- Depression?
- Physiologic factors
  - Hypertension
  - Hyperglycemia, insulin resistance, metabolic syndrome, and diabetes mellitus
  - ? Hyperlipidemia
- Concomitant clinical vascular disease
  - Coronary artery disease
  - Stroke
  - Chronic kidney disease

– Atrial fibrillation
– Peripheral arterial disease
– Low cardiac output

13.2 Mechanisms of Brain Injury and Vascular Distribution in VCI
(O'Brien et al., 2003; O'Brien, 2006; Román, 2003)

Mechanisms range from predominantly cortical to typically subcortical

13.2.1 Hemorrhagic

• Hypertension, cerebral amyloid angiopathy, subarachnoid hemorrhage, subdural hemorrhage

13.2.2 Ischemic

• Large vessel (usually acute)
  – Post-stroke
  – Multi-infarct dementia (cortical +/or subcortical)
  – Strategic single artery, e.g., posterior cerebral artery, anterior cerebral artery, angular gyrus
• Small vessel
  – Strategic single lacune, e.g., thalamic, head of caudate, genu of internal capsule
  – Subcortical ischemic
    ▪ Occlusion: lacunar
    ▪ Stenosis: Binswanger (most common type)
      - Cerebral autosomal-dominant arteriopathy with subcortical infarcts and leukoencephalopathy (CADASIL)
• Mixed

13.3 Selected Clinical Presentations

13.3.1 Lacunar Infarcts
(Norrving, 2008)

• Can cause clinically evident stroke at strategic sites
  – Pure motor hemiparesis
  – Pure sensory stroke
  – Sensorimotor stroke
  – Dysarthria-clumsy hand syndrome
  – Ataxic hemiparesis
• But > 25% of > 70 years have silent lacunar infarcts
  – > 90% subcortical
  – Associated with subtle declines in cognition
  – Increases risk of further vascular events, cognitive decline, dementia

13.3.2 Binswanger's Syndrome
(Chui, 2007; Swartz, Sahlas, & Black, 2003)

Combination of:
- Slowly progressive decline in cognition and gait, and early urinary incontinence
- Severe, confluent white matter changes
  - Diffuse atrophy and confluent white matter changes help differentiate from normal pressure hydrocephalus
  - Moderate or severe involvement of cholinergic pathways by white matter signal hyperintensities in 60% of subjects with probable vascular dementia
- Often vascular risk factors but no history of stroke or transient ischemic attack (TIA)
- Cognitive changes due to damage on neural feedback loop with frontal cortex and can mimic FTD:
  - Executive function ↓ without language impairment
  - Mild memory problems: retrieval deficits, cueing helps
  - Psychomotor retardation

Psychiatric manifestations:
- Late-life depression ("vascular depression"): less guilt, tearfulness, and suicidality
- Apathy
- Pseudobulbar palsy or "emotional incontinence"

Movement/gait disorders help differentiate from FTD and AD
- Parkinsonism, especially lower body
- Bilateral hyperreflexia, may have upgoing toes (positive Babinski?)
- "Frontal gait": feet stuck to floor

14. Dementias Due to Medical Conditions

DSM-5 has specific criteria for bolded conditions including "Another Medical Condition" (American Psychiatric Association, 2013)

- Neurologic: **Huntington's**, PSP, intracranial lesions, normal pressure hydrocephalus (NPH), **trauma**
- Metabolic disorders: toxic, metabolic, endocrine, nutritional
- Medications or other substances
- Inflammatory: multiple sclerosis, vasculitis
- Infectious processes: syphilis, **HIV**, other viral, fungal, **prion**
- Cancer: primary, metastatic, paraneoplastic
- Multiple etiologies

These may be reversible or stopped if recognized and treated early.

14.1 Clues Suggesting a Medical Cause
(Agronin, 2008)

- Sudden or rapid onset and/or progression of cognitive decline, including new confusion, delirium
- Younger age than expected

- Recent illness or chronic illness before onset: cancer, surgery, unexplained change
- History of trauma or toxic exposure, including substance abuse
- Predominant frontal and/or subcortical symptoms
- Onset of focal neurologic symptoms
- Family history of dementia subtype

15. Evaluation of Dementia
(Larson et al., 1986)

92.2% of diagnoses made by history, physical and neurological exam; improved accuracy with family interview

Main use of lab work-up was to identify coexisting illness

Screening for dementia
- No evidence for routine screening
- Perhaps best for > 70–75 years of age?
- Ask about changes in functioning (American Psychiatric Association 2013; Lawton & Brody, 1969)
- Basic ADL affected (DSM-5 moderate severity)
    - Dressing
    - Eating (weight loss)
    - Ambulation
    - Toileting
    - Transferring from bed or chair
    - Hygiene, grooming
- Instrumental ADL (DSM-5 mild severity)
    - **S**hopping (food or clothes)
    - **H**ousework/hobbies
    - **A**ccounting and managing finances
    - **F**ood preparation
    - **T**ransportation/telephone
        - Includes: driving problems and getting lost

Not due to other conditions…
- Delirium
- Drugs (recent changes): sedatives, anti-cholinergics
- Disease
    - Infections, especially urinary tract infection (UTI), upper respiratory tract
    - Pain (falls, fractures, ulcers)
    - Dehydration, weight loss
    - Incontinence or constipation
    - Sensory impairment
    - Hypothyroidism
- Depression or other psychiatric illness

15.1 Lab Testing and Imaging

15.1.1. Recommended Lab Testing
(Gauthier et al., 2012)

- Recommended tests in all:
    - Serum Na, K, Ca, fasting glucose
    - Complete blood count (CBC)
    - B12
    - Thyroid stimulating hormone (TSH)
- Additional tests depending on presentation
- Insufficient evidence to support serum homocysteine
- Biomarkers: none improve accuracy over clinical diagnosis, thus far

15.1.2 Image if...
(Gauthier et al., 2012)

- Age < 60
- Rapid unexplained decline (1–2 months) of cognition or function
- Short duration of dementia (< 2 years)
- Recent head trauma
- Unexplained central nervous system (CNS) symptom (new onset headaches, seizures, etc.)
- Past history of carcinoma
- Use of anticoagulants/history of bleeding disorder
- History of urinary incontinence and gait disorder early in course
- Any new localizing sign
- Unusual or atypical cognitive symptoms or presentation (e.g., progressive aphasia)
- Gait disturbance
- See Table 1.1.1 for the clinical uses of imaging

15.2 Other Testing

15.2.1 Neuropsychological Assessment
(Jacova et al., 2007)

- Should be used selectively in clinical settings as one element in the clinical work-up of dementia
- May aid in:
    - Distinction between normal aging, MCI, and early dementia
    - Addressing risk of progression from MCI to dementia
    - Differential diagnosis of dementia and other syndromes of cognitive impairment
    - Determining if there has been progression of cognitive impairment or development of new impairment(s) to assist in management

Table 1.1.1: Clinical Uses of Imaging

Clinical Situation	CT	MRI	SPECT/PET
MCI		Cortical and hippocampal atrophy (predictive of AD)	
AD	Cortical atrophy, medial temporal lobe atrophy (MTA: need special orientation) Cerebral amyloid angiopathy (CAA)	MTA – but not specific to AD Parietal atrophy Lobar microbleeds (MB): in cortical white-grey interface suggesting CAA	Bilateral temporoparietal hypometabolism
VCI	White matter changes: severity Lacunes Hemorrhages Rule out subdural hemorrhage (SDH)	White matter hyperintensities > 25% of white matter Lacunes, esp. if bilateral, in dominant hemisphere, and involving association cortex Non-lobar MB: in deep-brain structures Large vessel disease: territorial and watershed infarcts Serial MRI to track atrophy	
FTD		Specific atrophy patterns for bvFTD, nfPPA, svPPA	Differentiate from AD
Other	Rule out treatable causes, secondary dementias: neoplasms, SDH, NPH, infectious-inflammatory diseases of CNS	PSP Reduced ant-post diameter of midbrain Reduced volume of cerebral peduncles: hummingbird sign InflammationPrion disease	DLB: functional impairment of primary visual cortex PDD/DLB: Loss of dopamine uptake

AD = Alzheimer's disease; bvFTD = behavioural variant frontotemporal dementia; CNS = central nervous system; CT = computerized tomography (scan); DLB = dementia with Lewy bodies; FTD = frontotemporal dementia; MB = microbleeds; MCI = mild cognitive impairment; MRI = magnetic resonance imaging; nfPPA = non-fluent primary progressive aphasia; NPH = normal pressure hydrocephalus; PDD = Parkinson's disease dementia; PET = positron emission tomography; PSP = progressive supranuclear palsy; SPECT = single-photon emission computerized tomography; svPPA = semantic variant primary progressive aphasia; VCI = vascular cognitive impairment
Adapted from Herholz, 2011; Pasi, Poggesi, & Pantoni, 2011; Wattjes, 2011.

15.2.2 Predictive Genetic Testing
(Hsiung & Sadovnick, 2007)

- Predictive testing with pre- and post-test counselling can be offered to those "at risk" related to individual with mutation
  - 1st degree relatives: children and siblings
  - 1st cousins: if common ancestors (parents who were siblings) died before average age of onset of dementia in the family
  - Nieces or nephews: if common ancestors (parents who were siblings) died well before average age of onset of dementia in the family
- Not recommended for APOE screening due to low sensitivity/specificity

QUESTIONS

1. List five features that suggest a diagnosis other than Alzheimer's disease.
2. How would you differentiate between the four more common dementia syndromes, and what is the clinical impact of this differentiation?
3. List five atypical presentations of Alzheimer's disease and some practical reasons for identifying these variations.
4. List five features suggestive of behavioural variant frontotemporal dementia.
5. List five clues that suggest a medical "cause" of dementia.
6. List five reasons to order CT or MRI imaging in dementia.
7. What is episodic memory, how do you test for it, and why is it important?

ANSWERS

1. The table below provides a list of features suggesting a diagnosis other than Alzheimer's disease, in addition to the diagnostic consideration.

Feature	Diagnostic Consideration
Abrupt onset, stepwise deterioration	VaD
Prominent behaviour changes	FTD
Profound apathy	FTD
Prominent aphasia	FTD, VaD
Progressive gait disorder	VaD, NPH
Prominent fluctuations in levels of consciousness or cognitive abilities	Delirium; DLB; seizures
Hallucinations or delusions	Delirium; DLB
Extrapyramidal signs or gait	Parkinsonian syndromes, VaD
Eye-movement abnormalities	PSP, Wernicke's encephalopathy

DLB = dementia with Lewy bodies; FTD = frontotemporal dementia; NPH = normal pressure hydrocephalus; PSP = progressive supranuclear palsy; VaD = vascular dementia

2. In order to differentiate between the four more common dementia syndromes, the following features should be considered:
- Primarily cortical
    - Alzheimer's: episodic memory, word/way finding (visuospatial deficit)
    - Frontotemporal dementia: younger onset
        - *Behaviour*: bvFTD: behaviour, social-emotional skills deficits, early onset
        - *Language*: Primary progressive aphasia (2 types)
            - svPPA: deficit in semantic knowledge or emotional meaning
            - nfPPA: deficit in motor speech and language flency
        - Subcortical (or mixed)
            - PDD/DLB
                - PDD: dementia not early

      ◦ DLB: fluctuation in attention, visual hallucinations, parkinsonism
      - VaD: vascular risk factors, focal signs, temporal relationship
- The clinical importance: these disorders vary in terms of
  - Investigations
  - Genetic risk
  - Prognosis
  - Treatment

3. Atypical presentations of Alzheimer's disease include the following:
   - Posterior cortical atrophy (also known as visual or bi-parietal variant of AD):
     - Progressive decline in visuospatial and/or visuoperceptive abilities, literacy, and praxic skills in various combinations
     - Parieto-occipital atrophy with relative sparing of medial temporal lobes
     - F > M, low incidence of family history, present in middle age
     - Pathology: > 80% AD, some corticobasilar atrophy, DLB, prion diseases
   - Frontal AD:
     - Frontal > posterior deficits: more behavioural changes
     - Frontal, anterior temporal atrophy
     - Tend to be younger, M > F, strong family history
   - Logopenic variant primary progressive aphasia (lvPPA):
     - Prolonged word-finding pauses, impaired auditory verbal short-term memory → more difficulty in repeating and comprehending sentences than single words
     - Temporoparietal and posterior temporal atrophy
     - Pathology: > 60% AD, some FTD
   - Younger onset:
     - < 5% of AD
     - Usually more rapid progression
     - More severe visuospatial, attention, executive deficits
   - Rapid progressive AD: > 5 point ↓ MMSE/yr
     - 10% of AD
     - Severe cognitive impairment at onset
     - Medical problems: poor nutritional, DM
     - Neurologic: focal signs, seizures, signs of DLB
     - Psychotic symptoms: e.g., delusions, hallucinations (primarily visual)
     - Cortical signs: apraxia
     - Subcortical signs: e.g., apathy, deficits in executive function and attention
     - Behavioural: e.g., aggression, agitation, wandering
   - Rationale:
     - Atypical variants need a more in-depth evaluation than typical Alzheimer's and justify referral to specialized clinics if you don't feel comfortable in their management
     - Some provide rationale for genetic testing (early onset types) and family counselling

– Provides rationale for considering acetylcholinesterase inhibitors and possibly memantine

4. Features suggestive of behavioural variant frontotemporal dementia (bvFTD) include the following:

(Note that disinhibition and apathy/inertia are the common presentations. Stereotypies discriminate FTD well from non-FTD dementias.)

Early behavioural disinhibition
– Socially inappropriate behaviour
– Loss of manners or decorum
– Impulsive, rash, or careless actions

Early apathy or inertia
– Apathy
– Inertia

Early loss of sympathy or empathy
– Diminished response to other's needs and feelings
– Diminished social interest, interrelatedness, or personal warmth

Early perseverative, stereotyped, or compulsive/ritualistic behaviour
– Simple repetitive movements
– Complex, compulsive, or ritualistic behaviours
– Stereotypy of speech: repeating words/phrases

Hyperorality and dietary changes
– Altered food preferences
– Binge eating, increased consumption of alcohol or cigarettes
– Oral exploration or consumption of inedible objects

5. Clues suggesting a medical "cause" of dementia include the following:
   • Sudden or rapid onset and/or progression of cognitive decline, including new confusion, delirium
   • Younger age than expected
   • Recent illness or chronic illness before onset: cancer, surgery, unexplained change
   • History of trauma or toxic exposure, including substance abuse
   • Predominant frontal and/or subcortical symptoms
   • Onset of focal neurologic symptoms
   • Family history of dementia subtype

6. Reasons to order CT or MRI imaging include the following:
   • Age < 60
   • Rapid unexplained decline (1–2 months) of cognition or function
   • Short duration of dementia (< 2 years)
   • Recent head trauma
   • Unexplained CNS symptom (new onset headaches, seizures, etc.)
   • Past history of carcinoma

- Use of anticoagulants/history of bleeding disorder
- History of urinary incontinence and gait disorder early in course
- Any new localizing sign
- Unusual or atypical cognitive symptoms or presentation (e.g., progressive aphasia)
- Gait disturbance

7. Episodic memory refers to the explicit (associated with conscious awareness) and declarative (can be consciously recalled) memory system used to remember a particular episode of your life, such as sharing a meal with a friend.
    - Episodic memory has been largely defined by what patients with medial temporal lobe lesions cannot remember relative to healthy individuals.
    - The core of the episodic memory system is the medial temporal lobe (MTL) and the hippocampus.
    - The MTL receives a pattern from the cortex representing sight, sound, taste, emotion, and thoughts that is processed and transferred to the hippocampus, where context is assigned.
        - Can be tested with the five-word or three-word part of the Montreal Cognitive Assessment (MoCA) and MMSE respectively. This is actually mainly testing the dominant side. The three words–three shapes test includes a similar test of visual episodic memory (non-dominant).
    - The frontal lobes are the other important part of episodic memory. They are responsible for acquisition, registration, encoding, and retrieval of information.
        - When information is not remembered even with multiple rehearsals, and retrieval demands have been minimized with the use of a multiple-choice recognition, a primary failure of storage (frontal lobe) is present.
        - In the MMSE, testing is accomplished by going over the three words up to six times, and recording how often it took; MMSE does not include recognition.
        - In the MoCA, the list is repeated twice, which doesn't quite discriminate well enough, although you will get clues on frontal lobe function in other areas of the test; MoCA does include recognition.
    - Episodic memory is important because it is a key deficit in Alzheimer's disease.

CASE DISCUSSION

1. Although this patient has memory problems, the most prominent features are the behavioural and personality change. The CT was unremarkable. A reasonable differential diagnosis would include the following:
    - Behavioural variant frontotemporal dementia (bvFTD)
    - Atypical Alzheimer's, as this patient is older, and only about one-quarter of FTD cases present over age 65, though behavioural manifestations usually start in the moderate stage
    - Frontal/executive dysfunction can have subcortical etiologies, though most have some motor or gait abnormality; no mention is made here, so it is perhaps not a factor, or certainly not prominent
    - Dementia with Lewy bodies (DLB); but the "paranoia" sounds more like misinterpretation

- Other disorders affecting the frontal lobes:
  - Vascular dementia: though CT changes are not sufficient
  - Alcoholism: not mentioned though
- Bipolar disorder

The main point is that a wide net has to be cast in this case due to the atypical features.

2. A medical history and medication profile are needed to complete the picture as this may suggest other possibilities. A sexual history would be important, because his heightened sex drive may have resulted in unprotected sex and catching an exacerbating infection.

   Usual lab work as per consensus guidelines, as this could pick up exacerbating factors.

   The atypicality gives reason to go more into depth with the evaluation. Tests more sensitive to frontal changes such as the Trail Making Test Part B, or if available, neuropsychological assessment. An MRI may be more likely to pick up atrophy and if available a SPECT scan (it is unlikely a PET scan would be available, but this could be suggested).

RECOMMENDED RESOURCES FOR REVIEW

Although these resources may not be specifically cited in the text, their approach informed the contents of the chapter, and they are recommended as useful further reading.

Budson AE, Solomon PR. New diagnostic criteria for Alzheimer's disease and mild cognitive impairment for the practical neurologist. Pract Neurol. 2012;12(2):88–96. http://dx.doi.org/10.1136/practneurol-2011-000145. Medline:22450454

Schott JM, Warren JD. Alzheimer's disease: mimics and chameleons. Pract Neurol. 2012;12(6):358–66. http://dx.doi.org/10.1136/practneurol-2012-000315. Medline:23144298

Snowden JS, Thompson JC, Stopford CL, et al. The clinical diagnosis of early-onset dementias: diagnostic accuracy and clinicopathological relationships. Brain. 2011;134(9):2478–92. http://dx.doi.org/10.1093/brain/awr189. Medline:21840888

REFERENCES

Agronin ME. Alzheimer disease and other dementias: a practical guide. 2nd ed. Philadelphia: Wolters Kluwer Health/Lippincott Williams & Wilkins; 2008.

Albert MS, DeKosky ST, Dickson D, et al. The diagnosis of mild cognitive impairment due to Alzheimer's disease: recommendations from the National Institute on Aging- Alzheimer's Association workgroups on diagnostic guidelines for Alzheimer's disease. Alzheimers Dement. 2011;7(3):270–9. http://dx.doi.org/10.1016/j.jalz .2011.03.008. Medline:21514249

Alladi S, Xuereb J, Bak T, et al. Focal cortical presentations of Alzheimer's disease. Brain. 2007;130(10):2636–45. http://dx.doi.org/10.1093/brain/awm213. Medline:17898010

American Psychiatric Association. Diagnostic and statistical manual of mental disorders (DSM-5). 5th ed. Washington, DC: American Psychiatric Association; 2013.

Apostolova LG, Cummings JL. Neuropsychiatric manifestations in mild cognitive impairment: a systematic review of the literature. Dement Geriatr Cogn Disord. 2008;25(2):115–26. http://dx.doi.org/10.1159/000112509. Medline:18087152

Ballard C, Kahn Z, Corbett A. Treatment of dementia with Lewy bodies and Parkinson's disease dementia. Drugs Aging. 2011;28(10):769–77. http://dx.doi .org/10.2165/11594110-000000000-00000. Medline:21970305

Bertram L, Tanzi RE. Thirty years of Alzheimer's disease genetics: the implications of systematic meta-analyses. Nat Rev Neurosci. 2008;9(10):768–78. http://dx.doi.org/ 10.1038/nrn2494. Medline:18802446

Bugiani O. Aβ-related cerebral amyloid angiopathy. Neurol Sci. 2004;25(0 Suppl 1):S1–2. http://dx.doi.org/ 10.1007/s10072-004-0204-9. Medline:15045608

Canadian Study of Health and Aging. Canadian study of health and aging: study methods and prevalence of dementia. CMAJ. 1994;150(6):899–913. Medline:8131123

Canadian Study of Health and Aging Working Group. The incidence of dementia in Canada. Neurology. 2000;55(1):66–73. http://dx.doi.org/10.1212/WNL.55.1.66. Medline:10891908

Chare L, Hodges JR, Leyton CE, et al. New criteria for frontotemporal dementia syndromes: clinical and pathological diagnostic implications. J Neurol Neurosurg Psychiatry. 2014;85(8):865–70. http://dx.doi.org/ 10.1136/jnnp-2013-306948. Medline:24421286

Chui HC. Subcortical ischemic vascular dementia. [Abstract]. Neurol Clin. 2007;25(3):717–40, vi. http://dx.doi .org/10.1016/j.ncl.2007.04.003. Medline:17659187

Crutch SJ, Lehmann M, Schott JM, et al. Posterior cortical atrophy. Lancet Neurol. 2012;11(2):170–8. http:// dx.doi.org/10.1016/S1474-4422(11)70289-7. Medline:22265212

Dickson DW. Neuropathy of dementia. Presentation at the 5th Canadian Conference on Dementia (CCD), Toronto, ON, 1–3 October 2009a.

– Neuropathology of non-Alzheimer degenerative disorders. Int J Clin Exp Pathol. 2009b;3(1):1–23. Medline:19918325

Farlow MR. Alzheimer's disease. Continuum (Minneap Minn). 2007;13(2):39–68. http://dx.doi.org/ 10.1212/01.CON.0000267235.69379.07

Feldman H, Levy AR, Hsiung GY, et al.; ACCORD Study Group. A Canadian cohort study of cognitive impairment and related dementias (ACCORD): study methods and baseline results. Neuroepidemiology. 2003;22(5):265–74. http://dx.doi.org/ 10.1159/000071189. Medline:12902621

Freedman M. Frontotemporal dementia: recommendations for therapeutic studies, designs, and approaches. Can J Neurol Sci. 2007;34(Suppl 1):S118–24.

Galasko DR. Dementia with Lewy bodies. Continuum (Minneap Minn). 2007;13 (2 Dementia):69–86.

Gauthier S, Patterson C, Chertkow H, et al. Recommendations of the 4th Canadian Consensus Conference on the Diagnosis and Treatment of Dementia (CCCDTD4). Can Geriatr J. 2012;15(4):120–6. http://dx.doi.org/ 10.5770/cgj.15.49. Medline:23259025

Gauthier S, Vellas B, Farlow M, et al. Aggressive course of disease in dementia. Alzheimers Dement. 2006;2(3):210–7. http://dx.doi.org/10.1016/j.jalz.2006.03.002

Gorelick PB, Nyenhuis D. Understanding and treating vascular cognitive impairment. Continuum (Minneap Minn). 2013;19(2 Dementia):425–37. Medline:23558487

Haan MN, Shemanski L, Jagust WJ, et al. The role of APOE epsilon4 in modulating effects of other risk factors for cognitive decline in elderly persons. JAMA. 1999;282(1):40–6. http://dx.doi.org/10.1001/jama.282.1.40. Medline:10404910

Harada CN, Natelson Love MC, Triebel KL. Normal cognitive aging. Clin Geriatr Med. 2013;29(4):737–52. http://dx.doi.org/10.1016/j.cger.2013.07.002. Medline:24094294

Herholz K. Perfusion SPECT and FDG-PET. Int Psychogeriatr. 2011;23(S2 Suppl 2):S25–31. http://dx.doi.org/ 10.1017/S1041610211000937. Medline:21729421

Hsiung GY, Sadovnick AD. Genetics and dementia: risk factors, diagnosis, and management. Alzheimers Dement. 2007;3(4):418–27. http://dx.doi.org/10.1016/ j.jalz.2007.07.010

Huey ED, Putnam KT, Grafman J. A systematic review of neurotransmitter deficits and treatments in frontotemporal dementia. Neurology. 2006;66(1):17–22. http://dx.doi.org/10.1212/01.wnl.0000191304.55196.4d. Medline:16401839

Jacova C, Kertesz A, Blair M, et al. Neuropsychological testing and assessment for dementia. Alzheimers Dement. 2007;3(4):299–317. http://dx.doi.org/10.1016/ j.jalz.2007.07.011

Jaturapatporn D, Isaac MG, McCleery J, et al. Aspirin, steroidal and non-steroidal anti-inflammatory drugs for the treatment of Alzheimer's disease. Cochrane Database Syst Rev. 2012;2:CD006378. Medline:22336816

Kawas CH. Clinical practice. Early Alzheimer's disease. N Engl J Med. 2003; 349(11):1056–63. http://dx.doi .org/10.1056/NEJMcp022295. Medline:12968090

Kaye ED, Petrovic-Poljak A, Verhoeff NP, et al. Frontotemporal dementia and pharmacologic interventions. J Neuropsychiatry Clin Neurosci. 2010;22(1):19–29. http://dx.doi.org/10.1176/jnp.2010.22.1.19. Medline:20160206

Knopman DS, DeKosky ST, Cummings JL, et al. Practice parameter: diagnosis of dementia (an evidence-based review). Report of the Quality Standards Subcommittee of the American Academy of Neurology. Neurology. 2001;56(9):1143–53. http://dx.doi.org/10.1212/WNL.56.9.1143. Medline:11342678

Larson EB, Reifler BV, Sumi SM, et al. Diagnostic tests in the evaluation of dementia: a prospective study of 200 elderly outpatients. Arch Intern Med. 1986;146(10):1917–22. http://dx.doi.org/10.1001/archinte .1986.00360220061012. Medline:3767535

Lawton MP, Brody EM. Assessment of older people: self-maintaining and instrumental activities of daily living. Gerontologist. 1969;9(3 Part 1):179–86. http://dx.doi .org/10.1093/geront/9.3_Part_1.179. Medline:5349366

Lindsay J, Sykes E, McDowell I, et al. More than the epidemiology of Alzheimer's disease: contributions of the Canadian Study of Health and Aging. Can J Psychiatry. 2004;49(2):83–91. Medline:15065741

Loewenstein DA, Acevedo A, Small BJ, et al. Stability of different subtypes of mild cognitive impairment among the elderly over a 2- to 3-year follow-up period. Dement Geriatr Cogn Disord. 2009;27(5):418–23. http://dx.doi.org/10.1159/000211803. Medline:19365121

Loy CT, Schofield PR, Turner AM, et al. Genetics of dementia. Lancet. 2014; 383(9919):828–40. http://dx.doi .org/10.1016/S0140-6736(13)60603-3. Medline:23927914

Masellis M, Sherborn K, Neto P, et al. Early-onset dementias: diagnostic and etiological considerations. Alzheimers Res Ther. 2013;5(Suppl 1):S7. http://dx.doi .org/10.1186/alzrt197. Medline:24565469

Mathew R, Bak TH, Hodges JR. Diagnostic criteria for corticobasal syndrome: a comparative study. J Neurol Neurosurg Psychiatry. 2012;83(4):405–10. http://dx.doi.org/10.1136/jnnp-2011-300875. Medline:22019546

Mayeux R. Clinical practice. Early Alzheimer's disease. N Engl J Med. 2010;362(23):2194–201. http://dx.doi .org/10.1056/NEJMcp0910236. Medline:20558370

McKeith I. Dementia with Lewy bodies and Parkinson's disease with dementia: where two worlds collide. Pract Neurol. 2007;7(6):374–82. http://dx.doi.org/10.1136/jnnp.2007.134163. Medline:18024777

McKeith I, Mintzer J, Aarsland D, et al. Dementia with Lewy bodies. International Psychogeriatric Association Expert Meeting on DLB. Lancet Neurol. 2004;3(1): 19–28. PMID 14693108

McKeith IG, Dickson DW, Lowe J, et al.; Consortium on DLB. Diagnosis and management of dementia with Lewy bodies: third report of the DLB Consortium. Neurology. 2005;65(12):1863–72. http://dx.doi.org/ 10.1212/01.wnl.0000187889.17253.b1. Medline:16237129

McKhann GM, Knopman DS, Chertkow H, et al. The diagnosis of dementia due to Alzheimer's disease: recommendations from the National Institute on Aging-Alzheimer's Association workgroups on diagnostic guidelines for Alzheimer's disease. Alzheimers Dement. 2011;7(3): 263–9. http://dx.doi.org/10.1016/j.jalz .2011.03.005. Medline:21514250

Mendez MF, Joshi A, Tassniyom K, et al. Clinicopathologic differences among patients with behavioral variant frontotemporal dementia. Neurology. 2013;80(6):561–8. http://dx.doi.org/10.1212/WNL .0b013e3182815547. Medline:23325909

Mendez MF, Shapira JS, McMurtray A, et al. Accuracy of the clinical evaluation for frontotemporal dementia. Arch Neurol. 2007;64(6):830–5. http://dx.doi.org/ 10.1001/archneur.64.6.830. Medline:17562930

Molano J, Boeve B, Ferman T, et al. Mild cognitive impairment associated with limbic and neocortical Lewy body disease: a clinicopathological study. Brain. 2010;133(Pt 2):540–56. http://dx.doi.org/10.1093/brain/ awp280. PMID: 19889717

Neary D, Snowden J, Mann D. Frontotemporal dementia. Lancet Neurol. 2005;4(11):771–80. http://dx.doi.org/ 10.1016/S1474-4422(05)70223-4. Medline:16239184

Norrving B. Lacunar infarcts: no black holes in the brain are benign. Pract Neurol. 2008;8(4):222–8. http:// dx.doi.org/10.1136/jnnp.2008.153601. Medline:18644908

Norton S, Matthews FE, Barnes DE, et al. Potential for primary prevention of Alzheimer's disease: an analysis of population-based data. Lancet Neurol. 2014;13(8):788–94. http://dx.doi.org/10.1016/S1474-4422(14) 70136-X. Medline:25030513

O'Brien JT. Vascular cognitive impairment. Am J Geriatr Psychiatry. 2006;14(9):724–33. http://dx.doi.org/ 10.1097/01.JGP.0000231780.44684.7e. Medline:16943169

O'Brien JT, Erkinjuntti T, Reisberg B, et al. Vascular cognitive impairment. Lancet Neurol. 2003;2(2):89–98. http://dx.doi.org/10.1016/S1474-4422(03)00305-3. Medline:12849265

Panza F, Frisardi V, Capurso C, et al. Late-life depression, mild cognitive impairment, and dementia: possible continuum? Am J Geriatr Psychiatry. 2010;18(2):98–116. http://dx.doi.org/10.1097/JGP.0b013e3181b0fa13. Medline:20104067

Pasi M, Poggesi A, Pantoni L. The use of CT in dementia. Int Psychogeriatr. 2011;23(S2 Suppl 2):S6–12. http:// dx.doi.org/10.1017/S1041610211000950. Medline:21729420

Patterson C, Feightner J, Garcia A, et al. General risk factors for dementia: A systematic evidence review. Alzheimers Dement. 2007;3(4):341–7. http://dx.doi .org/10.1016/j.jalz.2007.07.001

Pendlebury ST, Rothwell PM. Prevalence, incidence, and factors associated with pre-stroke and post-stroke dementia: a systematic review and meta-analysis. Lancet Neurol. 2009;8(11):1006–18. http://dx.doi.org/ 10.1016/S1474-4422(09)70236-4. Medline:19782001

Pereira JM, Williams GB, Acosta-Cabronero J, et al. Atrophy patterns in histologic vs clinical groupings of frontotemporal lobar degeneration. Neurology. 2009;72(19):1653–60. http://dx.doi .org/10.1212/WNL.0b013e3181a55fa2. Medline:19433738

Perry EK, Tomlinson BE, Blessed G, et al. Correlation of cholinergic abnormalities with senile plaques and mental test scores in senile dementia. BMJ. 1978;2(6150):1457–9. http://dx.doi.org/ 10.1136/bmj.2.6150.1457. Medline:719462

Petersen RC. Clinical practice. Mild cognitive impairment. N Engl J Med. 2011;364(23):2227–34. http://dx.doi .org/10.1056/NEJMcp0910237. Medline:21651394

Petersen RC, Roberts RO, Knopman DS, et al. Mild cognitive impairment: ten years later. Arch Neurol. 2009;66(12):1447–55. http://dx.doi.org/10.1001/archneurol .2009.266. Medline:20008648

Piazza-Gardner AK, Gaffud TJ, Barry AE. The impact of alcohol on Alzheimer's disease: a systematic review. Aging Ment Health. 2013;17(2):133–46. http://dx.doi .org/10.1080/13607863.2012.742488. Medline:23171229

Rascovsky K, Hodges JR, Knopman D, et al. Sensitivity of revised diagnostic criteria for the behavioural variant of frontotemporal dementia. Brain. 2011;134(9):2456–77. http://dx.doi.org/10.1093/brain/awr179. Medline:21810890

Rodríguez-Puertas R, Pascual J, Vilaró T, et al. Autoradiographic distribution of M1, M2, M3, and M4 muscarinic receptor subtypes in Alzheimer's disease. Synapse. 1997;26(4):341–50. http://dx.doi.org/ 10.1002/(SICI)1098-2396(199708)26:4 <341::AID-SYN2>3.0.CO;2-6. Medline:9215593

Román GC. Vascular dementia: distinguishing characteristics, treatment, and prevention. J Am Geriatr Soc. 2003;51(5 Suppl Dementia):S296–304. http://dx.doi .org/10.1046/j.1532-5415.5155.x. Medline:12801386

Sahathevan R, Brodtmann A, Donnan GA. Dementia, stroke, and vascular risk factors; a review. Int J Stroke. 2012;7(1):61–73. http://dx.doi.org/10.1111/j.1747-4949.2011.00731.x. Medline:22188853

Schmidt C, Wolff M, Weitz M, et al. Rapidly progressive Alzheimer disease. Arch Neurol. 2011;68(9):1124–30. http://dx.doi.org/10.1001/archneurol.2011.189. Medline:21911694

Schneider JA, Arvanitakis Z, Bang W, et al. Mixed brain pathologies account for most dementia cases in community-dwelling older persons. Neurology. 2007;69(24):2197–204. http://dx.doi.org/10.1212/ 01.wnl.0000271090.28148.24. Medline:17568013

Seelaar H, Rohrer JD, Pijnenburg YA, et al. Clinical, genetic and pathological heterogeneity of frontotemporal dementia: a review. J Neurol Neurosurg Psychiatry. 2011;82(5):476–86. http://dx.doi.org/10.1136/jnnp .2010.212225. Medline:20971753

Snowden JS, Stopford CL, Julien CL, et al. Cognitive phenotypes in Alzheimer's disease and genetic risk. Cortex. 2007;43(7):835–45. http://dx.doi.org/10.1016/S0010-9452(08)70683-X. Medline:17941342

Stopford CL, Snowden JS, Thompson JC, et al. Distinct memory profiles in Alzheimer's disease. Cortex. 2007;43(7):846–57. http://dx.doi.org/10.1016/S0010-9452(08) 70684-1. Medline:17941343

Swartz RH, Sahlas DJ, Black SE. Strategic involvement of cholinergic pathways and executive dysfunction: does location of white matter signal hyperintensities matter? J Stroke Cerebrovasc Dis. 2003;12(1):29–36. http://dx.doi.org/10.1053/jscd.2003.5. Medline:17903901

Taipa R, Pinho J, Melo-Pires M. Clinico-pathological correlations of the most common neurodegenerative dementias. Front Neurol. 2012;3:68. http://dx.doi.org/10.3389/fneur.2012.00068. Medline:22557993

Teng E, Lu PH, Cummings JL. Neuropsychiatric symptoms are associated with progression from mild cognitive impairment to Alzheimer's disease. Dement Geriatr Cogn Disord. 2007;24(4):253–9. http://dx.doi.org/ 10.1159/000107100. Medline:17700021

Tröster AI. Neuropsychological characteristics of dementia with Lewy bodies and Parkinson's disease with dementia: differentiation, early detection, and implications for "mild cognitive impairment" and biomarkers. Neuropsychol Rev. 2008;18(1):103–19. http://dx.doi.org/10.1007/s11065-008-9055-0. Medline:18322801

Warren JD, Fletcher PD, Golden HL. The paradox of syndromic diversity in Alzheimer disease. Nat Rev Neurol. 2012;8(8):451–64. Medline:22801974

Wattjes MP. Structural MRI. Int Psychogeriatr. 2011;23(S2 Suppl 2):S13–24. http://dx.doi.org/10.1017/ S1041610211000913. Medline:21729419

Whitehouse PJ, Price DL, Struble RG, et al. Alzheimer's disease and senile dementia: loss of neurons in the basal forebrain. Science. 1982;215(4537):1237–9. http://dx.doi.org/10.1126/science.7058341. Medline:7058341

Williams JW, Plassman BL, Burke J, et al. Preventing Alzheimer's disease and cognitive decline. Evid Rep Technol Assess (Full Rep). 2010;(193):1–727. Medline:21500874

1.2 The Cognitive Examination in Geriatric Psychiatry

Mark Rapoport, MD, FRCPC

INTRODUCTION

In geriatric psychiatry, the cognitive exam is relevant across many diagnoses and contexts. It is important to adapt the tools that are used to the individual patient, diagnosis, and context. A detailed interview including obtaining collateral information is a critical first step, but will not be covered in this chapter. In teaching the cognitive examination to psychiatry residents at the University of Toronto over the last twelve years, I have recognized significant challenges in encouraging trainees to conduct even a basic cognitive screening assessment in routine clinical practice, rather than deferring it. Furthermore, when the screening assessments are done, these are often relied on as diagnostic rather than simply screening. This chapter is an overview of approaches to screening as well as more detailed testing to highlight cognitive patterns associated with different cognitive diagnoses. More sophisticated neuroimaging techniques cannot replace these basic bedside skills. I developed this chapter with a view to a practical approach, with evidence where available, and some modest discussion of the functional neuroanatomical bases of cognitive domains.

CASE SCENARIOS

Included here is a brief series of practical questions based on vignettes and challenges about Mini Mental State Examination (MMSE) interpretation that come up regularly in clinical practice.

Scenario 1. Your patient has English as a second language (ESL) and speaks little English, but fluent Italian. She has right hemiplegia and cannot use her right hand to write. She would never be able to say "no ifs ands or buts," even without cognitive impairment, and the examiner could not administer write, copy, or the three-stage command. She scores perfectly on all other measures, except that she lost a point for date. How would one report this?

Scenario 2. Your patient scored 0/3 on recall and 5/10 on orientation. The examiner wanted to double-check her ability to learn, so he/she told her the correct orientation information and asked her again a few minutes later. Her orientation score increased to 10. How would one score this?

Scenario 3. Your patient scored 2/2 on recall, but the examiner wanted to ensure she did not have aphasia, so he/she asked her to name 10 low-frequency words, and she got only 5. How would one score this?

Scenario 4. Your patient scored 24/30 on the MMSE, but had a grade 3 education and is 85 years old. How would one interpret this?

Scenario 5. Your patient scored 3 on serial 7s but 5 on WORLD backward. Which should be picked?

OVERVIEW

1. Choosing Tools

- Geriatric psychiatrists are increasingly using other tools beyond the MMSE.
- It is important for psychiatrists to have a full armamentarium of available cognitive examination skills that they can adapt to their patient encounters across diagnoses and contexts.
- Screening tools are a first step, usually at a first interview (and most geriatric psychiatrists believe they are necessary at every first interview), and then more detailed assessment will follow.

2. Introducing the Cognitive Exam

- Introducing the cognitive examination is a challenge and needs to be done skillfully.
- Using the word "test" makes many patients anxious.
- Try to use a natural transition to introduce the topic, tying in the patient's previous concerns that he/she have mentioned during the interview's history of present illness or review of symptoms (e.g., "I find I can't concentrate"), or starting with observations that you as interviewer have made during the interview (e.g., "I notice that you had trouble remembering how long it has been since your husband died.").
- To avoid the "test" word, you can simply introduce with a statement such as: "I'd like to look together with you at your (complaint about concentration) (ability to remember times)."
- Remember that if someone has significant cognitive difficulties during the history of present illness, you do not need to wait until the last 5–10 minutes to conduct a cognitive examination. Doing so earlier helps focus the interview.

3. Screening Tools

- It is important to note that in a first assessment with a patient, we are trying to make initial hypotheses about diagnoses and to minimize false positives and false negatives. Using the tools in this section is a practical way of doing this.
- In secondary, specialty care, the Mini-Cog netted optimal psychometric properties and a "grade A" recommendation for both screening and case-finding in a recent review by Mitchell and Malladi (2010).
- There are many other brief measures, and Mitchell and Malladi (2010) includes descriptions of their properties in community, primary care, and specialty settings. The sensitivity, specificity, positive and negative predictive values (PPV and NPV, respectively) vary significantly depending on prevalence, and hence across these settings.

3.1 MMSE

- Most psychiatrists have been taught to look for a specified MMSE cut-off across all patients, but this is problematic.
- Domains tested include orientation, memory, attention, language, and visuospatial.
- It is important to realize that in addition to setting and prevalence, the psychometric properties (sensitivity, specificity, PPV, and NPV) depend on age and education.
- It is important clinically to describe where the patient lost points, and if you had to adapt the tool to the patient's language or sensory limitations. Also describe if the score was obtained using serial 7s, WORLD backward, or both.
- Some clinicians use a denominator of 30 regardless of adaptations, and some correct the denominator to items that the patient is feasibly able to do with his/her limitations. One can move "beyond the MMSE" with other questions or cues, but these do not get scored.
- Practical tip:
  - *Scoring WORLD backward.* Follow Molloy's standardized sMMSE scoring (Molloy & Standish, 1997) to standardize: "Originally, Dr. Folstein advised that the score is 'the number of letters in the correct order.' We suggest the following method because it is so simple and foolproof. Score order not sequence. Simply write down the correct response: DLROW. Now place the last 5 letters the subject said below. Now draw lines between the same letters on the response given and DLROW. These lines may not cross. The person's score is the maximum # of lines that can be drawn, without crossing any."

3.1.1 Benefits of MMSE

Brief, widespread use; standardized with age and education norms; repeatable

3.1.2 Limitations of MMSE

Rough assessment of memory (floor and ceiling effects); arbitrary nature of several measures; language/culture/ESL issue; blindness/deafness issue; no assessment of executive functioning or visual memory; copyright

3.2 Clock Drawing Test (CDT)

The clock drawing test is a very brief screen of cognition. It is appealing for use when time is limited, or to supplement the use of the MMSE as a screen.

3.2.1 Advantages of CDT

Quick; ties in various domains of cognition, including visuospatial skills, attention, language and frontal-subcortical functioning; useful in detecting moderate or severe dementia; can help detect executive dysfunction among patients with higher MMSE scores; also useful to track change over time

3.2.2 Disadvantages of CDT

Non-specific in the functions that it tests, with numerous different scoring systems; less useful for detecting mild dementia or mild cognitive impairment (MCI)

3.2.3 Scoring the CDT

There is no conclusive evidence that the more elaborate scoring systems are better than simple judgments of "normal" vs "abnormal," and as such, I recommend making a global judgment. The rule for "normal" in the Mini-Cog score of the clock is a simple and practical way of doing this (Pinto & Peters, 2009; Shulman, 2000).

- If you conduct the MMSE and CDT, you are doing what the vast majority of geriatric psychiatrists internationally do "routinely and often," likely meeting the "standard of care"(Ismail et al., 2013; Shulman et al., 2006).
- However, this "standard" is likely substandard given the limitations of these tools, which were meant mainly for screening (Ismail et al., 2010).

3.3 Mini-Cog

Dr Soo Borson and colleagues (2000) developed the Mini-Cog as a way of establishing a screen for dementia that would be applicable to diverse language backgrounds and educational levels. It is much briefer than the MMSE, and incorporates the CDT. It compares favourably to MMSE as a screen, and in semi-literate and illiterate samples, has much fewer false positives (27%) than the MMSE (64%).

3.3.1 Administration and Scoring of Mini-Cog
(*Borson et al., 2000, 2006*)

Administration:
- "Instruct the patient to listen carefully to and remember 3 unrelated words, and then to repeat the words."
- "Instruct the patient to draw the face of a clock, either on a blank sheet or a sheet of paper, or on a sheet with the clock circle already drawn. After the patient puts the numbers on the clock face, ask him/her to draw the hands of the clock to read a specific time. These instructions can be repeated, but no additional instructions should be given. Give the patient as much time as needed to complete the task. The CDT serves as the recall distractor."
- "Ask the patient to repeat the 3 previously presented words."

Scoring: One point each is given for each recalled word to a maximum of 3.
- 0 words recalled is a positive screen for dementia.
- 3 words recalled is a negative screen for dementia.
- If the patient recalls 1–2 words, the result of the screen depends on the clock.
    - 1 or 2 word recall with a normal clock is a negative screen for dementia.
    - 1 or 2 word recall with an abnormal clock is a positive screen for dementia.
- Interpreting the clock: "The CDT is considered normal if all numbers are present in the correct sequence and the hands readably display the requested time."

3.4 Montreal Cognitive Assessment (MoCA)

The MoCA is a screening tool for cognitive impairment that was developed to overcome the limited sensitivity of the MMSE to milder degrees of cognitive impairment.

Domains: "visuospatial/executive" (modified trails, cube copy, and clock drawing), naming, memory, attention (digits forward and back, vigilance A test, serial 7s), language (repeat and F word registration), abstraction (similarities), recall (5 words), and orientation

The MoCA shows much greater differentiation between controls and patients with MCI and Alzheimer's disease (AD), and has greater sensitivity, compared with the MMSE. However, the trade-off is that, at least using the "normal >= 26/30" cut-off, the specificity drops off dramatically. In order to preserve the higher sensitivity, but keep a high degree of specificity, a cut-off of >= 23 is more optimal. Administration and scoring is carefully detailed on the primary document (Nasreddine et al., 2005; Smith, Gildeh, & Holmes, 2007; Luis, Keegan, & Mullan, 2009; mocatest.org).

3.5 Rowland Universal Dementia Assessment Scale (RUDAS)
(Basic et al., 2009; Rowland et al., 2006)

The RUDAS is another 30-item cognitive screen, developed in Australia, with similar goals to the MMSE, although meant to be less biased by issues pertaining to language, education, and culture.

Domains: visuospatial body orientation, praxis, visuoconstructional drawing, judgment, 4-word recall (supermarket items), and language (animal word list generation)

4. Going beyond Screening

- The domains tested in a cognitive examination are organized hierarchically.
    - For example, language testing is dependent on attention, which in turn is dependent on arousal/alertness.
- This section describes practical ways of doing qualitative and quantitative assessments of these domains, and presents evidence and ideas about functional neuroanatomy (where available).

4.1 Arousal

- This is the most fundamental requirement for cognitive testing.
- Making descriptive observations about arousal is likely the most helpful (e.g., "the patient was rousable but kept falling asleep as we were talking").
- In consultation-liaison or neurosurgical settings, a Glasgow Coma Scale (GCS) is often useful. The score ranges from 3 to 15, with scores of 1–4 for eye opening, 1–5 for best verbal response, and 1–6 for best motor response.

4.2 Attention

- Anatomically, attention is widely distributed. Intact attention requires an intact reticular activating system, pons, hippocampus, thalamus, prefrontal cortex, and right parietal cortex, as well as intact cholinergic and dopaminergic functioning, and optimal balance between the inhibitory (GABAergic) and the excitatory (glutamatergic) systems.
- Lesions causing increased intracranial pressure and sedating medications are common causes in medical settings of impaired attention.
- Again, qualitative descriptions of ability to focus, sustain, and shift attention, as well as the ability to resist interference/distractions, are necessary.
- For a more formal qualitative assessment, consider the Vigilance A test (an example of this is on the MoCA) or asking the patient to do a task backward.
- If you are trying to detect subtle attention deficits in an educated person who seems globally intact, consider alphabet backward (try this – it's hard!).

- If the person had trouble on the serial 7s on the MMSE/MoCA, you can try serial 3s, months backward, days backward, or (the easiest) counting backward from 20.
- *Digit Span.* For a more quantitative assessment of attention, consider digit span forward. To do this, present a series of 3 digits in a monotone at a one-digit-per-second pace, asking the patient to simply repeat; then do the same with 4 digits, 5 digits, etc. Once the patient fails, give him or her a try again with another set of digits of the same span. If the patient gets it, move up to a longer span; if not, the score is the span last achieved correctly. For example: if the patient gets a 4 digit span and fails a string of 5 digits once, but gets the second string of 5 digits, move upward to try 6 digits. If the patient fails the second string of 5 digits, his or her digit span is 4. Digit span backward is administered the same way as digit span forward, except the instructions are to repeat the digits backward. Digit span backward tests working memory as well as attention.
- *Trails A.* Trails A is a test of attention and psychomotor speed.

4.3 Language

An approach to language disturbance/aphasia is described here, and the categorization is summarized in Table 1.2.1.

Table 1.2.1: Categorization of Aphasia

Domain	Fluency	Repetition	Comprehension	Naming
1. Broca	Imp	Imp	N	Imp
2. Wernicke	N	Imp	Imp	Imp
3. Conduction	N	Imp	N	Imp
4. Transcortical motor	Imp	N	N	Imp
5. Transcortical sensory	N	N	Imp	Imp
6. Mixed transcortical	Imp	N	Imp	Imp
7. Global	Imp	Imp	Imp	Imp
8. Anomic	N	N	N	Imp

N = normal; Imp = impaired

4.3.1 Fluency

Informally we are assessing language fluency throughout the assessment with phrase length. It is important to document paraphasic errors. The animal naming test is both a test of language and executive function, and is described in more detail under the executive section below. Patients with long phrase length are generally considered "fluent." Non-fluent aphasias classically are related to Broca's area, and also include impaired repetition.

4.3.2 Naming

If a patient has an aphasia, by definition his or her naming is impaired. The examiner has likely already assessed high frequency naming on either the MMSE (pen, watch) or MoCA (lion, rhino, camel), but consider also asking low-frequency words (button, heel, frame, lens, etc.) for greater sensitivity.

4.3.3 Repetition

The items on MMSE are quite easy, whereas the MoCA items are more challenging. Easy words to repeat are "ball," "fall," "airplane." Harder are phrases such as "he is the one who said it," "the spy fled to Ireland," or "the orchestra played on and the audience applauded." Even more difficult is "Methodist Episcopalian." If the patient has an aphasia but repetition is intact, this means that the patient's pathology spares the arcuate fasciculus which connects Broca's with Wernicke's area. These aphasias are generally termed "transcortical" (motor if non-fluent, and sensory if fluent).

4.3.4 Comprehension

The three-stage command from MMSE partially tests comprehension but is also a motor task. As an examiner, you are generally informally assessing comprehension continuously, but consider asking about other simple commands, including ones that use syntax (e.g., put the pen in between the pencil and the paper). Fluent aphasias are ones in which fluency is not affected, so generally this reflects dysfunction of the posterior cortex, classically Wernicke's area and accompanied by poor comprehension.

4.3.5 Other

Reading is tested very simply on the MMSE; a longer paragraph can be used to assess both reading and comprehension. Writing is assessed on the MMSE. Prosody is not on the MMSE, but has both expressive and receptive components.

4.4 Memory

- Recent verbal memory is measured on the MMSE using orientation to time and place.
- It should be noted (although not for scoring) that college graduates tend to know the day or date or miss it by one day, whereas those with less than high school education may miss the day or date by two or three days.
- The MMSE has a fairly easy test of recent verbal memory of three-word recall after a short delay. One point is accorded for each correct reply on the first attempt.
- The MoCA contains a slightly harder task of five words after a somewhat longer delay. In both cases, if the patient cannot correctly recall the words, it is prudent to try semantic and then multiple-choice cueing. Although not scored, this is helpful diagnostically as I will describe shortly.
- Qualitatively, the interviewer will notice when patients have difficulty providing a history. Personal history taps long-term memory, whereas history of present illness probes shorter-term memory. The ability to remember accurately one's birthday, age, and address can be quickly established in the identifying data aspect of the history.
- The examiner can also ask for recall of recent events, names of four recent prime ministers, a short sentence (e.g., "Tom and Bill went fishing and caught three black trout") or name/address (e.g., "John McAdam, 75 Front St, Markham, Manitoba"), each of which contains seven items to remember in a context. These are qualitative or semi-quantitative assessments of verbal memory.
- For greater sensitivity, use the Rey Auditory Verbal Learning Test (RAVLT), in which 15 words are presented over five trials, and the patient is asked to freely recall them after a brief distractor list. Then, recognition cues are provided.

- In addition to greater sensitivity and a quantitative assessment, the tool allows one to differentiate between storage and retrieval problems. However, it is an enormously frustrating test for many.
- Differentiating between storage and retrieval can be done with the three words of the MMSE, the five words of the MoCA, and/or the short sentence or name/address provided above. This is why cueing is important.
- Patients with hippocampal damage (e.g., severe AD, Korsakoff syndrome, herpes simplex, or bilateral infarcts) generally are unable to benefit from cueing, and are thought to have true memory storage deficits.
- In contrast, patients with frontal-subcortical pathology (e.g., Parkinson's disease, traumatic brain injury, HIV, multiple sclerosis) tend to improve with cues, reflective of a retrieval deficit. This is a general rule, but there is overlap.
- Visual memory is not assessed by the screening tools discussed.
- The Rey-Osterrieth complex figure recall test is more sensitive, but requires specialized training and scoring. Clinicians generally assess this by recall of three figures (see the Baycrest behavioural neurology assessment [BNA] for examples; Darvesh et al., 2005) or by hiding objects in the room and asking the patient to recall what was hidden (verbal) and where it was hidden (visual).
- Anatomically, an intact medial temporal system is required for memory, and assigns affective valence to prioritize memories.
- The hippocampal formation with input from the amygdala is required to hold, integrate, and start encoding information via long-term potentiation, but memories are distributed in widespread networks (motor, sensory, association, limbic, paralimbic, and prefrontal regions).
- The frontal-subcortical circuits are responsible for organization and retrieval of the memories.

4.5 Visuospatial Skills

- Both the MMSE and MoCA have visuospatial components, in a limited fashion.
- The copy aspect of visual memory also tests visuospatial skills.
- A free drawn (or easier, copied) cube or daisy are alternate ways of assessing these skills.
- The clock drawing test tests visuospatial and executive functioning.
- Classically, these tools are testing right parietal functions, although with the auditory and visual components of the testing, other areas are involved.

4.6 Frontal-Subcortical Functioning

- Parallel circuits connect the frontal cortex to the basal ganglia, and thence to the thalamus.
- Circuits from the dorsolateral prefrontal cortex (DLPFC) are classically thought to be responsible for the deficits described in bedside "frontal" testing.
  - This means that lesions not just in the DLPFC, but also in the basal ganglia, thalamus, or in the white matter tracts connecting them, can yield similar deficits.
- Qualitatively, watch how errors are made in the history and in the rest of the cognitive examination.

- Other useful tests of executive or frontal-subcortical functioning are as follows:
  - The CDT described in 3.2 tests both visuospatial and executive functioning.
  - FAS test – patients are instructed to name as many words that start with the letter F as they can in one minute. The examiner counts these (not including repeats), and then the same is done with the letters A and S. The total count is tabulated and compared with published norms (Strauss et al., 2006).
  - Animals test – patients are instructed to name as many animals as they can ("anything that breathes" as a prompt) in one minute and the numbers are tabulated and compared with published norms. Some believe this is a better test of language than frontal-subcortical skills.
    - Generally speaking, in Alzheimer's disease FAS is usually better than animals (i.e., patients score better on FAS than they do on animals), while in vascular dementia (and likely other dementias affecting frontal-subcortical functioning), animals are better than FAS (i.e., patients score better on animals than they do on FAS). Furthermore, a score of less than 15 on animals is 20 times more likely in AD than in normal controls (Canning et al., 2004; Tierney et al., 2001).
  - Trails B generally tests both attention/psychomotor speed as well as executive functioning. Some authors suggest subtracting Trails B minus Trails A to get a more "executive" score.
  - The Frontal Assessment Battery (FAB) incorporates several clinically used assessments: similarities, s-word generation, go/no-go test, the Luria manoeuvre, grasp reflex. Patients with frontotemporal dementia (FTD) have worse (lower) scores on this than controls or patients with AD. Although not well studied, this is also true for patients with other frontal-subcortical pathology (Dubois et al., 2000; Slachevsky et al., 2004).
  - Please see section 4.4 re: retrieval aspects of memory as well.

4.7 Other

- Ideomotor praxis – lesions in the dominant frontal or parietal lobe, generally, although difficulty with imitation may be seen with lesions in the non-dominant hemisphere. Examples: blow out a candle, salute, wave, brush your teeth
- Neglect – can be seen in grooming, letter-cancellation tasks, and the clock drawing task, and generally reflect right frontal pathology
- Prosopagnosia (difficulty recognizing faces) – lesions in the temporal/occipital area
- "Head turning sign" (i.e., does the patient turn his/her head to the caregiver expecting help with an answer when the clinician asks a question?): in a memory clinic study of 207 participants, 133 had an informant. Of the total sample, 40% were cognitively impaired. The "head turning sign" had a sensitivity of 0.63, an NPV of 0.64, a specificity of 0.95, and a PPV of 0.94 (Larner, 2012).

5. How to Choose?

It is important as a clinician to develop your own approach to selecting cognitive tests, as there is no one-size-fits-all approach. For example, for an uncooperative patient, a more detailed assessment beyond a screen will be unrealistic. Conversely, for a university professor with mild cognitive complaints, a MMSE will be insufficiently sensitive for detection of deficits. Table 1.2.2 shows the author's approach to selecting such tests.

Table 1.2.2: Author's Approach to Choice of Cognitive Tests

Test	Scenario
Nothing (or GCS)	• Aggressive, hostile, combative, uncooperative, or comatose
CDT, or Mini-Cog +/– Orientation /10	• ESL • Significant sensory impairment • Examination or otherwise very short on time • Tracking cognition over time
MMSE	• English second language (and adjust) • Grade school or less education, although this changes the cut-off scores significantly • Screening where cognitive impairment is not primary reason for referral or "need to know"
RUDAS	• ESL • Grade school or less education
MoCA	• More than grade school education • Screening where cognition is a reason for referral or important comorbidity
More detailed assessment	• Beyond screening – honing a differential diagnosis for dementia or quantifying neuropsychological deficits in mood or psychotic disorder

CDT = clock drawing test; GCS = Glasgow Coma Scale; ESL = English as a second language; MMSE = Mini Mental State Examination; MoCA = Montreal Cognitive Assessment; RUDAS = Rowland University Dementia Assessment Scale

6. How to Interpret?

- Is the test performance valid?
    - Is this evidence of a true cognitive deficit?
    - Was there sufficient effort? Evidence of malingering?
    - Is the performance an artefact of anxiety, psychosis, depression, or medication?
- If the cognitive performance is a valid indicator of cognitive deficit:
    - What is the severity?
    - What is the pattern of deficits? (See chapter 3.5 for more details.)
        - Anterior vs posterior
        - Right vs left
        - Cortical vs subcortical

QUESTIONS

1. List four bedside tests of frontal-executive functioning.
2. List four threats to validity of bedside cognitive testing.

3. Describe two non-psychiatric psychosocial predictors of poor performance on bedside cognitive testing.

4. List two circumstances in which one would chose to use the MMSE instead of a more sensitive screen such as the MoCA?

ANSWERS

1. Bedside tests of frontal-executive functioning include the following:
   - Frontal Assessment Battery (and its sub-items – the go/no-go test, Luria manoeuvre, similarities, word list generation, and grasp reflex)
   - Trails B
   - Similarities
   - FAS/controlled oral word association test
   - Abstraction
   - CDT

2. Threats to validity of bedside cognitive testing include the following:
   - Anxiety
   - Agitation
   - Depression
   - Mania
   - Medication – anticholinergic, other sedating medications

3. A mismatch between age of patient and examiner, and knowledge of APOE-epsilon 4 allele status predict poorer performance (Lupien, 2011; Lineweaver et al., 2014).

4. Circumstances in which one would chose to use the MMSE instead of a more sensitive screen, such as the MoCA, include English as a second language (ESL), low education, delirium, and severe dementia.

CASE DISCUSSION

1. Option A: She scored 23/30 (but lost points for date, repeat, write, copy, and three-step due to her hemiplegia).

   Option B: She scored 23/24 (lost a point for date, did not administer repeat, write, copy, or three-step due to hemiplegia).

   Option C: Same as option B but correct to a denominator of 30. Corrected MMSE score = (23 x 30)/24 = 28.8/30, or rounding up 29/30. The key is describing the deficits.

2. One would code the recall score as 0/3 when calculating the total, but indicate improved to 3/3 with semantic cueing.

3. For the total score calculation, her naming is 2/2, and one would make a comment on the low-frequency naming challenge after the MMSE description.

4. Using the norms by from the Epidemiologic Catchment Area (ECA) study (Crum et al., 1993), we can see that the mean and SD MMSE for individuals 85 years old with a grade 3 education is 19 (SD 2.9). Calculate a Z-score: (patient's score – mean for age/

education) / SD for age/education. In this case, the Z-score is $(24-19)/2.9 = 1.72$. This means the patient is 1.72 SD above the mean for their age/education. Using a set cut-off for everyone is unfair.

5. Dr Folstein was silent about this in the original manuscript. Generally there should be a delay between registration and recall. A common practice is to administer both DLROW and serial 7s after presenting the three words for registration, and score the highest (noting both), then ask for recall. The key is describing what one has done so that others can compare scores.

RECOMMENDED RESOURCES FOR REVIEW

Although these resources may not be specifically cited in the text, their approach informed the contents of the chapter, and they are recommended as useful further reading.

Arciniegas, DB, Beresford, TP. Neuropsychiatry: an introductory approach. Cambridge, UK: Cambridge University Press; 2001.

Holsinger T, Deveau J, Boustani M, et al. Does this patient have dementia? JAMA. 2007;297(21):2391–404. http://dx.doi.org/10.1001/jama.297.21.2391. Medline:17551132

Kipps CM, Hodges JR. Cognitive assessment for clinicians. J Neurol Neurosurg Psychiatry. 2005;76(Suppl 1):i22–30. http://dx.doi.org/10.1136/jnnp.2004.059758. Medline:15718218

Strauss E, Sherman EM, Spreen O. A compendium of neuropsychological tests: administration and scoring. Oxford, UK: Oxford University Press; 2006.

Strubb RL, Black FW. The mental status examination in neurology. 4th ed. Philadelphia, PA: F.A. Davis Company; 1999.

REFERENCES

Basic D, Rowland JT, Conforti DA, et al. The validity of the Rowland Universal Dementia Assessment Scale (RUDAS) in a multicultural cohort of community-dwelling older persons with early dementia. Alzheimer Dis Assoc Disord. 2009;23(2):124–9. http://dx.doi.org/10.1097/WAD.0b013e31818ecc98. Medline:19484915

Borson S, Scanlan J, Brush M, et al. The mini-cog: a cognitive 'vital signs' measure for dementia screening in multi-lingual elderly. Int J Geriatr Psychiatry. 2000;15(11):1021–7. http://dx.doi.org/10.1002/1099-1166(200011)15:11<1021::AID-GPS234>3.0.CO;2-6. Medline:11113982

Borson S, Scanlan JM, Watanabe J, et al. Improving identification of cognitive impairment in primary care. Int J Geriatr Psychiatry. 2006;21(4):349–55. http://dx.doi.org/10.1002/gps.1470. Medline:16534774

Canning SJ, Leach L, Stuss D, et al. Diagnostic utility of abbreviated fluency measures in Alzheimer disease and vascular dementia. Neurology. 2004;62(4):556–62. http://dx.doi.org/10.1212/WNL.62.4.556. Medline:14981170

Crum RM, Anthony JC, Bassett SS, et al. Population-based norms for the Mini-Mental State Examination by age and educational level. JAMA. 1993;269(18):2386–91. http://dx.doi.org/10.1001/jama.1993.03500180078038. Medline:8479064

Ismail Z, Mulsant BH, Herrmann N, et al. Canadian academy of geriatric psychiatry survey of brief cognitive screening instruments. Can Geriatr J. 2013;16(2):54–60. http://dx.doi.org/10.5770/cgj.16.81. Medline:23737930

Ismail Z, Rajji TK, Shulman KI. Brief cognitive screening instruments: an update. Int J Geriatr Psychiatry. 2010;25(2):111–20. http://dx.doi.org/10.1002/gps.2306. Medline:19582756

Larner AJ. Head turning sign: pragmatic utility in clinical diagnosis of cognitive impairment. J Neurol Neurosurg Psychiatry. 2012;83(8):852–3. http://dx.doi.org/ 10.1136/jnnp-2011-301804. Medline:22338027

Lineweaver TT, Bondi MW, Galasko D, et al. Effect of knowledge of APOE genotype on subjective and objective memory performance in healthy older adults. Am J Psychiatry. 2014;171(2):201–8. http://dx.doi .org/10.1176/appi.ajp.2013.12121590. Medline:24170170

Luis CA, Keegan AP, Mullan M. Cross validation of the Montreal Cognitive Assessment in community dwelling older adults residing in the Southeastern US. Int J Geriatr Psychiatry. 2009;24(2):197–201. http:// dx.doi.org/10.1002/gps.2101. Medline:18850670

Mitchell AJ, Malladi S. Screening and case finding tools for the detection of dementia. Part I: evidence-based meta-analysis of multidomain tests. Am J Geriatr Psychiatry. 2010;18(9):759–82. http://dx.doi.org/10.1097/JGP.0b013e3181cdecb8. Medline:20808118

Molloy DW, Standish TI. A guide to the standardized Mini-Mental State Examination. Int Psychogeriatr. 1997;9(S1 Suppl 1):87–94, discussion 143–50. http://dx.doi .org/10.1017/S1041610297004754. Medline:9447431

Nasreddine ZS, Phillips NA, Bédirian V, et al. The Montreal Cognitive Assessment, MoCA: a brief screening tool for mild cognitive impairment. J Am Geriatr Soc. 2005;53(4):695–9. http://dx.doi.org/10.1111/j.1532-5415.2005.53221.x. Medline:15817019

Shulman KI, Herrmann N, Brodaty H, et al. IPA survey of brief cognitive screening instruments. Int Psychogeriatr. 2006;18(2):281–94. http://dx.doi.org/10.1017/S1041610205002693. Medline:16466586

Slachevsky A, Villalpando JM, Sarazin M, et al. Frontal assessment battery and differential diagnosis of frontotemporal dementia and Alzheimer disease. Arch Neurol. 2004;61(7):1104–7. http://dx.doi.org/10.1001/archneur.61.7.1104. Medline:15262742

Smith T, Gildeh N, Holmes C. The Montreal Cognitive Assessment: validity and utility in a memory clinic setting. Can J Psychiatry. 2007;52(5):329–32. Medline:17542384

Tierney MC, Black SE, Szalai JP, et al. Recognition memory and verbal fluency differentiate probable Alzheimer disease from subcortical ischemic vascular dementia. Arch Neurol. 2001;58(10):1654–9. http://dx.doi.org/10.1001/ archneur.58.10.1654. Medline:11594925

1.3 Neuropsychiatric Symptoms in Dementia

Dallas Seitz, MD, PhD, FRCPC

INTRODUCTION

Neuropsychiatric symptoms (NPS) associated with dementia are one of the most common and challenging clinical problems encountered by geriatric psychiatrists. One could argue that the assessment and management of NPS is the domain of geriatric psychiatrists and an area where geriatric psychiatrists have the greatest expertise when compared to other medical specialists involved in the care of older adults. Given the importance and complexity of NPS, several chapters in our review guide will centre on NPS. This chapter will focus on the phenomenology of NPS; additional chapters on the nonpharmacological and pharmacological management of NPS follow.

CASE SCENARIO

You are a geriatric psychiatrist consulting to a long-term care (LTC) facility and have recent received a referral. The referral indicates that the LTC home would like you to assess an 87-year-old woman with dementia who is "agitated and aggressive." The referral letter indicates that her last Mini Mental State Examination (MMSE) completed six months ago was 7/30. Her past medical history listed on your referral form includes diabetes mellitus, osteoarthritis, osteoporosis (history of hip fracture), macular degeneration, hearing impairment, and congestive heart failure. Her current medications include alendronate 70 mg weekly, vitamin D 800 IU, furosemide 40 mg daily, metformin 500 mg PO BID, and donepezil 10 mg PO OD. You are scheduled to meet with the patient, the patient's daughter, and nursing staff at the LTC home later this week. Please outline your approach to assessing neuropsychiatric symptoms in this patient.

OVERVIEW

1. Neuropsychiatric Symptoms
(Finkel et al., 1996)

- NPS are simply the non-cognitive symptoms associated with dementia.
- NPS are also known as behavioural and psychological symptoms of dementia (BPSD).
- International Psychogeriatric Association, 1996, defines NPS as "signs and symptoms of disturbed perception, thought content, mood, or behavior that frequently occur in patients with dementia."

- These symptoms are sometimes also referred to as "responsive behaviours," although this terminology is not commonly used in research literature.

1.1 What Are NPS?
(Cummings et al., 1994; Cohen-Mansfield, Marx, & Rosenthal, 1989)

NPS can include a variety of different symptoms; it is useful to be specific about the particular symptoms as the etiology, treatment, and prognosis associated with these symptoms can be different. Included within the terminology of NPS are the following:

- Delusions
- Hallucinations
- Anxiety
- Elevated mood
- Apathy

- Depression
- Irritability
- Sleep changes
- Agitation

1.2 Agitation

Agitation is a common term used when describing NPS. The term agitation may be used to describe a number of different symptoms:

- Restlessness
- Requests for help or repetitive questioning
- Screaming or vocalizations
- Hitting, pushing, kicking
- Sexually disinhibited behaviour

1.3 Clusters of NPS
(Cohen-Mansfield, Marx, & Rosenthal, 1989; Aalten et al., 2003)

Two commonly used measures of NPS include the Cohen-Mansfield Agitation Inventory (CMAI) and the Neuropsychiatric Inventory (NPI). Within these measures, certain groups or clusters of NPS tend to occur together within individuals:

- Cohen-Mansfield Agitation Inventory (CMAI):
  - Verbal agitation (yelling, repetitive vocalizations)
  - Non-aggressive physical agitation (restlessness, pacing)
  - Aggressive physical agitation
- Neuropsychiatric Inventory (NPI):
  - Psychotic symptoms (delusions, hallucinations)
  - Mood/apathy (depression, apathy, eating, sleep)
  - Hyperactivity (agitation, irritability, euphoria, disinhibition)

1.4 Alzheimer's Association Classification
(Cohen-Mansfield, Marx, & Rosenthal, 1989; Geda et al., 2013)

One clinically useful classification of NPS has been that proposed by the US Alzheimer's Association. Within this classification, five major groups of NPS are identified:

- Agitation
  - "Inappropriate verbal, vocal, or motor activity that is not an obvious expression of need or confusion"
- Psychosis
  - Delusions, hallucinations
- Depression
- Apathy
  - "Absence of responsiveness to stimuli as demonstrated by a lack of self-initiated action"
- Sleep

2. Depression in Dementia
(Byers & Yaffe, 2011; Starkstein et al., 2005)

Symptoms of depression are the most commonly observed NPS and can include depressive symptoms or major depressive disorder.

- Depression is a risk factor for development of Alzheimer's.
- Approximately 25% of older adults with dementia have comorbid depression.
- Depression is more common in vascular dementia (VaD) and dementia with Lewy bodies (DLB) than in Alzheimer's disease.

2.1 Diagnosing Depression in Dementia
(Teng et al., 2008)

Diagnosis is similar to diagnosing depression in individuals without dementia, with some minor proposed changes to the DSM criteria for major depression in individuals without dementia (although not incorporated into DSM-5).

A. Two week period of **three or more symptoms** of (one of first two required):
- Depressed mood
- Decreased positive affect or pleasure in response to social contacts and usual activities
- Disruption of sleep
- Disruption of appetite
- Psychomotor changes
- Irritability
- Fatigue or loss of energy
- Feelings of worthlessness, hopelessness, or excessive guilt
- Recurrent thoughts of death, suicidal ideation or plan

B. Criteria also met for dementia of the Alzheimer type
C. Symptoms cause distress and not caused by other conditions or substances

3. Psychosis in Dementia
(Jeste & Finkel, 2000)

Psychosis is also commonly observed in dementia. Proposed criteria for psychosis in Alzheimer's disease are:
- Either hallucinations or delusions are present.
- Diagnostic criteria for dementia are met.

- Psychotic symptoms were not continuously present prior to onset of dementia.
- Symptoms present for at least 1 month and cause distress for patient or others.
- Criteria for schizophrenia, mood disorder with psychotic features have never been met.
- Exclusion of delirium
- Exclusion of general medical condition (GMC)

Associated features:

- With agitation
- With negative symptoms
- With depression

4. Psychological Theories of NPS
(Hall & Buckwalter, 1987; Cohen-Mansfield, 2001, 2000)

Different psychological theories have been proposed to explain the development of NPS in persons with dementia. These theories may be helpful in treatment planning and understanding behaviours. Among these theories, learning theory and the unmet needs models both have some empirical support for treatments.

- Lowered stress threshold
- Learning theory
- Unmet needs → tailored interventions
    - Verbal agitation – depression, loneliness
    - Physically non-aggressive agitation – stimulation
    - Physically aggressive agitation – avoiding discomfort

5. TREA Approach
(Cohen-Mansfield, 2000)

One example of a treatment model based on the unmet needs model is the Treatment Routes for Exploring Agitation (TREA).

- Approach to assessment and management of behaviours is based on assumptions of unmet needs.

6. Understanding NPS
(Kitwood, 1993)

An approach to formulation of the causes and contributors of NPS in an individual is that proposed by Thomas Kitwood's personhood in dementia.

- Kitwood's framework for personhood in dementia can be expressed in an equation:
  SD = P + B + H + NI + SP
    - **SD** = clinical manifestation of dementia
    - **P**ersonality – previous coping strategies
    - **B**iography – other challenges presented in life
    - **H**ealth – sensory impairment
    - **N**europathological impairment – location, type, severity
    - **S**ocial **p**sychology – environmental effects on sense of safety, value, and personal being

7. Patient Correlates of NPS
(International Psychogeriatric Association, 2010)

- Demographics
  - Age: ↑ anxiety, depression with younger age
  - Gender:
    - Females: ↑ psychosis, verbal agitation, anxiety
    - Males: ↑ aggression
- Severity of cognitive impairment
- Increasing functional impairment
- Impaired communication/sensory

7.1 Environmental Correlates
(International Psychogeriatric Association, 2010)

- Single rooms may be helpful for reducing agitation.
- Smaller facility sizes may reduce aggression.
- High environment temperatures and physical discomfort are associated with verbal and non-aggressive physical agitation.

7.2 Biological Correlates
(International Psychogeriatric Association, 2010)

- Genetics and neurotransmitters
  - Serotonin HT2A T102C polymorphism and psychosis
  - Dopamine D1 and D3 polymorphisms and psychosis and agitation
  - Noradrenergic cell loss and increased noradrenaline postsynaptic sensitivity associated with aggression

7.3 Clinical Risk Factors for NPS
(International Psychogeriatric Association, 2010)

- Irritability may be more common in higher functioning groups.
- Early executive dysfunction increases risk of NPS and caregiver stress.
- Frontal symptoms associated agitation, aggression, depression, and severity of psychosis
- Higher degree of medical comorbidity increases risk of agitation, disinhibition, and irritability.

8. Diagnosis and Assessment of NPS
(International Psychogeriatric Association, 2010; Sink, Holden & Yaffe, 2005)

- Phenomenology the basis of diagnosis
- Direct interview
- Direct observation
- Proxy report

- Measurements and scales
- Need for accurate descriptions
- Think of physical illness
- Think of sensory impairment

Differential diagnosis:
- Delirium (medication-induced, other causes)
- Depression

- Pain or discomfort
- Other medical causes
- Environment causes

9. General Principles for Managing NPS
(International Psychogeriatric Association, 2010)

- Nonpharmacological treatments should be used first whenever available.
- Even when NPS are caused by specific etiologies (pain, depression, psychosis), nonpharmacological interventions should be used with medications.
- All nonpharmacological interventions work best when tailored to individual needs and background.
- Family and caregivers are key collaborators and need to be involved in treatment planning.

9.1 Serial Trial Intervention
(Kovach et al., 2006; Pieper et al., 2011)

One approach to assessment and management of NPS is the STI (Serial Trial Intervention) approach. At each step an assessment occurs with targeted interventions to address any identified contributors to NPS.

STEP 0: Basic care needs
- TARGET and if behaviour continues, proceed to STEP 1

STEP 1: Pain and physical needs
- TARGET and if behaviour continues, proceed to STEP 2

STEP 2: Affective needs
- TARGET and if behaviour continues, proceed to STEP 3

STEP 3: Trial nonpharmacological comfort interventions
- If behaviour continues, proceed to next step

STEP 4: Short trial of analgesia
- If behaviour continues, proceed to next step

STEP 5: Trial psychotropic drugs or consultation
- If behaviour continues, repeat STI!

10. Diagnosing Delirium
(Inouye et al., 1990)

For an approach to the assessment and management of delirium, please see the delirium chapter in this book (chapter 3.2).

11. Pain in Dementia
(Fox, Raina, & Jadad, 1999)

- Pain is common and undertreated in older adults.
  - 50–80% of individuals in LTC have pain.
- Assessment of pain in individuals with advanced dementia is particularly challenging:
  - Pain can present as agitation.
  - Language and communication difficulties
  - Recall of pain changes over time and poses an assessment challenge.

11.1 Assessment of Pain in Dementia
(Warden, Hurley, & Volicer, 2003)

- Several pain scales have been developed to measure pain in persons with dementia who may have limited verbal abilities:
    - Pain Assessment in Advanced Dementia (PAINAD) and the Pain Assessment Checklist for Seniors with Limited Ability to Communicate (PACSLAC) are two of the more common and better validated scales for measuring pain in persons with dementia.
    - Pain scales may misidentify emotional distress.

11.2 Four B's of Discomfort in Older Adults with Dementia
(Shah et al., 2011)

- **Bowels**: when was the patient's last bowel movement?
- **Bladder**: when did the patient last urinate? Any urinary symptoms?
- **Beverage**: is the patient hungry or thirsty? Has he/she been offered preferred beverages or food?
- **Bottom** (to top): visual survey for obvious precipitants of distress and agitation

12. Assessment of NPS

12.1 Assessment of Behaviours

- What are the risks associated with the behaviour?
    - To patient, caregivers/staff, other individuals
- What is the behaviour?
    - E.g., using instrument such as CMAI or NPI
- What type of dementia does the individual have?
- What is the stage of dementia?
- What are the goals of care?

12.2 Cohen-Mansfield Agitation Inventory (CMAI)

- 29-item scale commonly used as an outcome measure for agitation in dementia
- Informant ratings of the frequency of agitated behaviours in past 2 weeks
    - 1 = never
    - 3 = 1 to 2 times/week
    - 7 = several times per hour
- Score ranges from 29–203
- Can use total score, subscales, or ratings on individual items
- CMAI, subscales
    - Verbal agitation
    - Physically non-aggressive agitation
    - Physically aggressive agitation

12.3 Neuropsychiatric Inventory (NPI)
(Cummings et al., 1994)

- 12-item scale
- Assesses broad range of neuropsychiatric symptoms commonly observed in dementia
- Each item rated on frequency and severity
- Versions for use with caregivers, LTC staff or caregiver, patient interview, and clinician ratings

Neuropsychiatric Inventory (NPI) items:

- Delusions
- Hallucinations
- Agitation/aggression
- Depression
- Anxiety
- Apathy/indifference
- Elation/euphoria
- Disinhibition
- Irritability
- Aberrant motor behaviour
- Sleep and nighttime behaviour
- Appetite and eating disturbances

Using the NPI:

- Can be used to assess the type and severity of symptoms
- Identifies behaviours that are most important to target and monitor
- Frequency of behaviours
  - 1 = occasionally
  - 2 = often (1/week)
  - 3 = frequently (< than daily)
  - 4 = very frequently (daily)
- Severity
  - 1 = mild (little distress)
  - 2 = moderate (redirectable)
  - 3 = severe
- Distress associated with symptoms

12.4 Behavioural Pathology in Alzheimer's Disease (Behave-AD)
(Reisberg et al., 1987)

- Caregiver interview–based assessment of NPS
- 25 items categorized into 7 domains, preceding 2 weeks
  - Delusions
  - Hallucinations
  - Activity disturbances
  - Aggressiveness
  - Diurnal rhythm disturbance
  - Affective disturbance
  - Anxiety and phobias

Each domain rated from 0 (not present) to 3 (severe)
Global severity rating by caregiver 0–3

12.5 ABC (Antecedents, Behaviours, Consequences) Approach

Behavioural analysis approach to understanding dementia, based on learning theory

- **A**ntecedents to the behaviour (i.e., during care)
- **B**ehaviours (what was the behaviour?)

- Consequences (what was the response to the behaviour)
- Behavioural charting using Dementia Observation System (DOS)
- Charting of behaviours over several days
- Helps to identify patterns and precipitants of NPS
- Frequency of behaviours over days
- Informs timing of interventions
- Activities or medications

12.6 Measuring Depression in Dementia
(Alexopoulos et al., 1988)

- Cornell Scale for Depression in Dementia (CSDD)
- Based on informant interview and patient observation over the preceding week
- Items scored from 0 = absent, 1 = mild, 2 = severe
- 19 items
- Items include mood-related items, behavioural changes, physical changes, activity cycle, and negative ideation

13. Prevalence of NPS in Alzheimer's Disease

Neuropsychiatric symptoms are common among individuals with dementia, and the prevalence of various types of behaviours varies (Figure 1.3.1).

Figure 1.3.1: Prevalence of NPS among Individuals with Alzheimer's Disease

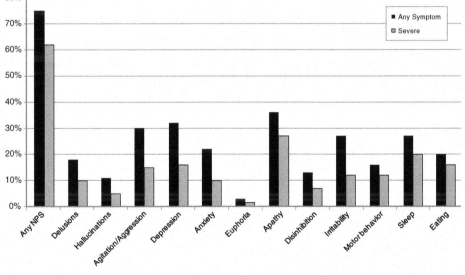

NPS = neuropsychiatric symptom
Adapted from Lyketsos et al., 2002.

13.1 Prevalence of NPS in Long-Term Care

(Seitz, Purandare, & Conn, 2010; Zuidema, Koopmans, & Verhey, 2007)

- 60% of individuals in LTC settings have dementia

Overall prevalence of NPS:

- Median prevalence of any NPS: 78%

Prevalence of NPS:

- Psychosis: 15–30%
- Depression: 30–50%
- Physical agitation: 30%
- Aggression: 10–20%

The overall prevalence of specific NPS in one LTC study using the BEHAVE-AD scale is summarized in Table 1.3.1.

Table 1.3.1: Prevalence of NPS in Long-Term Care

BEHAVE-AD Symptoms	Prevalence (%)
Delusions	54
Hallucinations	33
Psychosis	60
Aggression	77
Activity disturbance	53
Diurnal disturbance	47
Affective disturbance	60
Anxiety	69
Any BEHAVE-AD symptom	92

BEHAVE-AD = behavioural pathology in Alzheimer's disease; NPS = neuropsychiatric symptoms
Adapted from Brodaty et al., 2001; International Psychogeriatric Association, 2011.

13.2 Associations with Stage of Illness

Certain NPS are more common at different stages of Alzheimer's disease than at other stages (see Figure 1.3.2).

13.3 Persistence of NPS

(Steinberg et al., 2004; Aalten et al., 2005)

- Neuropsychiatric symptoms are often chronic.
    - More likely to persist: delusions, depression, aberrant motor behaviour
    - Less likely to persist: hallucinations, disinhibition

13.4 Prevalence of NPS in Mild Cognitive Impairment (MCI)

NPS are also common among older adults with mild cognitive impairment (Figure 1.3.3).

Figure 1.3.2: Prevalence of NPS by Stage of Dementia

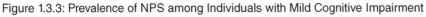

Adapted from Chen et al., 2000.

Figure 1.3.3: Prevalence of NPS among Individuals with Mild Cognitive Impairment

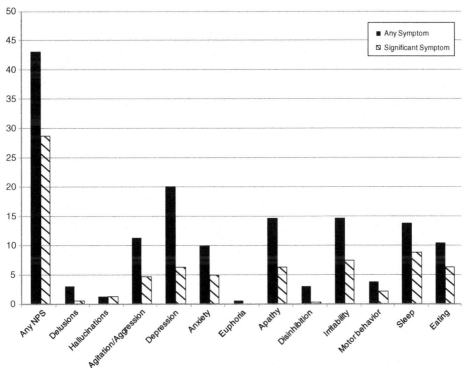

NPS = neuropsychiatric symptom
Adapted from Lyketsos et al., 2002.

NPS in MCI and AD conversion (Palmer et al., 2007; Palmer et al., 2010; Gabryelewicz et al., 2007)

- Each symptom of anxiety in MCI increases risk of AD conversion by HR = 1.8
- Persistent worrying (HR = 5.3), decision making (HR = 5.6)
- MCI conversion over 3 years:
  - No anxiety: 40.9%
  - Anxiety: 83.3%
- MCI with apathy associated with 6.9X increased risk of conversion
- Depression also a predictor of conversion in MCI

13.5 NPS in Different Types of Dementia

When compared to Alzheimer's disease, other types of dementia may have patterns of NPS that tend to differ.

13.5.1 Vascular Dementia
(Fuh, Wang, & Cummings, 2005)

- Overall, patterns of NPS for cortical and subcortical vascular dementia are similar to AD.
- Cortical vascular dementia is associated with higher rates of apathy and sleep disturbance when compared to AD.

13.5.2 Frontotemporal Dementia
(Srikanth, Nagaraja, & Ratnavalli, 2005)

- Higher rates of NPS for a given severity of dementia
- Compared to AD, higher rates of delusions (18% vs 10%), disinhibition (82% vs 45%), abnormal motor behaviour (74% vs 21%)
- Significant abnormal eating behaviours only occurred in frontotemporal dementia (FTD) group (22%)

13.5.3 Dementia with Lewy Bodies and Parkinson's Disease Dementia
(Noe et al., 2004; Ballard et al., 1999; Aarsland et al., 2001)

- Psychosis at illness presentation is more common with DLB (31.3%) compared to AD (6.3%).
- DLB patient is more likely to have hallucinations (75% vs 38%), depression (48% vs 17%) than AD patient.
- Delusions and hallucinations are more common in DLB (57%, 76%) than PDD (29%, 54%).

14. Impact of NPS
(Banerjee et al., 2006)

- Increased patient and caregiver distress
- Increased risk for institutionalization
- More rapid functional decline
- Increased risk of mortality
- Economic costs

15. More General Principles for Managing NPS
(International Psychogeriatric Association, 2010)

15.1 General Behavioural Interventions

- Reduce isolation, distract person from frustration.
- Identify precipitants to the behaviours.
- Experiment with targeted changes to schedule and environment.
- Provide reassurance.
- Allow patient to wander if safe to do so.
- Encourage pleasant experiences.

15.2 Understanding the Person with Dementia

- Social history
- Marital status, family, religion, country of birth, religion, first language, occupation
- Personal preferences:
    - Food, hobbies, music, conversational topics
- Daily routines:
    - Sleeping, eating, meal preparation, activities
- Personal priorities
- Functional abilities
- Cognitive severity

15.3 Care Environments and NPS

- Long-term care
    - Severity of dementia
    - Environmental challenges
    - Resource availability
    - Medical comorbidity
- Community
    - Availability of caregivers
    - Unstructured environment
    - Access to medical care or allied health professionals
- See also chapter 4.5.

15.4 Environmental Correlates of NPS

- Single rooms may be helpful for reducing agitation.
- Smaller facility sizes may reduce aggression.
- High environment temperatures and physical discomfort are associated with verbal and non-aggressive physical agitation.

15.5 Structuring the Environment

- Provide predictable routines.
- Promote a safe environment.

- Use a night light.
- Provide orienting stimuli.
- Ensure bright enough daytime lighting.
- Separate noisy and disruptive individuals from quieter persons.
- Ensure adequate space.

QUESTIONS

1. List three major psychological theories that are used to conceptualize the development of NPS.
2. List five clinical patient factors which may contribute to the development of NPS.
3. List five different major clusters of NPS commonly encountered in dementia.
4. Are all NPS in dementia due to unmet needs?

ANSWERS

1. Major psychological theories that are used to conceptualize the development of NPS include:
   - Lower stress threshold
   - Learning theory
   - Unmet needs

2. Clinical patient factors which may contribute to the development of NPS include:
   - Pain
   - Sensory impairment
   - Severity of cognitive impairment
   - Type of dementia
   - Premorbid personality

3. Major clusters of NPS in dementia include:
   - Apathy
   - Sleep
   - Depression
   - Psychosis
   - Agitation/aggression

4. Are all NPS in dementia due to unmet needs? This model seems to work best to explain most behaviours except psychosis and aggression, where it is acknowledged that other factors may play a more important role in explaining these behaviours. Even with the optimal care environment and knowledgeable staff, neuropsychiatric symptoms continue to be highly prevalent, suggesting that unmet needs are not necessarily easily identified in many cases. The authors of the unmet needs model acknowledge that not all behaviours are due to unmet needs, although many may be.

CASE DISCUSSION

Additional history concerning the details of the symptoms is required, starting with the onset of symptoms. Sudden onset of symptoms may suggest a delirium, medication-related problems, or medical contributors to the symptoms.

A risk assessment needs to be completed, looking at any safety concerns for the patient, staff, and co-residents. Review of staff- or family-related stress associated with the behaviours is important.

History from the staff, family, and patient (if possible) should be sought to further describe the behaviour. Behavioural charting with an instrument such as the Dementia Observation System or similar tool could be used to better understand when and where the behaviours are occurring and to identify potential environmental or interpersonal contributors to the behaviour. A more detailed history of the "agitation and aggression" should be sought, and consideration given to using a tool such as a Cohen-Mansfield Agitation Inventory to further detail the frequency of the agitation and aggression. Other potential neuropsychiatric symptoms, including psychosis, depression, apathy, and sleep patterns, should be reviewed.

Following this more detailed description of the behaviours, investigations should be completed to determine potential contributors to behaviours. These investigations should include a review of medications for potential side effects. The potential for pain as a contributor to behaviours should be considered, along with pain charting using a tool for dementia (such as PAINAD). Medical history and psychiatric history should be reviewed for potential contributors to the current symptoms. The severity of cognitive impairment, functional limitations, and sensory deficits should be assessed. A psychosocial history should be completed, evaluating for potential environmental factors that may exacerbate behaviours or serve as potential areas for interventions (e.g., identifying previously enjoyed activities).

RECOMMENDED RESOURCES FOR REVIEW

Although these resources may not be specifically cited in the text, their approach informed the contents of the chapter, and they are recommended as useful further reading.

Canadian Coalition for Seniors' Mental Health. The assessment and treatment of mental health issues in long-term care homes (focus on mood and behaviour symptoms). Toronto: Canadian Coalition for Seniors' Mental Health; 2006, updated 2014. http://www.ccsmh.ca/en/projects/ltc.cfm

Lyketsos CG, Lopez O, Jones B, et al. Prevalence of neuropsychiatric symptoms in dementia and mild cognitive impairment: results from the cardiovascular health study. JAMA. 2002;288(12):1475–83. http://dx.doi.org/10.1001/jama.288.12.1475. Medline:12243634

Zuidema S, Koopmans R, Verhey F. Prevalence and predictors of neuropsychiatric symptoms in cognitively impaired nursing home patients. J Geriatr Psychiatry Neurol. 2007;20(1):41–9. http://dx.doi.org/10.1177/0891988706292762. Medline:17341770

REFERENCES

Aalten P, de Vugt ME, Jaspers N, et al. The course of neuropsychiatric symptoms in dementia. Part I: findings from the two-year longitudinal Maasbed study. Int J Geriatr Psychiatry. 2005;20(6):523–30. http://dx.doi.org/10.1002/gps.1316. Medline:15920712

Aalten P, de Vugt ME, Lousberg R, et al. Behavioral problems in dementia: a factor analysis of the neuropsychiatric inventory. Dement Geriatr Cogn Disord. 2003;15(2):99–105. http://dx.doi.org/10.1159/000067972. Medline:12566599

Aarsland D, Andersen K, Larsen JP, et al. Risk of dementia in Parkinson's disease: a community-based, prospective study. Neurology. 2001;56(6):730–6. http://dx.doi .org/10.1212/WNL.56.6.730. Medline:11274306

Alexopoulos GS, Abrams RC, Young RC, et al. Cornell scale for depression in dementia. Biol Psychiatry. 1988;23(3):271–84. http://dx.doi.org/10.1016/ 0006-3223(88)90038-8. Medline:3337862

Ballard C, Holmes C, McKeith I, et al. Psychiatric morbidity in dementia with Lewy bodies: a prospective clinical and neuropathological comparative study with Alzheimer's disease. Am J Psychiatry. 1999;156(7):1039–45. Medline:10401449

Banerjee S, Smith SC, Lamping DL, et al. Quality of life in dementia: more than just cognition. An analysis of associations with quality of life in dementia. J Neurol Neurosurg Psychiatry. 2006;77(2):146–8. http:// dx.doi.org/10.1136/jnnp.2005 .072983. Medline:16421113

Brodaty H, Luscombe G, Parker G, et al. Early and late onset depression in old age: different aetiologies, same phenomenology. J Affect Disord. 2001;66(2-3):225–36. http://dx.doi.org/10.1016/S0165-0327(00)00317-7. Medline:11578676

Byers AL, Yaffe K. Depression and risk of developing dementia. Nat Rev Neurol. 2011;7(6):323–31. http:// dx.doi.org/10.1038/nrneurol.2011.60. Medline:21537355

Chen P, Ratcliff G, Belle SH, et al. Cognitive tests that best discriminate between presymptomatic AD and those who remain nondemented. Neurology. 2000;55(12):1847–53. http://dx.doi.org/10.1212/WNL.55.12.1847. Medline:11134384

Cohen-Mansfield J. Theoretical frameworks for behavioral problems in dementia. Alzheimer's Care Quarterly. 2000;1(4):8–21.

– Nonpharmacologic interventions for inappropriate behaviors in dementia: a review, summary, and critique. Am J Geriatr Psychiatry. 2001;9(4):361–81. http://dx.doi .org/10.1097/00019442-200111000-00005. Medline:11739063

Cohen-Mansfield J, Marx MS, Rosenthal AS. A description of agitation in a nursing home. J Gerontol. 1989;44(3):M77–84. http://dx.doi.org/10.1093/geronj/44.3.M77. Medline:2715584

Cummings JL, Mega M, Gray K, et al. The Neuropsychiatric Inventory: comprehensive assessment of psychopathology in dementia. Neurology. 1994;44(12):2308–14. http://dx.doi.org/10.1212/WNL .44.12.2308. Medline:7991117

Finkel SI, Costa e Silva J, Cohen G, et al. Behavioral and psychological signs and symptoms of dementia: a consensus statement on current knowledge and implications for research and treatment. Int Psychogeriatr. 1996;8(S3):497–500. http://dx.doi.org/10.1017/S1041610297003943. Medline:9154615

Fox PL, Raina P, Jadad AR. Prevalence and treatment of pain in older adults in nursing homes and other long-term care institutions: a systematic review. CMAJ. 1999;160(3):329–33. Medline:10065074

Fuh JL, Wang SJ, Cummings JL. Neuropsychiatric profiles in patients with Alzheimer's disease and vascular dementia. J Neurol Neurosurg Psychiatry. 2005;76(10):1337–41. http://dx.doi.org/10.1136/jnnp.2004 .056408. Medline:16170072

Gabryelewicz T, Styczynska M, Luczywek E, et al. The rate of conversion of mild cognitive impairment to dementia: predictive role of depression. Int J Geriatr Psychiatry. 2007;22(6):563–7. http://dx.doi.org/ 10.1002/gps.1716. Medline:17136705

Geda YE, Schneider LS, Gitlin LN, et al. Neuropsychiatric symptoms in Alzheimer's disease: past progress and anticipation of the future. Alzheimer Dement. 2013;9(5)602–8. http://dx.doi.org/10.1016/j.jalz.2012.12.001. Medline:23562430

Hall GR, Buckwalter KC. Progressively lowered stress threshold: a conceptual model for care of adults with Alzheimer's disease. Arch Psychiatr Nurs. 1987;1(6):399–406. Medline:3426250

Inouye SK, van Dyck CH, Alessi CA, et al. Clarifying confusion: the confusion assessment method. A new method for detection of delirium. Ann Intern Med. 1990;113(12):941–8. http://dx.doi.org/10.7326/0003-4819-113-12-941. Medline:2240918

International Psychogeriatric Association. The IPA complete guides to behavioral andpsychological symptoms of dementia. Milwaukee, WI: International Psychogeriatric Association; 2010. http://www.ipa-online.org/ publications/guides-to-bpsd

Jeste DV, Finkel SI. Psychosis of Alzheimer's disease and related dementias: diagnostic criteria for a distinct syndrome. Am J Geriatr Psychiatry. 2000;8(1):29–34. http://dx.doi.org/10.1097/00019442-200002000-00004. Medline:10648292

Kitwood T. Person and process in dementia. Int J Geriatr Psychiatry. 1993;8(7):541–5. http://dx.doi.org/ 10.1002/gps.930080702

Kovach CR, Logan BR, Noonan PE, et al. Effects of the Serial Trial Intervention on discomfort and behavior of nursing home residents with dementia. Am J Alzheimers Dis Other Demen. 2006;21(3): 147–55. Medline:16869334

Noe E, Marder K, Bell KL, et al. Comparison of dementia with Lewy bodies to Alzheimer's disease and Parkinson's disease with dementia. Mov Disord. 2004;19(1):60–7. http://dx.doi.org/10.1002/mds.10633. Medline:14743362

Palmer K, Berger AK, Monastero R, et al. Predictors of progression from mild cognitive impairment to Alzheimer disease. Neurology. 2007;68(19):1596–602. http://dx.doi.org/10.1212/01.wnl.0000260968 .92345.3f. Medline:17485646

Palmer K, Di Iulio F, Varsi AE, et al. Neuropsychiatric predictors of progression from amnestic-mild cognitive impairment to Alzheimer's disease: the role of depression and apathy. J Alzheimers Dis. 2010;20(1):175–83. Medline:20164594

Pieper MJ, Achterberg WP, Francke AL, et al. The implementation of the serial trial intervention for pain and challenging behaviour in advanced dementia patients (STA OP!): a clustered randomized controlled trial. BMC Geriatr. 2011;11(1):12. http://dx.doi.org/10.1186/1471-2318-11-12. Medline:21435251

Reisberg B, Borenstein J, Salob SP, et al. Behavioral symptoms in Alzheimer's disease: phenomenology and treatment. J Clin Psychiatry. 1987;48(Suppl):9–15. Medline:3553166

Seitz D, Purandare N, Conn D. Prevalence of psychiatric disorders among older adults in long-term care homes: a systematic review. Int Psychogeriatr. 2010;22(7):1025–39. http://dx.doi.org/10.1017/S1041610210000608 . Medline:20522279

Shah SM, Carey IM, Harris T, et al. Quality of chronic disease care for older people in care homes and the community in a primary care pay for performance system: retrospective study. BMJ. 2011;342:d912. http://dx.doi.org/10.1136/bmj.d912. Medline:21385803

Sink KM, Holden KF, Yaffe K. Pharmacological treatment of neuropsychiatric symptoms of dementia: a review of the evidence. JAMA. 2005;293(5):596–608. http://dx.doi.org/10.1001/jama.293.5.596. Medline:15687315

Srikanth S, Nagaraja AV, Ratnavalli E. Neuropsychiatric symptoms in dementia-frequency, relationship to dementia severity and comparison in Alzheimer's disease, vascular dementia and frontotemporal dementia. J Neurol Sci. 2005;236 (1-2):43–8. http://dx.doi.org/10.1016/j.jns.2005.04.014. Medline:15964021

Starkstein SE, Jorge R, Mizrahi R, et al. The construct of minor and major depression in Alzheimer's disease. Am J Psychiatry. 2005;162(11):2086–93. http://dx.doi.org/ 10.1176/appi.ajp.162.11.2086. Medline:16263848

Steinberg M, Tschanz JT, Corcoran C, et al. The persistence of neuropsychiatric symptoms in dementia: the Cache County Study. Int J Geriatr Psychiatry. 2004;19(1):19–26. http://dx.doi .org/10.1002/gps.1025. Medline:14716695

Teng E, Ringman JM, Ross LK, et al.; Alzheimer's Disease Research Centers of California–Depression in Alzheimer's Disease Investigators. Diagnosing depression in Alzheimer disease with the national institute of mental health provisional criteria. Am J Geriatr Psychiatry. 2008;16(6):469–77. http://dx.doi.org/10.1097/ JGP.0b013e318165dbae. Medline:18515691

Warden V, Hurley AC, Volicer L. Development and psychometric evaluation of the Pain Assessment in Advanced Dementia (PAINAD) scale. J Am Med Dir Assoc. 2003;4(1):9–15. http://dx.doi.org/10.1097/ 01.JAM.0000043422.31640.F7. Medline:12807591

1.4 Nonpharmacological Management of Neuropsychiatric Symptoms of Dementia

Dallas Seitz, MD, PhD, FRCPC

INTRODUCTION

Nonpharmacological interventions, sometimes referred to as psychosocial interventions, are generally recommended as the first-line treatments for the management of neuropsychiatric symptoms (NPS) associated with dementia. These interventions include a broad range of treatment modalities delivered in either community or long-term care (LTC) settings. To effectively practice geriatric psychiatry, knowledge of the evidence-based nonpharmacological treatments is required, along with clinical experience in delivering these approaches, which often involve educating family members or caregivers. There is increasing evidence to support many of these therapies which form the cornerstone of managing NPS.

CASE SCENARIO

You have completed your assessment of the 87-year-old patient described in chapter 1.3. No immediate safety concerns have been identified. The symptoms have been present for the last year, but have gradually worsened in severity over the past six months following a hip fracture. There have been no recent medication changes, recent bloodwork is unremarkable, and clinically the patient does not have symptoms or signs of delirium. Behavioural assessment indicates that the patient tends to have verbal agitation frequently throughout the day (yelling out, "Come here, come here!"), particularly when seated in her wheelchair and when she is alone. She can be physically aggressive when staff try to provide direct care such as changing or bathing her. Pain observation indicates that she displays nonverbal indicators that are possibly consistent with pain (facial grimacing, laboured breathing, guarding during movement). Staff do not report symptoms of psychosis, persistent signs of depression, or major sleep changes. She is unable to transfer on her own and spends most of her time in a wheelchair, either in her room or at the nursing station. Her vision is very limited, although her hearing is adequate for communication. Social history indicates that she has two daughters who visit infrequently. The patient used to enjoy cats and attending church prior to her admission to LTC several years ago. With this information, outline a potential nonpharmacological management plan.

OVERVIEW

There are several evidence-based interventions that can be beneficial for NPS (Cohen-Mansfield, 2001; Livingston et al., 2005; Seitz et al., 2012). Most nonpharmacological interventions can be broadly classified into the categories of interventions listed below. These interventions have the greatest evidence for reducing symptoms of agitation. The evidence for interventions targeting other NPS (e.g., depression, apathy) is presented separately.

- Training caregivers or staff in behavioural management strategies and communication
- Mental health consultations
- Participation in pleasant events
- Exercise
- Music
- Sensory stimulation (e.g., touch, Snoezelen, aromatherapy)

1. Training Caregivers and Staff

(McCallion et al., 1999; Chenoweth et al., 2009; Testad et al., 2010)

Of the different nonpharmacological approaches for the management of NPS, training of caregivers (either nursing staff or family caregivers) has the most extensive and consistent evidence.

- Some staff and caregiver training approaches effective in reducing NPS
- Also referred to as patient-centred care
- Most training programs involve psychoeducation about dementia symptoms
- Communication strategies to avoid confrontation
- Strategies for redirection and distraction
- Often incorporate personalized pleasant events into interactions

1.1 Caregiver Training Approaches

1.1.1 The Caring for Aged in Dementia Care Resident Study (CADRES)
(Chenoweth et al., 2009)

- Randomized controlled trial (RCT) of two models of person-centred care (PCC); PCC and dementia care mapping compared to usual care
- 15 LTC facilities in Australia, N = 298
- Evaluated outcomes at 4, 8 months
- Significant reductions on the Cohen-Mansfield Agitation Inventory (CMAI) with either dementia care mapping or person-centred model of care when compared to usual care
- Neuropsychiatric Inventory (NPI): PCC showed reduction in NPI score
- Quality of life not significantly impacted by either PCC or dementia care mapping

1.1.2 Other Caregiver Training Approaches

- In Canada, programs or resources that would be most comparable to that used in the CADRES study would include the Gentle Persuasive Approach and related programs.
- Gentle Persuasive Approach: https://www.ageinc.ca/
- Murray Alzheimer Research and Education Program: https://uwaterloo.ca/murray-alzheimer-research-and-education-program/
    - Dementia Care Education Series: https://uwaterloo.ca/murray-alzheimer-research-and-education-program/education-and-knowledge-translation/products-education-tools/dementia-care-education-series

– Managing and Accommodating Responsive Behaviours in Dementia Care: https://uwaterloo.ca/murray-alzheimer-research-and-education-program/education-and-knowledge-translation/products-education-tools/managing-and-accomodating-responsive-behaviours-dementia

1.2 Caregiver Training Compared to Medications
(Teri et al., 2000)

- Relatively few interventions comparing caregiver training approaches to other treatments such as medications
- One study by Teri et al. (2000) in community-dwelling persons with dementia treated with either haloperidol, trazodone, behavioural management therapy (BMT), or placebo for 16 weeks (n = 148)
- BMT consisted of eight sessions involving psychoeducation, strategies for reducing agitation
- Overall, no difference noted in changes in behaviours between the groups
- 34% improved overall; 20% had no change
- BMT less likely to drop out due to adverse events, although dropout rates due to caregiver difficulties was higher in the BMT group
- Medications associated ↓ activities of daily living (ADLs) and Mini Mental State Examination (MMSE)

2. Care Management for Dementia
(Callahan et al., 2006)

- Dementia nursing care management vs usual care in primary care
- Care managers reviewed memory and behavioural symptoms at visits
- Implemented protocol-delivered interventions for behaviours (e.g., sleep, delusions)
- NPI scores reduced with care management
- Intervention had no effect on depression, ADL, cognition

3. Mental Health Consultation
(Rovner et al., 1996; Cohen-Mansfield, Libin, & Marx, 2007)

- Referral to geriatric providers (e.g., psychiatrists, psychologists, geriatricians) for NPS effective in reducing NPS
- Evaluations focus on the following:
    – Assessing for treatable causes of behavioural changes including pain and delirium
    – Patient-centred nonpharmacological interventions for NPS
    – Working with staff and physicians to optimize care and environment

4. TREA Approach
(Cohen-Mansfield, 2000; Cohen-Mansfield et al., 2012)

- Treatment Routes for Exploring Agitation (TREA)
- Approach to assessment and management of behaviours based on assumptions of unmet needs
- RCT in 11 LTC homes in the United States; participants received activities to address unmet needs (N = 89) or usual care (N = 36)

- Unmet needs conceptualized as loneliness/depression, boredom, or discomfort
- Unmet needs identified from nursing staff, family members, and physicians
- Separate algorithms for verbal agitation, physically non-aggressive agitation, aggressive agitation

4.1 TREA Intervention

- Each participant had interventions from algorithms trailed over 3-week period prior to intervention time period.
- Interventions implemented daily for 4 hours when person most agitated
- Primary outcome: observed agitation at the end of 2 weeks

4.2 TREA Outcomes

- Individuals in the TREA program had significant reductions in physically non-aggressive agitation and verbal agitation, and increases in pleasure and interest when compared to those in the usual care group.

5. Participation in Pleasant Events
(Lichtenberg et al., 2005; Toseland et al., 1997)

- One-to-one interaction with personalized pleasant events has been demonstrated to reduce NPS.
  - Given 3X/week: 20–30 minutes/session
- Participation in group "validation therapy" may also be beneficial.

5.1 SMILE Program
(Low et al., 2013)

- Sydney Multisite Intervention for LaughterBosses and ElderClowns (SMILE) is a recent example of pleasant events intervention.
- RCT in 36 LTC facilities, 18 SMILE (N = 189), 18 control (N = 209)
- Intervention: humour therapy delivered by professional therapists (ElderClowns), training of LTC staff in humour therapy (LaughterBosses)
- Primary outcome: change in depression; secondary outcomes: change in agitation, other NPS

5.1.1 SMILE Outcomes

- No significant difference on primary outcome of depression using Cornell scale.
- Sample did not have high levels of depression at start.
- Agitation as measured on CMAI was significantly reduced at week 13 (endpoint) and week 26 (follow-up).
- Quality of life and other NPS were not affected by intervention.

5.1.2 SMILE Facility and Resident Predictors of Outcomes
(Brodaty et al., 2014)

- Participants with more committed LaughterBoss had significant reduction in depression.
- Management buy-in facilitated LaughterBoss participation.

6. Exercise
(Alessi et al., 1999; Landi, Russo, & Bernabei, 2004; Williams & Tappen, 2007; Teri et al., 2003)

- Exercise programs have been demonstrated to reduce NPS in LTC residents.
- Training caregivers in behavioural management and exercise programs improved physical functioning of patients with dementia and depressive symptoms.
- 30 minutes/day was recommended.
- Exercise program included strength, flexibility, aerobic activity, balance.

7. Music
(Sung et al., 2006; Raglio et al., 2008)

- Group music with movement and/or individualized music therapy is effective in reducing NPS.
- 30 minutes, 2–3 times/ week
- May use prior to times of increased agitation
- *Personalized* music more effective than generic music

8. Sensory Stimulation
(Hawranik, Johnston, & Deatrich, 2008; Woods, Craven, & Whitney, 2005; van Weert et al., 2005; Ballard et al., 2002; Burns et al., 2011; Fung, Tsang, & Chung, 2012)

- Therapeutic touch or gentle massage may relieve symptoms of agitation.
- Snoezelen (multisensory stimulation) providing tactile, light, olfactory, or auditory stimulation
- Aromatherapy may be effective although additional research is required.

8.1 Montessori for Dementia
(Orsulic-Jeras, Judge, & Camp, 2000; Lin et al., 2009)

- Montessori-based activities focus on sensory stimulation and activities associated with daily living. Montessori-based activities use activities based on functional ability to provide meaningful activities and stimulation for people with dementia while also attempting to preserve cognitive and functional abilities. Some activities that may be included in Montessori include scooping, pouring, squeezing, and fine motor activities facilitated by a staff member familiar with Montessori techniques.
- Some small studies of Montessori-based activities for dementia suggest improved engagement, affect, and agitation with activities.

8.1.1 Montessori for Agitation
(van der Ploeg et al., 2013)

- Randomized crossover trial in Australian nursing homes (n = 44) over 4 weeks
- Received either Montessori sessions or non-specific interaction twice weekly for 30 minutes
- Primary outcome of physically agitated behaviours
- Unmet need for stimulation
- Ruled out significant depression, pain, psychosis
- Examined effects of participants primary language

- Intervention can be delivered nonverbally.
- Intervention group had 50% reduction in agitation; 42% reduction in control group.
- Behaviours returned after sessions ended.
- Small effect on positive affect noted with Montessori during sessions.
- Non-English speaking participants had the greatest benefit from the program.

9. Interventions for Depression
(Goldwasser, Auerbach, & Harkins, 1987; Buettner & Fitzsimmons, 2002; Buettner, 1999; Teri et al., 1997; Teri et al., 2003)

- Staff training approaches to improve engagement in pleasant activities
- Small RCTs of reminiscence therapy, validation therapy for LTC residents
- AD-Venture, wheelchair bicycling for LTC residents with dementia and depression
- "Simple Pleasures" interventions improved affect and engagement in dementia.
- Training family caregivers in behavioural therapy in either pleasant event scheduling or problem-solving approaches reduces depression in both patients and caregivers.
- Caregiver training in behavioural management and regular exercise (Reducing Disability in Alzheimer Disease) reduces depression and improves function.

10. Interventions for Sleep
(McCurry et al., 2003; McCurry et al., 2005; McCurry et al., 2011; Skjerve et al., 2004; Forbes et al., 2014)

- Combination of exercise and sleep hygiene delivered to caregivers of persons with dementia
- Consistent wake time and bedtime, discourage napping, assess and reduce physiologic and environmental contributors
- Exercise (e.g., walking) for a target time of 30 minutes daily
- Some bright light therapy as part of treatment protocol
- Improvements in sleep outcomes (number of awakenings, time awake), and patient depression
- Adherence to program is strong predictor of outcome
- Inconsistent results for bright light therapy alone

11. Interventions for Apathy
(Brodaty & Burns, 2012; Baker et al., 2001)

- Therapeutic activities have greatest support for treatment of apathy.
- Reality orientation may improve apathy and engagement in environment.
- Snoezelen improves interaction with environment during sessions.
- Some evidence for exercise, music, animal-assisted therapy

12. Supporting Caregivers
(Mittelman et al., 1996)

- Components of effective spouse-caregiver intervention
    - Individualized counselling (2 sessions)
    - Family therapy (4 sessions)

  – Support group participation
  – Availability of counsellor for support and management
- Intervention prolonged time to LTC placement by > 300 days
- Impact of intervention greatest in male caregivers and care recipients with mild-to-moderate dementia (compared to more severe depression)

12.1 Caregiver Training and Psychoeducation
(Thomson et al., 2007)

The following strategies have been shown to reduce caregiver distress:
  – Referral to local Alzheimer's Society (www.alzheimer.ca)
  – Psychoeducation
  – Behavioural and communication strategies
  – Peer support

13. Interventions for Other NPS
(International Psychogeriatric Association, 2010, 2015)

- Wandering
  – Limited evidence for mirrors, wandering gardens, barriers
- Sexually inappropriate behaviours
  – Small studies have suggested that multidisciplinary assessment and strategies employing redirection and improved communication can decrease some behaviours.
- Bathing
  – Bed baths may reduce agitation; no adverse effects on health or hygiene.
- Eating
  – Music played during mealtimes can reduce agitation and improve oral intake.

14. Some General Limitations of Nonpharmacological Strategies for NPS

- Modest effects of treatments
- Effect size = 0.2–0.5 for many interventions
- Effectiveness for aggression and psychosis may be limited.
- Agitation, depressive symptoms, apathy may be more likely to respond.
- May require prolonged and sustained implementation for effects to be realized
- Many interventions have only been evaluated in small studies; methodological quality is limited.

15. Safety of Nonpharmacological Interventions
(Seitz et al., 2011)

Review of nonpharmacological interventions for NPS in LTC populations

- Risk of trial withdrawal and mortality associated with nonpharmacological interventions
- Trial withdrawals reported in 17/40 (43%) studies, and mortality reported in 11/40 (25%) studies
- Trial withdrawal: OR = 0.99 (95% CI: 0.8–1.2, $p = 0.9$)
- Mortality: OR = 0.88 (95% CI: 0.6–1.2, $p = 0.4$)

16. Feasibility of Nonpharmacological Interventions

- Some potential barriers to the use of nonpharmacological interventions include requirements for specialized staffing, significant staff time to implement the intervention, and monetary costs.
- A summary of some of the feasibility issues with nonpharmacological interventions is presented in Figure 1.4.1 (Note: high, medium, and low refer to high, medium, and low feasibility in typical LTC settings).

Figure 1.4.1: Feasibility of Nonpharmacological Interventions for NPS in Long-Term Care

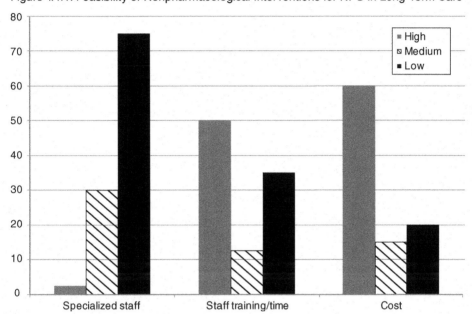

NPS = neuropsychiatric symptoms
Adapted from Seitz et al., 2012.

17. Evidence Summary

The evidence for different types of nonpharmacological interventions for specific NPS is variable (Table 1.4.1).

18. NPS Guidelines
(Vickland et al., 2012)

Multiple guidelines from different organizations have been created for the management of NPS. Several of the guidelines are listed in Table 1.4.2.

19. Conclusions

- NPS are common in dementia and have an important impact on patients and caregivers.
- A comprehensive assessment of NPS is important and informs treatment strategies.
- Nonpharmacological interventions have an important role in the management of NPS.

Table 1.4.1: Evidence for Nonpharmacological Treatments for Specific NPS

Intervention	Global NPS	Agitation/ Aggression	Psychosis	Depression	Apathy	Sleep
Staff or caregiver training	✓	✓		✓	✓	
Mental health assessment		✓				
Psychosocial interventions/ Pleasant events	✓	✓		✓	✓	
Exercise		✓		✓	✓	✓
Music	✓			✓	✓	
Sensory stimulation	✓			✓	✓	
Light therapy				?		?

NPS = neuropsychiatric symptoms

Table 1.4.2: Guidelines for the Management of NPS

Alexopoulos et al., 2007	Herrmann & Gauthier, 2008
American Association for Geriatric Psychiatry: Lyketsos et al., 2006	National Institute for Health and Clinical Excellence (NICE)/Social Care Institute for Excellence (SCIE), 2007 (UK)
American Psychiatric Association, 2007 (online)	Royal Australian and New Zealand College of General Practitioners, 2006
Benoit et al., 2006	Royal Australian and New Zealand College of Psychiatrists, 2009
Guidelines and Protocols Advisory Committee (GPAC); British Columbia Ministry of Health; Doctors of BC (DOBC), 2014	Royal College of Psychiatrists, 2005 (UK)
Canadian Coalition for Seniors' Mental Health, 2006, updated 2014	Salzman et al., 2008
Dettmore, Kolanowski, & Boustani, 2009	Scottish Intercollegiate Guidelines Network, 2006
Fletcher, 2008	

NPS = neuropsychiatric symptoms

QUESTIONS

1. List five different types of evidence-based nonpharmacological interventions for the treatment of neuropsychiatric symptoms.

2. List four barriers to the implementation of nonpharmacological interventions for NPS in long-term care settings.

3. Should nonpharmacological interventions always be used before pharmacological interventions?

ANSWERS

1. Evidence-based nonpharmacological interventions for the treatment of neuropsychiatric symptoms in dementia include:
   - Caregiver training or education
   - Exercise
   - Sensory stimulation (Snoezelen, therapeutic touch)
   - Music therapy
   - Scheduled pleasant events

2. Barriers to the implementation of nonpharmacological interventions for NPS in long-term care settings include, but are not limited to:
   - Costs of some treatments
   - Limited access to specialist services
   - Time required to implement interventions
   - Lack of patient cooperation

3. The question of whether nonpharmacological interventions should always be used before pharmacological interventions depends on the situation and the nonpharmacological intervention. The evidence base for nonpharmacological interventions for aggression and significant psychotic symptoms is limited at the present time, although training caregivers and nursing staff in person-centred approaches to care may help to minimize the impact of these behaviours. While it is never a bad idea to try to implement nonpharmacological interventions, persons with dementia may not cooperate with them, which can limit the utility of some nonpharmacological interventions in some settings.

CASE DISCUSSION

Nonpharmacological strategies for behavioural symptoms involve identifying and removing triggers along with other specific strategies such as staff education, pleasant events, music, exercise, and sensory stimulation.

First steps may include education for the staff, including strategies for effective communication such as speaking in a calm, friendly voice and using simple sentences. Staff training strategies such as the Gentle Persuasive Approach could be recommended if not already available at the home.

Pain seems to be a potential contributor this patient's presentation, given the temporal relationship to hip fracture, pain charting, and patterns of behaviour associated with movement. Recommendations for a trial of analgesia might be appropriate (such as Tylenol 650 mg PO QID) or other interventions such as occupational therapy reassessment to see if repositioning of wheelchairs may be helpful.

After these assessments for potential contributors, a number of nonpharmacological strategies could be considered. Recreation staff, family, or volunteers may be able to provide individualized activities based on past interests. In this particular patient, conversation about past pleasant events such as a discussion about family members, past hobbies (e.g., cats), or activities (such as church) could be trialled, depending on availability of resources for this. Music, personalized to the patient's known preferences, could be considered as an intervention during periods of distress to see if this reduces behaviours. Some forms of sensory stimulation (e.g., presences of a simulated cat) may also be considered for this patient.

Changes to her daily routine, such as trying to have the patient in a well-lit area of the LTC home where other residents and staff are present (in a common area or near the nursing station), may help to reduce potentially fears of being alone and provide more stimulation, which may reduce some behaviours.

RECOMMENDED RESOURCES FOR REVIEW

Although these resources may not be specifically cited in the text, their approach informed the contents of the chapter, and they are recommended as useful further reading.

Gitlin LN, Kales HC, Lyketsos CG. Nonpharmacologic management of behavioral symptoms in dementia. JAMA. 2012;308(19):2020–9. http://dx.doi.org/10.1001/jama.2012.36918. Medline:23168825

Pieper MJ, Achterberg WP, Francke AL, et al. The implementation of the serial trial intervention for pain and challenging behaviour in advanced dementia patients (STA OP!): a clustered randomized controlled trial. BMC Geriatr. 2011;11(1):12. http://dx.doi.org/10.1186/1471-2318-11-12. Medline:21435251

REFERENCES

Alessi CA, Yoon EJ, Schnelle JF, et al. A randomized trial of a combined physical activity and environmental intervention in nursing home residents: do sleep and agitation improve? J Am Geriatr Soc. 1999;47(7):784–91. http://dx.doi.org/10.1111/j.1532-5415.1999.tb03833.x. Medline:10404920

Alexopoulos GS, Jeste DV, Chung H, et al. Treatment of dementia and agitation: a guide for families and caregivers. J Psychiatr Pract. 2007;13(3):207–16. http://dx.doi.org/10.1097/01.pra.0000271667.53717.9f

American Psychiatric Association. Practice guideline for the treatment of people with Alzheimer's disease and other dementias. 2nd. ed. Arlington, VA: American Psychiatric Association; 2007. http://psychiatryonline.com/pracGuide/ pracGuideTopic_3.aspx

Baker R, Bell S, Baker E, et al. A randomized controlled trial of the effects of multi-sensory stimulation (MSS) for people with dementia. Br J Clin Psychol. 2001;40(Pt 1):81–96. Medline:11317951

Ballard CG, O'Brien JT, Reichelt K, et al. Aromatherapy as a safe and effective treatment for the management of agitation in severe dementia: the results of a double-blind, placebo-controlled trial with Melissa. J Clin Psychiatry. 2002;63(7):553–8. http://dx.doi.org/10.4088/JCP.v63n0703. Medline:12143909

Benoit M, Arbus C, Blanchard F, et al. Professional consensus on the treatment of agitation, aggressive behaviour, oppositional behaviour and psychotic disturbances in dementia. J Nutr Health Aging. 2006;10(5):410–5. Medline:17066213

Brodaty H, Burns K. Nonpharmacological management of apathy in dementia: a systematic review. Am J Geriatr Psychiatry. 2012;20(7):549–64. http://dx.doi.org/ 10.1097/JGP.0b013e31822be242. Medline:21860324

Brodaty H, Low LF, Liu Z, et al. Successful ingredients in the SMILE study: resident, staff, and management factors influence the effects of humor therapy in residential aged care. Am J Geriatr Psychiatry. 2014;22(12):1427–37. Medline:24119859

Buettner LL. Simple pleasures: a multilevel sensorimotor intervention for nursing home residents with dementia. Am J Alzheimers Dis (Columbia). 1999;14(1):41–52. http://dx.doi.org/10.1177/153331759901400103

Buettner LL, Fitzsimmons S. AD-venture program: therapeutic biking for the treatment of depression in long-term care residents with dementia. Am J Alzheimers Dis Other Demen. 2002;17(2):121–7. http://dx.doi.org/10.1177/ 153331750201700205. Medline:11954670

Burns A, Perry E, Holmes C, et al. A double-blind placebo-controlled randomized trial of *Melissa officinalis* oil and donepezil for the treatment of agitation in Alzheimer's disease. Dement Geriatr Cogn Disord. 2011;31(2):158–64. http://dx.doi.org/ 10.1159/000324438. Medline:21335973

Callahan CM, Boustani MA, Unverzagt FW, et al. Effectiveness of collaborative care for older adults with Alzheimer disease in primary care: a randomized controlled trial. JAMA. 2006;295(18):2148–57. http://dx.doi.org/10.1001/jama.295.18.2148. Medline:16684985

Canadian Coalition for Seniors' Mental Health. The assessment and treatment of mental health issues in long-term care homes (focus on mood and behaviour symptoms). Toronto: Canadian Coalition for Seniors' Mental Health; 2006, updated 2014. http://www.ccsmh.ca/en/projects/ltc.cfm

Chenoweth L, King MT, Jeon YH, et al. Caring for Aged Dementia Care Resident Study (CADRES) of person-centred care, dementia-care mapping, and usual care in dementia: a cluster-randomised trial. Lancet Neurol. 2009;8(4):317–25. http://dx.doi.org/10.1016/S1474-4422(09)70045-6. Medline:19282246

Cohen-Mansfield J. Theoretical frameworks for behavioral problems in dementia. Alzheimer's Care Quarterly. 2000;1(4):8–21.

– Nonpharmacologic interventions for inappropriate behaviors in dementia: a review, summary, and critique. Am J Geriatr Psychiatry. 2001;9(4):361–81. http://dx.doi .org/10.1097/00019442-200111000-00005. Medline:11739063

Cohen-Mansfield J, Libin A, Marx MS. Nonpharmacological treatment of agitation: a controlled trial of systematic individualized intervention. J Gerontol A Biol Sci Med Sci. 2007;62(8):908–16. http://dx.doi.org/10.1093/gerona/62.8.908. Medline:17702884

Cohen-Mansfield J, Thein K, Marx MS, et al. Efficacy of nonpharmacologic interventions for agitation in advanced dementia: a randomized, placebo-controlled trial. J Clin Psychiatry. 2012;73(9):1255–61. http://dx.doi.org/10.4088/JCP.12m07918. Medline:23059151

Dettmore D, Kolanowski A, Boustani M. Aggression in persons with dementia: use of nursing theory to guide clinical practice. Geriatr Nurs. 2009;30(1):8–17. http://dx.doi.org/10.1016/j.gerinurse.2008.03.001. Medline:19215808

Fletcher K. Dementia. In Capezuti E, Zwicker D, Mezey M, et al., editors. Evidence-based geriatric nursing protocols for best practice. 3rd ed. New York: Springer; 2008. p. 83–109.

Forbes D, Blake CM, Thiessen EJ, et al. Light therapy for improving cognition, activities of daily living, sleep, challenging behaviour, and psychiatric disturbances in dementia. Cochrane Database Syst Rev. 2014;(2):CD003946. http://dx.doi .org/10.1002/14651858.CD003946.pub4

Fung JKKM, Tsang HWH, Chung RCK. A systematic review of the use of aromatherapy in treatment of behavioral problems in dementia. Geriatr Gerontol Int. 2012;12(3):372–82. http://dx.doi.org/10.1111/j.1447-0594.2012.00849.x. Medline:22433025

Goldwasser AN, Auerbach SM, Harkins SW. Cognitive, affective, and behavioral effects of reminiscence group therapy on demented elderly. Int J Aging Hum Dev. 1987;25(3):209–22. http://dx.doi.org/10.2190/8UX8-68VC-RDYF-VK4F. Medline:3429043

Guidelines and Protocols Advisory Committee (GPAC); British Columbia Ministry of Health; Doctors of BC (DOBC). Cognitive impairment – recognition, diagnosis and management in primary care. Victoria, BC: GPAC; 2014. http://www2.gov.bc.ca/gov/content/health/practitioner-professional-resources/bc-guidelines/cognitive- impairment

Hawranik P, Johnston P, Deatrich J. Therapeutic touch and agitation in individuals with Alzheimer's disease. West J Nurs Res. 2008;30(4):417–34. http://dx.doi.org/10.1177/0193945907305126. Medline:18272750

Herrmann N, Gauthier S. Diagnosis and treatment of dementia: 6. Management of severe Alzheimer disease. CMAJ. 2008;179(12):1279–87. http://dx.doi.org/ 10.1503/cmaj.070804. Medline:19047609

International Psychogeriatric Association. The IPA complete guides to behavioral and psychological symptoms of dementia. Milwaukee, WI: International Psychogeriatric Association; 2010, rev. 2015. http://www.ipa-online.org/publications/guides-to-bpsd

Landi F, Russo A, Bernabei R. Physical activity and behavior in the elderly: a pilot study. Arch Gerontol Geriatr Suppl. 2004;38(9):235–41. http://dx.doi.org/10.1016/ j.archger.2004.04.033. Medline:15207420

Lichtenberg PA, Kemp-Havican J, Macneill SE, et al. Pilot study of behavioral treatment in dementia care units. Gerontologist. 2005;45(3):406–10. http://dx.doi .org/10.1093/geront/45.3.406. Medline:15933281

Lin LC, Yang MH, Kao CC, et al. Using acupressure and Montessori-based activities to decrease agitation for residents with dementia: a cross-over trial. J Am Geriatr Soc. 2009;57(6):1022–9. http://dx.doi.org/10.1111/j.1532-5415.2009.02271.x. Medline:19507295

Livingston G, Johnston K, Katona C, et al.; Old Age Task Force of the World Federation of Biological Psychiatry. Systematic review of psychological approaches to the management of neuropsychiatric symptoms of dementia. Am J Psychiatry. 2005;162(11):1996–2021. http://dx.doi.org/10.1176/appi.ajp.162.11.1996. Medline:16263837

Low LF, Brodaty H, Goodenough B, et al. The Sydney Multisite Intervention of LaughterBosses and ElderClowns (SMILE) study: cluster randomised trial of humour therapy in nursing homes. BMJ Open. 2013;3(1):e002072. http://dx.doi .org/10.1136/bmjopen-2012-002072. Medline:23315520

Lyketsos CG, Colenda CC, Beck C, et al.; Task Force of American Association for Geriatric Psychiatry. Position statement of the American Association for Geriatric Psychiatry regarding principles of care for patients with dementia resulting from Alzheimer disease. Am J Geriatr Psychiatry. 2006;14(7):561–72. http://dx.doi.org/10.1097/01.JGP.0000221334.65330.55. Medline:16816009

McCallion P, Toseland RW, Lacey D, et al. Educating nursing assistants to communicate more effectively with nursing home residents with dementia. Gerontologist. 1999;39(5):546–58. http://dx.doi.org/10.1093/geront/39.5.546. Medline:10568079

McCurry SM, Gibbons LE, Logsdon RG, et al. Training caregivers to change the sleep hygiene practices of patients with dementia: the NITE-AD project. J Am Geriatr Soc. 2003;51(10):1455–60. http://dx.doi.org/10.1046/j.1532-5415.2003.51466.x. Medline:14511168

– Nighttime insomnia treatment and education for Alzheimer's disease: a randomized, controlled trial. J Am Geriatr Soc. 2005;53(5):793–802. http://dx.doi.org/10.1111/j.1532-5415.2005.53252.x. Medline:15877554

McCurry SM, Pike KC, Vitiello MV, et al. Increasing walking and bright light exposure to improve sleep in community-dwelling persons with Alzheimer's disease: results of a randomized, controlled trial. J Am Geriatr Soc. 2011;59(8):1393–402. http://dx.doi.org/10.1111/j.1532-5415.2011.03519.x. Medline:21797835

Mittelman MS, Ferris SH, Shulman E, et al. A family intervention to delay nursing home placement of patients with Alzheimer disease: a randomized controlled trial. JAMA. 1996;276(21):1725–31. http://dx.doi.org/10.1001/jama.1996.03540210033030. Medline:8940320

National Institute for Health and Clinical Excellence (NICE); Social Care Institute for Excellence (SCIE). Dementia: the NICE-SCIE guideline on supporting people with dementia and their carers in health and social care. Clinical Guideline 42. London, UK: NICE-SCIE; 2007.

Orsulic-Jeras S, Judge KS, Camp CJ. Montessori-based activities for long-term care residents with advanced dementia: effects on engagement and affect. Gerontologist. 2000;40(1):107–11. http://dx.doi.org/10.1093/geront/40.1.107. Medline:10750318

Raglio A, Bellelli G, Traficante D, et al. Efficacy of music therapy in the treatment of behavioral and psychiatric symptoms of dementia. Alzheimer Dis Assoc Disord. 2008;22(2):158–62. http://dx.doi.org/10.1097/WAD.0b013e3181630b6f. Medline:18525288

Rovner BW, Steele CD, Shmuely Y, et al. A randomized trial of dementia care in nursing homes. J Am Geriatr Soc. 1996;44(1):7–13. http://dx.doi.org/10.1111/j.1532-5415.1996.tb05631.x. Medline:8537594

Royal Australian and New Zealand College of General Practitioners. Dementia in medical care of older persons in residential aged care facilities. 4th ed. Melbourne: The Royal Australian and New Zealand College of General Practitioners; 2006.

Royal Australian and New Zealand College of Psychiatrists. Practice guideline 10: antipsychotic medications as a treatment of behavioural and psychological symptoms of dementia. Melbourne: Royal Australian and New Zealand College of Psychiatrists; 2009. https://www.ranzcp.org/Publications/Guidelines-and-resources-for-practice.aspx

Royal College of Psychiatrists. Forgetful but not forgotten: assessment and aspects of treatment of people with dementia by a specialist old age psychiatry service: Council Report. London: Royal College of Psychiatrists; 2005.

Salzman C, Jeste DV, Meyer RE, et al. Elderly patients with dementia-related symptoms of severe agitation and aggression: consensus statement on treatment options, clinical trials methodology, and policy. J Clin Psychiatry. 2008;69(6):889–98. http://dx.doi.org/10.4088/JCP.v69n0602. Medline:18494535

Scottish Intercollegiate Guidelines Network (SIGN). Management of patients with dementia: a national clinical guideline. Sign Publication No. 86. Edinburgh: SIGN; 2006. http://www.sign.ac.uk/guidelines/fulltext/86/

Seitz DP, Brisbin S, Herrmann N, et al. Efficacy and feasibility of nonpharmacological interventions for neuropsychiatric symptoms of dementia in long term care: a systematic review. J Am Med Dir Assoc. 2012;13(6):503–506.e2. http://dx.doi.org/10.1016/j.jamda.2011.12.059. Medline:22342481

Seitz D, Rines J, Brisbin S, et al. Safety of non-pharmacological interventions for neuropsychiatric symptoms of dementia in long-term care: a systematic review and meta-snalysis. 6th Canadian Conference on Dementia, Montreal, QC, 27–9 October 2011.

Skjerve A, Holsten F, Aarsland D, et al. Improvement in behavioral symptoms and advance of activity acrophase after short-term bright light treatment in severe dementia. Psychiatry Clin Neurosci. 2004;58(4):343–7. http://dx.doi.org/10.1111/j.1440-1819.2004.01265.x. Medline:15298644

Sung HC, Chang SM, Lee WL, et al. The effects of group music with movement intervention on agitated behaviours of institutionalized elders with dementia in Taiwan. Complement Ther Med. 2006;14(2):113–9. http://dx.doi.org/10.1016/j.ctim.2006.03.002. Medline:16765849

Teri L, Gibbons LE, McCurry SM, et al. Exercise plus behavioral management in patients with Alzheimer disease: a randomized controlled trial. JAMA. 2003;290(15):2015–22. http://dx.doi.org/10.1001/jama.290.15.2015. Medline:14559955

Teri L, Logsdon RG, Peskind E, et al.; Alzheimer's Disease Cooperative Study. Treatment of agitation in AD: a randomized, placebo-controlled clinical trial. Neurology. 2000;55(9):1271–8. Medline:11087767

Teri L, Logsdon RG, Uomoto J, et al. Behavioral treatment of depression in dementia patients: a controlled clinical trial. J Gerontol B Psychol Sci Soc Sci. 1997;52B(4):P159–66. http://dx.doi.org/10.1093/geronb/52B.4.P159. Medline:9224439

Testad I, Ballard C, Brønnick K, et al. The effect of staff training on agitation and use of restraint in nursing home residents with dementia: a single-blind, randomized controlled trial. J Clin Psychiatry. 2010;71(1):80–6. http://dx.doi.org/10.4088/JCP.09m05486oli. Medline:20129008

Thompson CA, Spilsbury K, Hall J, et al. Systematic review of information and support interventions for caregivers of people with dementia. BMC Geriatr. 2007;7:18. http://dx.doi.org/10.1186/1471-2318-7-18. Medline:17662119

Toseland RW, Diehl M, Freeman K, et al. The impact of validation group therapy on nursing home residents with dementia. J Appl Gerontol. 1997;16(1):31–50. http://dx.doi.org/10.1177/073346489701600102

van der Ploeg ES, Eppingstall B, Camp CJ, et al. A randomized crossover trial to study the effect of personalized, one-to-one interaction using Montessori-based activities on agitation, affect, and engagement in nursing home residents with dementia. Int Psychogeriatr. 2013;25(4):565–75. http://dx.doi.org/10.1017/S1041610212002128. Medline:23237211

van Weert JC, van Dulmen AM, Spreeuwenberg PM, et al. Behavioral and mood effects of snoezelen integrated into 24-hour dementia care. J Am Geriatr Soc. 2005;53(1):24–33. http://dx.doi.org/10.1111/j.1532-5415.2005.53006.x. Medline:15667372

Vickland V, Chilko N, Draper B, et al. Individualized guidelines for the management of aggression in dementia – Part 2: appraisal of current guidelines. Int Psychogeriatr. 2012;24(7):1125–32. http://dx.doi.org/10.1017/S104161021200004X. Medline:22420860

Williams CL, Tappen RM. Effect of exercise on mood in nursing home residents with Alzheimer's disease. Am J Alzheimers Dis Other Demen. 2007;22(5):389–97. http://dx.doi.org/10.1177/1533317507305588. Medline:17959874

Woods DL, Craven RF, Whitney J. The effect of therapeutic touch on behavioral symptoms of persons with dementia. Altern Ther Health Med. 2005;11(1):66–74. Medline:15712768

ADDITIONAL E-RESOURCES

Alzheimer Society Canada: www.alzheimer.ca

brainXchange: http://brainxchange.ca/public/home.aspx

Canadian Coalition for Seniors Mental Health: www.ccsmh.ca

Educational slides: Behavioural and psychological symptoms of dementia (BPSD); International Psychogeriatric Association, 2011

International Psychogeriatric Association BPSD Guides: http://www.ipa-online.org/publications/guides-to-bpsd

University of Iowa Geriatric Education Centre: http://www.healthcare.uiowa.edu/igec/

1.5 Pharmacologic Treatment of Dementia: The Cognitive Enhancers

Andrew Wiens, MD, FRCPC

INTRODUCTION

Pharmacologic treatment of dementia is a key difference between geriatric psychiatry and most other areas of psychiatry, and overlaps with geriatric medicine and neurology. Despite extensive research in this area, the range of treatments available to clinicians remains limited. For the most part, these medications are safe, and their relatively infrequent side effects are, when present, bothersome rather than dangerous. In this chapter, I review the evidence on the choice of agent, how to monitor treatment, deal with side effects, and decide if, and when, to discontinue these agents, based on evidence in the literature.

CASE SCENARIO

Mr S., an 80-year-old man, is brought to you for an assessment by his daughter. She says he was found lying on the ground in his apartment and was quite confused about a month earlier. He was admitted to hospital and was found to be in acute renal failure due to rhabdomyolysis. He had been living on his own since the death of his wife a month before that, and his daughter says her mother had not told anyone how impaired her father was. On discharge he scored 10 on a Mini Mental State Examination (MMSE). The note from his family doctor says Mr S. rarely came to see him in the past and has not been on a cognitive enhancer. He asks for assistance in treatment given a history of renal failure and a slow heart rate. When you take his pulse, it is 55. He lives with his daughter presently. He is frequently incontinent and needs assistance for bathing and dressing. He does little most of the day. He believes his wife is still alive and is shopping, and he sometimes tries to leave the house to go pick her up, but he has not otherwise exhibited behaviour problems. His daughter says things have been easier since her father was given a "mild sedative" to help him sleep at night. She is quite anxious for her father to be treated, as he has a twin bother with Alzheimer's disease (AD) who has responded well to a "dementia medication." He is on the following medication: oxybutynin 2.5 mg BID, zopiclone 5 mg QHS, metoprolol 12.5 mg BID, and takes multivitamins.

1. How would you decide which cognitive enhancer to prescribe to this man?
2. How would you monitor response, and what indicators would you use to alter or stop treatment?

OVERVIEW

1. Cognitive Enhancers: What Are They?
(Gauthier, 2002; Lipton & Rosenberg, 1994)

Medications that affect one of two main neurotransmitter changes
- Abnormally low levels of acetylcholine (acetylcholinesterase inhibitors [AChEI])
- Elevated levels of the excitatory neurotransmitter glutamate (memantine)

2. Summary of Effectiveness: AD
(Raina et al., 2008; Trinh et al., 2003)

- Are considered symptomatic treatments as they ↓ symptoms but do not alter clinical course overall

AChEIs:
- Display statistically significant, but clinically marginal benefits (Raina et al., 2008)
- Behaviour: ↓ appearance, no evidence of effect on pre-existing agitation (Trinh et al., 2003)
- Global function/quality of life: consistent but small effect (Trinh et al., 2003)

Memantine:
- Displays statistically significant effect on cognition and global function, but effect is clinically marginal (Raina et al., 2008)

3. Typical Effects of Dementia Medications
(Raskind et al., 2000)

- Maximum effect at 13 weeks
- Open-label studies suggest possibility of:
  - Return to treatment baseline at 52 weeks
  - Delaying start of treatment: improvement does not catch up to where an earlier start would have given

4. When to Start
(Hogan, 2009)

- When diagnosis of a treatable dementia is made
- No absolute contraindications:
  - AChEI relative contraindications:
    - Cardiac: bradycardia (< 50), left bundle branch block (LBBB)
    - Other diseases: peptic ulcer disease, chronic obstructive pulmonary disease (COPD)? (no evidence in mild and moderate) (Stephenson et al., 2012)
    - Medications: anticholinergic medications
    - Provincial formularies pay when MMSE 10–26, based on early pivotal trials; later studies show benefit in moderately severe Alzheimer's
  - Memantine: creatinine clearance < 30 mL/min

5. Cardiac Safety of AChEI
(Gill et al., 2009; Rowland et al., 2007)

- Due to vagal influences
- Incidence of problems is rare:
  - Heart block: 0.001–0.1%
  - Sinus bradycardia: 6.9 per 1000 person years (versus 4.4)
  - Syncope: 31.5 per 1000 person years (versus 18.6)
- No significant changes found in randomized controlled trials (RCTs) or open-label studies.
  - Electrocardiograms (ECGs) in trials were not predictive of adverse events.
  - There are no high risk groups on whom to target screening.
- Guidelines suggested to minimize risk (Rowland et al., 2007):
  - If HR < 50 or symptomatic (e.g., syncope, dizziness), stop AChEI and assess cause.
    - If unrelated to drug, or pacemaker inserted, restart AChEI.
    - Conduct routine pulse checks at baseline, during titration, and at 6-monthly intervals thereafter.
    - Consider consulting a cardiologist.
  - If HR 50–60 and asymptomatic, check pulse again 1 week after starting or after each dose increase.

6. Patients Started on AChEIs

- Are more likely to subsequently be started on anticholinergic (Gill et al., 2005)
- Combination seen in about 30% (Carnahan et al., 2004)

7. Which One to Start
(Herrmann, Lanctôt, & Hogan, 2013; Schwarz, Froelich, & Burns, 2012; Zekry & Gold, 2010)

- Treat based on diagnosis based to be predominant contributing cause (see Table 1.5.1)
- RCTs: statistically, but not necessarily clinically significant effect on cognition in dementia

8. How to Start: Acetylcholinesterase Inhibitors
(Blennow, de Leon, & Zetterberg, 2006; Massoud, Desmarais, & Gauthier, 2011)

Table 1.5.2 outlines the pharmacology of acetylcholinesterase inhibitors.

9. How to Start: Memantine
(Danysz et al., 2000; Jones et al., 2007; Livingston & Katona, 2004)

- N-methyl-D-aspartate (NMDA) receptor channel blocker
- Blocks effect of glutamate
- Reduces excessive neuronal activity that interferes with synaptic transmission
Dosage:
  - Week 1: 5 mg QAM
  - Week 2: 5 mg BID (highest dose for creatinine clearance [CrCl] 5–30)

Table 1.5.1: Randomized Controlled Trials of Acetylcholinesterase Inhibitor and Memantine in the Treatment of Dementia

Clinical Situation	AChEI	Memantine	Notes
Mild cognitive impairment	~	~	There are a number of negative studies and even a possible risk of increased mortality in the galantamine study.
Mild-to-moderate Alzheimer's disease	✔	*Memantine has evidence for moderate but not mild Alzheimer's disease.	All 3 AChEIs show efficacy. Methodologically limited direct comparison studies show similar benefits, so choice should be based on side-effect profile, ease of use, and familiarity.
Severe Alzheimer's disease	✔	✔	All 3 AChEIs and memantine show efficacy. No comparisons between medications to guide choice.
Alzheimer's disease with cerebrovascular disease	✔	No studies	In AChEI studies it is felt that most of the improvement comes from response of Alzheimer's disease component, so there is no reason to assume one AChEI better.
Vascular dementia	~	~	No effect shown for galantamine or donepezil. Rivastigmine only showed effects on older patients who were felt to also have Alzheimer's disease.
Dementia with Lewy bodies	~	~	Evidence for AChEI unclear; minimal for memantine.
Parkinson's disease dementia	✔	~	RCT evidence best for rivastigmine, inconclusive for the other two AChEIs, and lacking for memantine.
Dementia in Down syndrome	~	~	No recommendation can be made for AChEIs; a good RCT with memantine failed to demonstrate effects.
Neuropsychiatric symptoms	~	~	No evidence as a primary outcome.
Combination therapy		~	Combination safe, but conflicting results on available studies suggests insufficient evidence for or against combination.

✔ = recommended; ~ = insufficient or inconsistent evidence

AChEI = acetylcholinesterase inhibitor; AD = Alzheimer's disease; RCT = randomized controlled trial

- – Week 3: 10 mg QAM/5 mg QPM
- – Week 4: 10 mg BID (most effective)

Effect of food: none

10. How to Monitor Treatment

- Use the strategies from RCTs (Budson & Solomon, 2011).
- Use a measure of cognition, e.g., MMSE, MoCA, Mini-Cog, GPCOG.

Table 1.5.2: Pharmacology of Acetylcholinesterase Inhibitors

	Donepezil	Galantamine ER	Rivastigmine	
Inhibition	**AChE**		**AChE and BuChE**	
			Oral	Transdermal
Half-life	70 hours	7–8 hours	1–2 hours	
Doses per day	1		2	1
Starting dose	5 mg QAM	8 mg QAM	1.5 mg BID	4.8 mg
Monthly increment	5 mg	8 mg	1.5 mg BID	To 9.5 mg size
Maximum	10 mg	24 mg	6 mg BID	9.5 mg
2D6/3A4 metabolite		Yes	No	
Given with food	Irrelevant	Recommended	↑ bio-availability	
Elimination	Liver	Liver & kidneys	Kidneys	

AChE = acetylcholinesterase; BID = twice daily; BuChE = butyrylcholinesterase;
QAM = daily before noon

- Use a global measure of overall function: interview patient and caregiver about cognition, mood/behaviour, and function and "rate":
  - Marked improvement
  - Moderate improvement
  - Mild improvement
  - Unchanged
  - Mild worsening
  - Moderate worsening
  - Marked worsening
- Consider using a target symptom approach (Global Attainment Scaling); the following have been found responsive to donepezil (Rockwood & Lussier, 2007):
  - Being "present," "in tune," being "themselves"
  - Withdrawal, lack of interest
  - Participation in family discussion, sociability, interest in others
  - Keeps attention focused (e.g., follows TV program)
  - Willingness to do activities
  - Playing cards, knitting, writing a card or letter
  - Depression, emotional lability, irritability
  - Fetching mail, newspaper, taking out garbage, vacuuming, preparing snacks
  - Repetitive questioning
- Use other ideas from *Dementia Guide*'s symptom library, available at www.dementia guide.com/symptomlibrary/.

11. Adherence to Medication
(Arlt et al., 2008; Small & Bullock, 2011)

Non-compliance is the most important factor for lack of effectiveness.

Majority of patients or their caregivers discontinue treatment after 4–5 months because of:
- Perceived lack of effectiveness
- Side effects
- Poor knowledge, understanding, too complex, low education

- Cognitive dysfunction: forgetfulness, reduced insight, dementia
- Depression
- Health beliefs
- Conflict with caregivers (physician, family, etc.)

11.1 Ways to Improve Compliance

- Better instructions: verbal, written, visual
- Counselling patient and caregivers on disease, importance of treatment, effects of no treatment
- Telephone follow-up (including automated)
- Simplified dosing, reduce overall number of pills
- Involving patients in care: self-monitoring
- Reminders
- Tailoring to daily habits, e.g., self-care routine
- Reminder posters or charts
- Medication organizers: blister packs, dated pillbox
- Rewards: reducing need for frequent follow-up
- Different formulation: transdermal rather than oral
- Community support, home visits (including pharmacies)

12. Side Effects: Acetylcholinesterase Inhibitors
(Bentué-Ferrer et al., 2003; Cummings, 2003; Kim et al., 2011; Small & Bullock, 2011)

- Mainly gastrointestinal (GI), tend to be early: nausea, vomiting, diarrhea, anorexia; more common with:
    - Rivastigmine (oral) and especially nausea and vomiting in Parkinson's disease dementia (PDD) (Emre et al., 2004)
    - Patients weighing < 50 kg
- Sleep: insomnia, nightmares (especially donepezil)
- Neuromuscular: muscle cramps, weakness, tremors (especially rivastigmine in PDD: consider alternate if tremor-dominant PD)
- Cardiac: dizziness; caution in LBBB
- Bradycardia, syncope (both higher with rivastigmine and galantamine (World Health Organization, 2004)); ↑ consequential permanent pacemaker insertion and hip fractures (Gill et al., 2009)
- Respiratory: bronchospasm (caution in asthma, COPD; no evidence in mild-to-moderate cases) (Stephenson et al., 2012))
- Urogenital: incontinence
- Rhinorrhea
- Psychiatric: agitation, panic-like state, depression
- May lower seizure threshold and exaggerate effect of succinylcholine type muscle relaxants

13. Side Effects: Memantine
(Robinson & Keating, 2006)

- Neuropsychiatric: agitation, confusion, sleepiness

- Neurologic: headache
- GI: constipation, diarrhea
- Other:
    - Dizziness
    - Influenza-like symptoms
    - Hypertension
    - Urinary incontinence
    - Peripheral edema
    - Insomnia

14. What to Do about Side Effects
(Hogan et al., 2007; Massoud & Léger, 2011)

If disabling and/or dangerous: discontinue
If minor in severity:
- Decrease dose.
- Consider later option to retry higher dose in 2 to 4 weeks if lower dose is tolerated.
- Consider slower titration.

GI (nausea, vomiting, anorexia, weight loss):
- Wait: more common at onset or when dose is increased.
- Decrease titration rate.
- Decrease dose.
- Get caregiver to administer: e.g., if evidence of unintentional overdose.
- Take with food (especially rivastigmine).
- Switch to rivastigmine patch (3x fewer GI side effects).
- Discontinue.
- Antiemetics can be used but many are anticholinergic.

Table 1.5.3 shows several common side effects of treatment medications and suggests strategies for managing them.

Table 1.5.3: Selected Strategies for Dealing with Side Effects of Acetylcholinesterase Inhibitors

Side Effect	What to Do
Dizziness	Assess for bradycardia; review: BP, postural BP, urinalysis, CBC, ECG; if disabling ↓ dose
Sleep disturbances	Take in a.m., ↓ dose; if donepezil, switch to another AChEI
Headache	↓ dose
Rhinorrhea	↓ dose
Salivation	↓ dose
Muscle cramps	↑ water intake, ↑ electrolytes (e.g., bananas for potassium), OTC magnesium oxide, ↓ dose
Rash	Discontinue; may be able to try another AChEI
Seizure	Single, brief: ↓ dose; Multiple or prolonged: discontinue

AChEI = acetylcholinesterase inhibitor; BP = blood pressure; CBC = complete blood count; ECG = electrocardiogram; OTC = over-the-counter drug

Source: Budson & Solomon, 2011.

Beware of the "prescribing cascade": misinterpretation of an adverse reaction to one drug followed by the prescription of a potentially inappropriate second drug (Gill et al., 2005; Hogan et al., 2007; Stahl et al., 2003).

- Patients on donepezil
  - 1.55 × risk of being started on an anticholinergic drug
    - To treat urinary incontinence (both a possible side effect of acetylcholinesterase inhibitors and related to frailty as well as dementia)
  - Odds 3.34 × greater of being started on a hypnotic

15. Frequency of Switching
(Massoud, Desmarais, & Gauthier, 2011)

- Rates vary considerably between studies:
  - Donepezil: 3.3–21.9%
  - Rivastigmine: 4.7–40.5%
  - Galantamine: 2–32.3%

16. Details of Switching
(Massoud, Desmarais, & Gauthier, 2011)

- Based on open-label or retrospective trials
- Duration to initiation varied from overnight to several weeks
- Several methods described:
  - If intolerant of side effect (S/E): wait to start new agent when side effects subside.
  - For others, specific methods studied
    - Switch to rivastigmine patch overnight resulted in more asymptomatic bradycardia and GI S/E than waiting 7 days.
    - Switch to another tablet (here donepezil to galantamine) resulted in more GI S/E 4 weeks after 7-day delay than 4-day delay.
      - This may be due to greater decrease in AChEI levels after longer delay.

16.1 Switching Due to Intolerance
(Hogan et al., 2007; MacKnight, 2007; Massoud & Léger, 2011; Massoud, Desmarais, & Gauthier, 2011; Winblad & Machado, 2008)

- Individual pharmacological properties suggest switching is possible.
- Try first to deal with side effects as previously described.
- Inform patients and caregivers that switching can lead to deterioration.
- Stop the original acetylcholinesterase inhibitor and wait until all side effects leading to switching have ended.
- Switch to new cognitive enhancer (acetylcholinesterase inhibitor or memantine) and use according to recommended titration schedule:
  - < 50% tolerated second agent
- Consider using rivastigmine patch, especially for nausea, vomiting, weight loss, and dizziness.

16.2 Switching Due to Lack of Benefit
(Massoud, Desmarais, & Gauthier, 2011)

- Ensure patient was compliant.
- Make sure patient has tried maximum dose for at least 3 months.
- > 50% show improvement with switch of one AChEI to another.
- Make sure lack of response is well defined, e.g.:
    - Decline > 2 on MMSE over 12 months
    - Well-documented deterioration in functional autonomy, global impression, or behaviour within past 6–12 months
- Switching can likely be done overnight: initiate at recommended dose, increase twice as fast to avoid possible deterioration during switch.

16.3 Switching Due to Loss of Response
(MacKnight, 2007; Massoud, Desmarais, & Gauthier, 2011)

- Very hard to define
- May be due to disease progression or new lack of compliance
- Assess for:
    - Compliance to treatment
    - Side effect or interaction with new drug
    - Delirium, depression
    - Need for more services by overburdened caregivers
- Switching to another AChEI generally unsatisfactory in this situation
    - Consider adding or switching to memantine
    - Best evidence in moderate-to-severe Alzheimer's disease study

17. When to Stop
(Herrmann, Lanctôt, & Hogan, 2013)

Consider stopping if:
- Patient/caregiver want to and understand risks and benefits of continuing and of stopping
- Nonadherence
- Rate of decline greater than before treatment
- Intolerable side effects
- Comorbidities make treatment risky or futile
- Global deterioration scale = 7

Don't necessarily consider stopping in the following circumstances:
- Based on MMSE alone
- When patient institutionalized
- Based on adverse events that may have multiple possible causes (falls)

18. Vascular Prevention for All
(Massoud & Léger, 2011; Zekry & Gold, 2010)

- Mid-life hypertension
    - Primary prevention:

- ▪ Optimal treatment may be associated with better cognitive outcome
- ▪ But no reduction in incidence of dementia
  - – Secondary prevention (post stroke): ↓ cognitive decline and dementia
- Cholesterol: no cognitive benefits associated with cholesterol-lowering agents
- Results may be due to short follow-up and crude cognitive measures.
- Longitudinal observations in tertiary memory clinic suggest slower decline of AD with treatment of vascular risk factors.

19. Pharmacotherapy of Mild Cognitive Impairment (MCI)

(Herrmann, Lanctôt, & Hogan, 2013; Petersen, 2011)

- AChEIs: no clear benefit
- No evidence for non-steroidal anti-inflammatory drugs (NSAIDs), prednisone, estrogen, ginkgo biloba, vitamin E or COX-2 inhibitors (↑ rate of decline)

20. Pharmacotherapy of Frontotemporal Dementia (FTD)

(Kaye et al., 2010; Kertesz et al., 2008; UCSF Memory and Aging Centre, 2016)

Disease modifying
- Research stage: no specific treatments

Clinicians have used the following strategies:
- Treatments used in Alzheimer's
- Treating individual behavioural symptoms
- Medications used in similar psychiatric disorders
- Targeting neurotransmitter deficits: mainly serotonergic
- Most studies are small and show no improvement or unclear benefits
  - – Rivastigmine: some effect but patients were 10 years older than the average FTD and had significant cognitive impairment, suggesting they had AD
  - – Galantamine: improved word production in non-fluent primary progressive aphasia (nfPPA)
  - – Memantine: inconsistent results – positive in case series of 3, negative in a small study of 16

Problems:
- No neuropathologic evidence of a cholinergic deficit
- Reports of worse disinhibition and compulsive or stereotypical acts
- In FTD with motor neuron disease (FTD-MND) increased oral secretions may be dangerous.
- Note: because frontal-variant AD can be hard to distinguish from FTD, acetylcholinesterase inhibitors and memantine warrant consideration.

20.1 FTD: Individual Behaviours

(Kaye et al., 2010; Portugal, Marinho, & Laks, 2011; UCSF Memory and Aging Centre, 2016)

Mostly small studies with limited descriptions of diagnosis and evaluation

- Disinhibition: trazodone, selective serotonin reuptake inhibitors (SSRIs), moclobemide, selegiline

- In refractory cases: quetiapine, risperidone – but FTD patients may have ↑ risk extrapyramidal symptoms (EPS)
- Risk-taking: methylphenidate
- Inappropriate sexual behaviour: fluvoxamine
- Apathy-inertia: dextroamphetamine, memantine
- Perseverative, stereotyped, or compulsive/ritualistic behaviour: sertraline, fluvoxamine, paroxetine
- Hyperorality and dietary changes: SSRIs
- Mood disorders: SSRIs, moclobemide
- svPPA: SSRI for compulsive behaviours
- nfPPA: SSRI for depression (↑ risk due to preserved insight)

21. Pharmacotherapy of PDD/DLB

(Galasko, 2013; McKeith et al., 2005; Rolinski et al., 2012)

Motor symptoms:
- Low dose L-dopa: more useful in Parkinson's; risk of psychosis, agitation
- No anti-cholinergics in dementia with Lewy bodies (DLB)

Neuropsychiatric symptoms:
- Fluctuations, hallucinations: acetylcholinesterase inhibitors (DLB may have better response than AD)
- Psychosis:
    – Try to lower dopamine agonists
    – Consider quetiapine, clozapine, aripiprazole
    – Highly sensitive to typical antipsychotics
- Depressive symptoms: SSRIs, serotonin norepinephrine reuptake inhibitors (SNRIs)

Cognitive changes:
- ChEI with a positive impact on global assessment, cognitive function, behavioural disturbance, and activities of daily living (ADLs)
- Memantine: improved global assessment and behaviour in DLB; not in PDD
- May be due to greater overlap of DLB with AD

REM sleep behaviour disorder:
- Rule out obstructive sleep apnea (OSA); clonazepam +/− melatonin

QUESTIONS

1. List five potential contraindications to using cognitive enhancers.
2. Describe five strategies that can be used to deal with gastrointestinal side effects of acetylcholinesterase inhibitors.
3. List some ways to assess treatment response with cognitive enhancers.
4. Compliance is a significant cause of poor response to treatments. List five ways to improve compliance with cognitive enhancers.
5. What would be your approach with intolerance to a cognitive enhancer? In this situation, how would you switch to another cognitive enhancer?
6. What would be your approach with lack of response to a cognitive enhancer? In this situation, how would you switch to another cognitive enhancer?

7. List reasons for stopping a cognitive enhancer.
8. What would affect your decision to choose one cognitive enhancer over another?
9. How would you explain the use of a cognitive enhancer to a power of attorney (POA) who is reluctant to consider this treatment in their relative who has Alzheimer's?

ANSWERS

1. Contraindications to using cognitive enhancers include the following:
   - Medical contraindications:
     - Acetylcholinesterase inhibitors:
       - Cardiac: bradycardia (< 50), LBBB, syncope (more common with rivastigmine and galantamine)
       - Other diseases: peptic ulcer disease, COPD (no evidence in mild and moderate), seizure disorder, liver disease (especially galantamine), renal insufficiency (especially rivastigmine)
       - Medications: anticholinergic medications, beta blockers
     - Memantine: creatinine clearance < 30 mL/min (dose should be max 10 mg/d at CrCl 5–30)
   - Psychosocial "contraindications"
     - Cost of medications where they are not covered
     - POA/ substitute decision maker (SDM) or patient (if capable) not in agreement: may need more psychosocial education
     - Patient refuses to take oral meds: consider patch
2. Strategies for gastrointestinal side effects of acetylcholinesterase inhibitors include:
   - Wait: these are more common at treatment onset or when dose is increased, and tend to be transient.
   - Slow titration rate.
   - Lower dose.
   - Get caregiver to administer: e.g., if evidence of unintentional overdose.
   - Take with food (especially rivastigmine).
   - Switch to rivastigmine patch (3x fewer GI side effects).
   - Discontinue.
   - Although antiemetics can be used, many have anticholinergic properties.
   - Note: nausea, vomiting, diarrhea, anorexia; more common with:
     - Rivastigmine, and especially nausea and vomiting in PDD
     - Patients weighing < 50 kg
3. In order to assess treatment response with cognitive enhancers:
   - Use the strategies from RCTs.
   - Use a measure of cognition.
     - e.g., MMSE, MoCA, Mini-Cog, GPCOG
   - Use a global measure of overall function: interview patient and caregiver about cognition, mood/behaviour, and function and "rate":
     - Marked improvement
     - Moderate improvement
     - Mild improvement

- – Unchanged
- – Mild worsening
- – Moderate worsening
- – Marked worsening
- Use symptom check lists:
  - – Budson & Solomon, 2011
    - ▪ Forgetting information over short periods
    - ▪ Repeating stories or questions
    - ▪ Difficulty handling finances
    - ▪ Problems with judgment
    - ▪ Disorientation to time
    - ▪ Bewildered in familiar settings
    - ▪ Difficulty learning something new
    - ▪ Social withdrawal
    - ▪ Loss of interest in usual activities
    - ▪ Difficulty with everyday activities
  - – Rockwood et al., 2007; Rockwood & Lussier, 2007
    - ▪ Consider using a target symptom approach: the following have been found responsive to donepezil:
      - - Being "present," "in tune," being "themselves"
      - - Withdrawal, lack of interest
      - - Participation in family discussion, sociability, interest in others
      - - Keeps attention focused (e.g., follows TV program)
      - - Willingness to do activities
      - - Playing cards, knitting, writing a card or letter
      - - Depression, emotional lability, irritability
      - - Fetching mail, newspaper, taking out garbage, vacuuming, preparing snacks
      - - Repetitive questioning
    - ▪ Use ideas from the *Dementia Guide*'s symptom library, available at www.dementiaguide.com/symptomlibrary/.

4. Compliance with cognitive enhancers can be improved with:
   - Better instructions: verbal, written, visual
   - Counselling patient and caregivers on disease, importance of treatment, effects of no treatment, importance of follow-up to manage potential side effects
   - Telephone follow-up (including automated)
   - Simplified dosing, reduce overall number of pills
   - Involving patients in care: self-monitoring
   - Reminders:
     - – Tailoring to daily habits, e.g., self-care routine
     - – Reminder posters or charts
   - Medication organizers: blister packs, dated pillbox
   - Rewards: reducing need for frequent follow-up

- Different formulation: transdermal rather than oral
- Community support, home visits (including pharmacies)

5. Approach to intolerance:
   - Individual pharmacological properties suggest switching is possible.
   - Try first to deal with side effects and/or decrease the dose.
   - Inform patients and caregivers that decreasing the dose or switching can lead to deterioration.
   - In order to switch:
     - Stop the original acetylcholinesterase inhibitor and wait until all side effects leading to switching have ended.
     - Switch to new cognitive enhancer and use according to recommended titration schedule.
       - Note: < 50% tolerated second agent
     - Consider using rivastigmine patch, especially for nausea, vomiting, weight loss, and dizziness.

6. Approach to non-response:
   - Ensure patient was compliant.
   - Make sure patient has tried maximum dose for at least 3 months.
   - > 50% show improvement with switch of one AChEI to another.
   - Make sure lack of response is well defined, e.g.:
     - Decline > 2 on MMSE over 12 months
     - Well-documented deterioration in functional autonomy, global impression, or behaviour within past 6–12 months
   - Switching can be done quickly: initiate at recommended dose, increase twice as fast to avoid possible deterioration during switch.
     - Switch to rivastigmine patch overnight resulted in more asymptomatic bradycardia and GI S/E than waiting 7 days.
     - Switch to another tablet (here donepezil to galantamine) resulted in more GI S/E 4 weeks after 7-day delay than 4-day delay.
       - May be due greater decrease in AChEI levels after longer delay

7. Consider stopping an acetylcholinesterase inhibitor if:
   - Patient/caregiver wants to and understands risks and benefits of continuing and of stopping.
   - Rate of decline is greater than before treatment.
   - Global deterioration scale = 7
   - Patient experiences swallowing difficulties.
   - Significant GI adverse events (nausea, vomiting, distressing loose stools, anorexia with weight loss)
   - Don't necessarily consider stopping in the following circumstances:
     - Based on MMSE alone
     - When patient institutionalized
     - Based on adverse events that may have multiple possible causes (falls)

8. Regarding choice of specific cognitive enhancer:
   - Evidence in literature: note that memantine has less evidence in less severely ill patients

Clinical Situation	AChEI	Memantine
Mild cognitive impairment	~	~
Mild-to-moderate Alzheimer's disease	✔	~
Severe Alzheimer's disease	✔	✔
Alzheimer's disease with cerebrovascular disease	✔	No studies
Vascular dementia	~	~
Dementia with Lewy bodies	~	~
Parkinson's disease dementia	✔	~
Neuropsychiatric symptoms	~	~
Combination therapy		~

✔ = recommended; ~ = insufficient or inconsistent evidence
AChEI = acetylcholinesterase inhibitor

- Potential contraindications: see questions #1 and 2 above
- Administration schedule and impact: once-a-day, BID, patch
- Consider drug-specific side effects: e.g., donepezil and insomnia. Others are listed in questions #1 and 2 above

9. An approach to explaining the use of a cognitive enhancer to a reluctant POA should include the following:
    - First explain that the treatment is not disease modifying (neurodegenerative process will go on).
    - Explain mechanism of action on acetylcholine and its role in cognition.
    - Explain secondary effects.
    - State that benefice is modest but sustained and significant.
    - Explain that the effect can be improving of cognition, behaviour, global, for mild to severe dementia.

Approach would explain realistic goals:
    - Stabilization, slower progression rather than improvement
    - Lost functions will not be regained
    - Maximal global improvement at 3 months
    - Could prevent the apparition of new behavioural symptoms (mainly depression, apathy, anxiety)
    - Could diminish caregiver burden and time given for caring for patient
    - Could delay institutionalization

(Acknowledgement: Dr Nancy Vasil, 2012–2013 Study Group member)

CASE DISCUSSION

1. In picking a cognitive enhancer for this man:
    - Ensure you are not dealing with depression or delirium.
    - Find out what medication the brother took: although we don't have trials that use this information to see if it helps, it seems to make sense to try (if appropriate) what a genetically related family member took for a similar/same illness.

In cooperation with family doctor:

- Try to decrease or stop ditropan, zopiclone due to cognitive side effects, and metoprolol due to bradycardia.
- Assess current kidney function: it may determine first choice.
- Assess severity: MMSE and symptom profile (by FAST) suggests he is in moderately severe stage – this doesn't exclude potential benefit for memantine.
- Slow pulse rate suggests caution with AChE; although if asymptomatic, it may still be possible: an enquiry about light-headedness, syncope, etc. should occur.
- Note: ECGs on the RCTs did not help identify patients at higher risk of cardiac side effects.
- Is there any symptom that could be worsened by a cognitive enhancer? Here, the only one seems to be insomnia, which suggests donepezil may not be the first choice. One would have to enquire about other things too:
  - GI symptoms (especially if Parkinsonian) or weight less than 50 kg? Rivastigmine less good as first choice
  - Tremor-dominant Parkinson's? Rivastigmine more likely to exacerbate
  - Syncope: higher with rivastigmine and galantamine

In this man:

- If not depressed, or delirious
- If kidneys now okay, memantine perhaps safest
- If some renal insufficiency:
  - Perhaps memantine, but < 10 mg/day (especially if anticholinergic "couldn't" be stopped), or
- If no treatable/unstable cardiac problem, careful (slow) administration of rivastigmine or galantamine (due to problematic insomnia that could be worsened with donepezil)

2. In monitoring his response:

- Cognitive screens will become less useful as we approach the floor for these tools.
- At this stage, the thrust is on preserving function and, hopefully, delaying appearance of behavioural problems.
- The symptom check lists in the response to question 3 above could be helpful.
- Use tools that evaluate function and track behaviour.
- Question #7 above and the reference by Herrmann, Lanctôt, & Hogan, 2013, listed below, provides a helpful approach to decision making about stopping acetylcholinesterase inhibitors.

RECOMMENDED RESOURCES FOR REVIEW

Although these resources may not be specifically cited in the text, their approach informed the contents of the chapter, and they are recommended as useful further reading.

Massoud F, Léger GC. Pharmacological treatment of Alzheimer disease. Can J Psychiatry. 2011;56(10):579–88. Medline:22014690

Raina P, Santaguida P, Ismaila A, et al. Effectiveness of cholinesterase inhibitors and memantine for treating dementia: evidence review for a clinical practice guideline. Ann Intern Med. 2008;148(5):379–97. http://dx.doi.org/10.7326/0003-4819-148-5-200803040-00009. Medline:18316756

REFERENCES

Arlt S, Lindner R, Rösler A, et al. Adherence to medication in patients with dementia: predictors and strategies for improvement. Drugs Aging. 2008;25(12):1033–47. http://dx.doi.org/10.2165/0002512-200825120-00005. Medline:19021302

Bentué-Ferrer D, Tribut O, Polard E, et al. Clinically significant drug interactions with cholinesterase inhibitors: a guide for neurologists. CNS Drugs. 2003;17(13):947–63. http://dx.doi.org/10.2165/00023210-200317130-00002. Medline:14533945

Blennow K, de Leon MJ, Zetterberg H. Alzheimer's disease. Lancet. 2006;368(9533):387–403. http://dx.doi.org/10.1016/S0140-6736(06)69113-7. Medline:16876668

Budson AE, Solomon PR. Memory loss: a practical guide for clinicians. Edinburgh: Elsevier Saunders; 2011.

Carnahan RM, Lund BC, Perry PJ, et al. The concurrent use of anticholinergics and cholinesterase inhibitors: rare event or common practice? J Am Geriatr Soc. 2004;52(12):2082–7. http://dx.doi.org/10.1111/j.1532-5415.2004.52563.x. Medline:15571547

Cummings JL. Use of cholinesterase inhibitors in clinical practice: evidence-based recommendations. Am J Geriatr Psychiatry. 2003;11(2):131–45. http://dx.doi.org/10.1097/00019442-200303000-00004. Medline:12611743

Danysz W, Parsons CG, Mobius HJ, et al. Neuroprotective and symptomatological action of memantine relevant for Alzheimer's disease–a unified glutamatergic hypothesis on the mechanism of action. Neurotox Res. 2000;2(2-3):85–97. http://dx.doi.org/10.1007/BF03033787. Medline:16787834

Emre M, Aarsland D, Albanese A, et al. Rivastigmine for dementia associated with Parkinson's disease. N Engl J Med. 2004;351(24):2509–18. http://dx.doi.org/10.1056/NEJMoa041470. Medline:15590953

Galasko D. The diagnostic evaluation of a patient with dementia. Continuum (Minneap Minn). 2013;19(2 Dementia):397–410. PMID 23558485

Gauthier S. Advances in the pharmacotherapy of Alzheimer's disease. CMAJ. 2002;166(5):616–23. Medline:11898943

Gill SS, Anderson GM, Fischer HD, et al. Syncope and its consequences in patients with dementia receiving cholinesterase inhibitors: a population-based cohort study. Arch Intern Med. 2009;169(9):867–73. http://dx.doi.org/10.1001/archinternmed.2009.43. Medline:19433698

Gill SS, Mamdani M, Naglie G, et al. A prescribing cascade involving cholinesterase inhibitors and anticholinergic drugs. Arch Intern Med. 2005;165(7):808–13. http://dx.doi.org/10.1001/archinte.165.7.808. Medline:15824303

Herrmann N, Lanctôt KL, Hogan DB. Pharmacological recommendations for the symptomatic treatment of dementia: the Canadian Consensus Conference on the Diagnosis and Treatment of Dementia 2012. Alzheimers Res Ther. 2013;5(Suppl 1):S5. http://dx.doi.org/10.1186/alzrt201. Medline:24565367

Hogan DB. Practical approach to the use of cholinesterase inhibitors in patients with early Alzheimer's disease. Geriatr Aging. 2009;12(4):202–7.

Hogan DB, Bailey P, Carswell A, et al. Management of mild to moderate Alzheimer's disease and dementia. Alzheimers Dement . 2007;3(4):355–84. http://dx.doi.org/10.1016/j.jalz.2007.07.006. PMID:19595958

Jones RW, Bayer A, Inglis F, et al. Safety and tolerability of once-daily versus twice-daily memantine: a randomised, double-blind study in moderate to severe Alzheimer's disease. Int J Geriatr Psychiatry. 2007;22(3):258–62. http://dx.doi.org/10.1002/gps.1752. Medline:17243195

Kaye ED, Petrovic-Poljak A, Verhoeff NP, et al. Frontotemporal dementia and pharmacologic interventions. J Neuropsychiatry Clin Neurosci. 2010;22(1):19–29. http://dx.doi.org/10.1176/jnp.2010.22.1.19. Medline:20160206

Kertesz A, Morlog D, Light M, et al. Galantamine in frontotemporal dementia and primary progressive aphasia. Dement Geriatr Cogn Disord. 2008;25(2):178–85. http://dx.doi.org/10.1159/000113034. Medline:18196898

Kim DH, Brown RT, Ding EL, et al. Dementia medications and risk of falls, syncope, and related adverse events: meta-analysis of randomized controlled trials. J Am Geriatr Soc. 2011;59(6):1019–31. http://dx.doi.org/10.1111/j.1532-5415.2011.03450.x. Medline:21649634

Lipton SA, Rosenberg PA. Excitatory amino acids as a final common pathway for neurologic disorders. N Engl J Med. 1994;330(9):613–22. http://dx.doi.org/10.1056/NEJM199403033300907. PMID:7905600

Livingston G, Katona C. The place of memantine in the treatment of Alzheimer's disease: a number needed to treat analysis. Int J Geriatr Psychiatry. 2004;19(10):919–25. http://dx.doi.org/10.1002/gps.1166. Medline:15449303

MacKnight C. Switching cholinesterase inhibitors: when and how. Geriatr Aging. 2007;10(3):158–61.

Massoud F, Desmarais JE, Gauthier S. Switching cholinesterase inhibitors in older adults with dementia. Int Psychogeriatr. 2011;23(3):372–8. http://dx.doi.org/10.1017/S1041610210001985. Medline:21044399

McKeith IG, Dickson DW, Lowe J, et al.; Consortium on DLB. Diagnosis and management of dementia with Lewy bodies: third report of the DLB Consortium. Neurology. 2005;65(12):1863–72. http://dx.doi.org/10.1212/01.wnl.0000187889.17253.b1. Medline:16237129

Petersen RC. Clinical practice: mild cognitive impairment. N Engl J Med. 2011;364(23):2227–34. http://dx.doi.org/10.1056/NEJMcp0910237. Medline:21651394

Portugal MG, Marinho V, Laks J. Pharmacological treatment of frontotemporal lobar degeneration: systematic review. Rev Bras Psiquiatr. 2011;33(1):81–90. http://dx.doi.org/10.1590/S1516-44462011000100016. Medline:21537725

Raskind MA, Peskind ER, Wessel T, et al.; Galantamine USA-1 Study Group. Galantamine in AD: a 6-month randomized, placebo-controlled trial with a 6-month extension. Neurology. 2000;54(12):2261–8. http://dx.doi.org/10.1212/WNL.54.12.2261. Medline:10881250

Robinson DM, Keating GM. Memantine: a review of its use in Alzheimer's disease. Drugs 2006;66(11):1515–34. PMID:16906789

Rockwood K, Fay S, Jarrett P, et al. Effect of galantamine on verbal repetition in AD: a secondary analysis of the VISTA trial. Neurology. 2007;68(14):1116–21. http://dx.doi.org/10.1212/01.wnl.0000258661.61577.b7. Medline:17404193

Rockwood K, Lussier I. Which effects do physicians look for in evaluating whether donepezil treatment is beneficial? Canadian Review of Alzheimer's Disease and Other Dementias. 2007;10(2):22–6.

Rolinski M, Fox C, Maidment I, et al. Cholinesterase inhibitors for dementia with Lewy bodies, Parkinson's disease dementia and cognitive impairment in Parkinson's disease. Cochrane Database Syst Rev. 2012;3:CD006504. Medline:22419314

Rowland R, Rigby J, Harper AC, et al. Cardiovascular monitoring with acetylcholinesterase inhibitors: a clinical protocol. Adv Psychiatr Treat. 2007;13(3):178–84. http://dx.doi.org/10.1192/apt.bp.106.002725

Schwarz S, Froelich L, Burns A. Pharmacological treatment of dementia. Curr Opin Psychiatry. 2012;25(6):542–50. http://dx.doi.org/10.1097/YCO.0b013e328358e4f2. Medline:22992546

Small G, Bullock R. Defining optimal treatment with cholinesterase inhibitors in Alzheimer's disease. Alzheimers Dement. 2011;7(2):177–84. http://dx.doi.org/10.1016/j.jalz.2010.03.016

Stahl SM, Markowitz JS, Gutterman EM, et al. Co-use of donepezil and hypnotics among Alzheimer's disease patients living in the community. J Clin Psychiatry. 2003;64(4):466–72. http://dx.doi.org/10.4088/JCP.v64n0418. Medline:12716251

Stephenson A, Seitz DP, Fischer HD, et al. Cholinesterase inhibitors and adverse pulmonary events in older people with chronic obstructive pulmonary disease and concomitant dementia: a population-based, cohort study. Drugs Aging. 2012;29(3):213–23. http://dx.doi.org/10.2165/11599480-000000000-00000. Medline:22332932

Trinh NH, Hoblyn J, Mohanty S, et al. Efficacy of cholinesterase inhibitors in the treatment of neuropsychiatric symptoms and functional impairment in Alzheimer disease: a meta-analysis. JAMA. 2003;289(2):210–6. http://dx.doi.org/10.1001/jama.289.2.210. Medline:12517232

UCSF Memory and Aging Centre. [Internet]. San Francisco, CA: University of California; 2016. Frontotemporal dementia. http://memory.ucsf.edu/ftd/

Winblad B, Machado JC. Use of rivastigmine transdermal patch in the treatment of Alzheimer's disease. Expert Opin Drug Deliv. 2008;5(12):1377–86. http://dx.doi.org/10.1517/17425240802542690. Medline:19040398

World Health Organization. Cholinesterase inhibitors and cardiac arrhythmias. WHO Drug Information. 2004;18(4):273–4.

Zekry D, Gold G. Management of mixed dementia. Drugs Aging. 2010;27(9):715–28. http://dx.doi.org/10.2165/11538250-000000000-00000. Medline:20809662

ADDITIONAL E-RESOURCE

Dementia Guide [Internet]. Halifax, NS: Dementia Guide Inc.; 2014. Symptom library; 2016 April 4. http://www.dementiaguide.com/symptomlibrary/

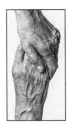

SECTION 2:
MOOD AND ANXIETY DISORDERS

2.1 Recognition and Assessment of Depression in Older Adults

Benoit H. Mulsant, MD, MS, FRCPC

INTRODUCTION

Major depression is one of the cornerstone diagnoses in geriatric psychiatry, and the approach to the diagnosis and assessment is far more complex in older adults than in younger adults. Dr Mulsant takes a scholarly and pragmatic approach, highlighting some of these differences and suggesting ways of overcoming barriers in order to ensure that older adults in need of care can be appropriately identified. He provides an approach to delineating depression from dementia and other medical conditions, and describes strategies for screening.

CASE SCENARIO

An 82-year-old man who has slow-progressing prostatic cancer with bone metastasis presents to you with anhedonia, insomnia, anergia, a 30-pound weight loss, and a passive death wish. He denies being depressed and attributes his insomnia to bone pain and the rest of his symptoms to his cancer. When confronted about his death wish, he replies that he is lonely, tired of living, and ready to die.

1. What element would increase your confidence in a diagnosis of major depressive episode?
2. What laboratory tests should be considered for this patient?
3. What could you reply to his son if he points out that "anybody would be depressed in similar circumstances"?

OVERVIEW

1. Differential Diagnosis of Depression in Older Adults

- Major depressive disorder (MDD)
- Bipolar disorder
- Other specified depressive disorder, depressive episode with insufficient symptoms ("minor depression")
- Bereavement
- Adjustment disorders
- Mood disorder due to another medical condition

- Substance-induced mood disorder
- Neurocognitive disorder ("dementia") with depressed mood

2. Approach to Diagnosis of Depression in Older Adults

Step 1: Is there a major depressive episode (MDE)?
Step 2: Assess context:
      Current comorbid conditions, e.g.:
- Substance misuse
- General medical conditions
- Dementia

      Death of a loved one; other stressors
      Past history: recurrent MDD, bipolar
Step 3: If no MDE, but distress or impairment:
      Adjustment disorder vs minor depression

3. Depression as a Manifestation of a Physical Illness (General Medical Condition)

DSM-IV-TR lists only a few specific medical conditions that "cause" a mood disorder:
- Degenerative neurological conditions (e.g., Parkinson's disease)
- Cerebrovascular disease (e.g., stroke)
- Metabolic conditions (e.g., B12 deficiency)
- Endocrine conditions (e.g., thyroid and adrenal diseases)
- Autoimmune conditions (e.g., systemic lupus erythematosus)
- Viral and other infections (e.g., hepatitis, mononucleosis, HIV)
- Certain cancers (e.g., pancreatic)

DSM-5 calls any of these conditions "another medical condition" instead of "general medical condition."

4. Core DSM Features of a Major Depressive Episode

(1) Depressed mood or (2) loss of pleasure/interest
At least four other symptoms [three, if both (1) and (2) are present]:
- Loss of appetite or weight (or increase)
- Insomnia or hypersomnia
- Psychomotor retardation or agitation (observable by others)
- Fatigue or loss of energy
- Worthlessness or guilt
- Diminished ability to think, concentrate, or make decisions
- Recurrent thoughts of death, passive or active suicidal ideas

≥ 2 weeks with symptoms most of the time, nearly every day
Symptoms distressing or interfering with functioning

5. Challenges in Diagnostic Features: The Overlaps
(Blazer, 2003)

DSM criteria for a major depressive episode
- Loss of pleasure/interest → apathy of dementia, other neurological illness
- Loss of appetite or weight → physical illness, dementia
- Insomnia → chronic pain, physical illness
    or hypersomnia → physical illness, opioids
- Psychomotor retardation → neurological illnesses
- Fatigue/loss of energy → physical or neurological illness
- Inability to think, concentrate, or make decisions → dementia
- Worthlessness; thoughts of death → end of life, terminal illness
- Symptoms distressing or interfering with functioning → disability associated with physical illness

6. Four Approaches to Diagnosing Depression in the Context of Comorbid Medical Conditions

- Exclusive approach
    Neurovegetative symptoms are not considered towards diagnosis.
- Substitutive approach
    Neurovegetative symptoms are replaced by additional psychological symptoms.
- Etiologic approach
    Each symptom is evaluated separately and a clinical judgment is made regarding attribution.
- Inclusive approach
    All depressive symptoms present are counted regardless of their (multiple) potential causes.

These approaches are used to diagnose an MDE that putatively requires pharmacologic treatment in patients with physical illnesses (e.g., cancer, renal failure, etc.). With the exclusive approach, a depressive symptom is not counted towards a diagnosis of an MDE if it could be due to another medical condition. For example, insomnia with sleep continuity disturbance would not be counted in a patient with prostatism and nocturia; weight loss would not be counted in a patient with cancer; fatigue/anergia would not be counted in a patient with anaemia. In contrast, the inclusive approach considers all depressive symptoms, regardless of their potential etiology.

Two other approaches have been proposed. With the etiologic approach, a clinical judgment about the etiology of the symptoms is made. For example, fatigue in a patient with anaemia could still count towards a diagnosis of depression if the anaemia is considered chronic but the fatigue is recent. The substitutive approach requires five depressive symptoms for a diagnosis of MDE, but the somatic symptoms are disregarded; weight loss and anergia are replaced by psychological symptoms such as helplessness and hopelessness. The etiologic approach is unreliable: clinicians cannot reliably determine whether a somatic symptom is due to a depression or a comorbid medical issue. The difficulty with the substitutive approach is that somatic symptoms are an integral part of a depressive syndrome in an older adult. Like the exclusive approach, this approach leads to underdiagnosis and undertreatment of late-life depression.

Some clinicians are concerned by the possibility of overdiagnosing and overtreating late-life depression. While there are some older patients who are prescribed antidepressants for no clear reasons, most epidemiologic studies point to the opposite problem. Approximately 50% of clinically significant depressions (i.e., those that require and benefit from treatment) in late life are missed. Of those that are diagnosed, only about 50% are treated, and at most 50% of the treated cases receive appropriate treatment. Studies comparing the "utility" of the inclusive versus the exclusive approach have found that more patients who would potentially benefit from treatment are diagnosed when the inclusive approach is used (Hendrie et al., 1995; Koenig et al., 1997).

7. Features that Distinguish Major Depression in Younger and Older Patients

7.1 In Older Adults, Depression Amplifies

- Dysfunction, suffering
- Physical symptoms (somatization)
- Cognitive impairment
- Disability
- Utilization of healthcare resources
- Medical mortality and suicide

7.2 Specific Features of Depression in Older Adults

- Symptoms and context – increased complexity
- Cognitive impairment – more common
- Age of onset – risk of dementia increased in later onset
- Comorbid physical illness – more common
- Psychotic features – more common

7.3 Low Detection of Depression

- Other medical conditions confuse the diagnosis.
- Older adults are more likely to present with somatic symptoms (Hegeman et al., 2012).
- Older adults are less likely to use the word "depressed" or to endorse low mood or guilt (but they or an informant will report anhedonia if asked) (Davison, McCabe, & Mellor, 2009).
- US primary care data from the National Ambulatory Medical Care Surveys (NAMCS) show a lower likelihood of diagnosis of depression *after controlling for presenting symptoms* (Harman et al., 2001):
  - In older patients (56% less likely)
  - In African-Americans (37% less likely)
  - With poverty (35% less likely)
- Family physicians are 65% more likely to record a diagnosis than internists.

7.4 Clues to Depression

- Help-seeking, persistent complaints of pain, headache, fatigue, insomnia, gastrointestinal symptoms, "arthritis," multiple diffuse symptoms, weight loss
- Frequent calls and visits to family doctor
- High utilization of services

7.5 Additional Clues in Hospitalized Patients

- Coronary artery bypass graft (CABG)
- Myocardial infarction (MI)
- Stroke
- Hip fracture
- Delayed recovery
- Treatment refusal
- Discharge refusal

7.6 Additional Clues in Nursing Home

- Apathy, withdrawal, isolation
- Failure to thrive
- Agitation
- Delayed rehabilitation

7.7 Somatic Symptoms in Late-Life Depression
(Mulsant, Ganguli, & Seaberg, 1997; Schulberg et al., 1998; Drayer et al., 2005)

In older patients with depression and physical illness, somatic symptoms are more strongly associated with depression than with physical illness.

8. Depressive Symptoms and Dementia: What Are the Links?
(Butters et al., 2008)

8.1 "Post-Depression Dementia"

- Depression as a risk factor for dementia
- Depression as a prodrome of dementia
- Depression as a presenting symptom of dementia

8.2 "Post-Dementia Depression"

- Depression as one of the behavioural syndromes associated with dementia

8.3 Cognitive Impairment and Late-Life Depression

A bidirectional relationship:
- Depressive symptoms and clinical depression are common in patients with dementia ("post-dementia depression").
- Cognitive impairment and dementia are common in patients with clinical depression ("post-depression dementia").

8.4 Cross-Sectional Prevalence of Clinical Depression in Various Dementing Diseases

Table 2.1.1 shows the prevalence of clinical depression associated with various neurologic diseases and in people aged 65 years and older.

8.5 Alzheimer Disease vs Depression: Contrasting Presenting Symptoms

- Apathy, agitation vs anhedonia, anxiety
- Sundowning vs insomnia
- Weight loss without loss of appetite vs weight loss with loss of appetite

Table 2.1.1: Prevalence of Clinical Depression in Various Neurologic Diseases

Disease	Prevalence (%)
Alzheimer's disease	20
Stroke	20
Huntington disease	38
Parkinson's disease	50
Older population	4

- Minimizing of cognitive deficit despite impaired memory and executive function vs subjective complaints of cognitive impairment that exceed objective deficits
- Guesses and wrong answers during testing vs "I don't know, I can't"
- Aphasia and apraxia vs language and motor skills clinically intact

8.6 Cognitive Deficits in Older Patients with Major Depression Are Common and Broad-Based
(Butters et al., 2004)

- Information processing speed
- Visuospatial ability
- Episodic memory
- Executive functions
- Language

9. Late-Onset Depression: Various Mechanisms

- Lower likelihood of family history
- A prodrome to Alzheimer's disease (due to loss of noradrenergic neurons in locus ceruleus)
- A manifestation of cerebrovascular disease (vascular depression [VaD])
- Caused by other general medical conditions (e.g., hypothyroidism, stroke)
- Psychosocial context – end of life

9.1 How Does Depression Result from Other Medical Conditions?
(Whyte & Mulsant, 2002)

Various mechanisms hypothesized:

- Direct disruption of neurotransmitters or neural circuits (e.g., stroke, Parkinson's, Alzheimer's)
- Physiologic stress (e.g., post-CABG, post-MI)
- Functional disability (e.g., hip fracture, renal failure)
- Psychosocial stress (e.g., bereavement)
    DOES NOT MATTER FOR TREATMENT!

10. Assessing Depression and Suicidality in Late Life

See also chapter 2.8

10.1 Suicide in Older Adults
(Szanto et al., 2002)

- Most tragic consequence of late-life depression
- Can be active or passive, e.g., refusing treatment
- Elderly have one of the highest rates of suicide in North America (largely due to older white males).
- Higher intent and likelihood to complete suicide when they attempt
- Violent methods (e.g., hanging, firearms) more common than non-violent methods
- Higher risks of dying when overdosing on own medications
- Slow but worrisome increase in combined murder-suicide

10.2 Two Screening Questions for Depression:
Patient Health Questionnaire-2 (PHQ-2)
(Kroenke, Spitzer, & Williams, 2003)

- Over the past two weeks, how often have you been bothered by the following problems:
    - Little interest or pleasure in doing things?
    - Feeling down, depressed, or hopeless?
  0 = not at all; 1 = several days; 2 = more than half the days; 3 = nearly every day
- Clinically significant depression based on total score:
  1+: 37%; 2+: 48%; 3+: 75%; 4+: 81%; 5+: 85%; 6: 93%

10.3 Four Screening Questions for Suicidality: Suicidal Ideation Scale (SIS)
(Beck, Kovacs, & Weissman, 1979)

- Do you care if you live or die?
- Do you want to die now?
- Do you think that your reasons for staying alive are better than your reasons for dying?
- Do you want to kill yourself now?

Any "positive" answer requires full exploration of suicidality.

10.4 A Hierarchy of Questions for Suicidality

- Life is empty, not worth living: do you feel that your life is empty or not worth living?
- Thoughts of death: have you been feeling so bad lately that you have been thinking about death or dying?
- Passive death wish: do you ever feel so bad that you wish you would fall asleep and not wake up?
- Suicidal ideation: have you been feeling so bad that you have been thinking about taking your own life?
- Suicidal plan: if you decided to kill yourself, how would you do it?
- Suicidal intent, access to means, reasons for living vs dying

10.5 Indirect Self-Destructive Behaviours (ISDB)

- Food refusal, non-compliance with medical care, carelessness
- In nursing homes, deaths from ISDB five times more common than from suicide (80 vs 16 per 100 000).
- Almost always associated with depression and hopelessness
- Can be explored with SIS questions:
    - Right now, would you deliberately ignore taking care of your health?
    - Do you feel like trying to die by eating or drinking too little, or by not taking needed medications?
    - Have you thought that it might be good to leave life or death to chance; for example, carelessly crossing a busy street, driving recklessly, or even walking alone at night in a rough part of town?

11. Conclusions: Depression in Older Adults

- Common
- Associated with disability and morbidity
- Diagnosable
- Treatable
- DO NOT GIVE UP!

QUESTIONS

1. List two questions that can be used to screen for depression in older adults.
2. List two symptoms that favour a diagnosis of a major depressive disorder when depression occurs in the context of bereavement.
3. Among the nine DSM symptoms of a major depressive episode, which ones are more common or less common in older adults than in younger adults?
4. List three possible etiologic pathways linking cognitive disorders and depression in older adults.
5. List two rating scales that have been developed to assess depression in older adults.
6. List and discuss three blood tests that can be useful when assessing an older person with a depressive syndrome.
7. Discuss the main reasons a diagnosis of depression may be missed in an older primary care patient.
8. Describe the advantages and disadvantages of using an inclusive vs exclusive approach when assessing depressive symptoms in late life.

ANSWERS

1. To screen for depression in older adults:
    - Over the past two weeks, how often have you been bothered by the following problems:
        - Little interest or pleasure in doing things?
        - Feeling down, depressed, or hopeless?

2. Symptoms that favour a diagnosis of a major depressive disorder when depression occurs in the context of bereavement include:
   - Persistent depressed mood
   - Inability to anticipate happiness or pleasure
   - Depressed mood not associated with specific thoughts or preoccupations
   - Pervasive unhappiness and misery
   - Self-critical and pessimistic ruminations
   - Worthlessness, self-loathing
   - Thoughts of ending one's life because of worthlessness, undeserving of life, psychic pain

3. Regarding age-related differences in the presentation of major depressive episode, the following symptoms are more common or less common in older adults compared to younger adults:

More Common	Less Common
• Anhedonia	• Depressed mood
• Diminished ability to think, concentrate, or make decisions	• Feelings of worthlessness or guilt

4. Possible etiologic pathways linking cognitive disorders and depression in older adults include:
   - Depression as an early psychological reaction to (subclinical) cognitive decline due to an incipient dementia (i.e., a "grief reaction to the loss of self")
   - Depression directly causes cognitive impairment and lowers "threshold" for diagnosis of dementia.
   - Cerebrovascular pathology leading to both vascular depression and VaD/AD
   - Loss of noradrenergic neurons due to AD pathology, which manifests as prodromal depression at the onset of dementia
   - Depression causes neuropathology (e.g., loss of hippocampal volume) that in turn causes cognitive impairment.
   - Other interaction between depression and AD neuropathology
   - Chronic hypercortisolaemia leading to hippocampal atrophy and AD pathology
   - Systemic inflammation associated with late-life depression may also contribute to pathogenesis of AD pathology.

5. Two rating scales that have been developed specifically to assess depression in an older population in whom physical symptoms or cognitive impairment are prevalent are:
   - Geriatric Depression Scale (GDS)
   - Cornell Scale for Depression in Dementia (CSDD)

6. Blood tests that can be useful when assessing an older person with a depressive syndrome include:
    - TSH (to rule out hypothyroidism that can cause a depressive syndrome)
    - B12 (to rule out low B12 that can cause a depressive syndrome)
    - Folates level (to rule out low folates that can cause a depressive syndrome)
    - CBC with differential (to rule out anaemia and some cancers that can present with fatigue, weight loss, and other depressive symptoms)
    - Sodium (to rule out hyponatremia that can present with fatigue, poor concentration, and other depressive symptoms)
    - Liver function tests (to rule out liver pathology that can present with fatigue, weight loss, and other depressive symptoms, and for indirect evidence of alcoholism that can present with low mood, weight loss, and other depressive symptoms)
    - Glucose (to rule out diabetes that can present with fatigue, weight loss, and other depressive symptoms)
    - Creatinine (to rule out renal disease that can present with fatigue, weight loss, poor concentration, and other depressive symptoms)
    - VDRL test (to rule out syphilis that can cause a depressive syndrome)
    - HIV test (to rule out HIV infection that can present with fatigue, weight loss, and other depressive symptoms)
    - Serum albumin (to assess nutritional status and rule out diseases that can present with depressive symptoms)
    - Parathyroid hormone (PTH) and vitamin D (because increased PTH and decreased vitamin D may be associated with depressive symptoms)

7. The main reasons a diagnosis of depression may be missed in an older primary care patient are:
    - Older patient does not report or denies a depressed mood/depression (e.g., "I have nothing to be depressed about").
    - Older patients focus on somatic symptoms.
    - Physician suspects depression but does not pursue it because he/she focuses on what he/she considers to be more urgent physical problems (i.e., competing demands for his or her attention).
    - Physician identifies depressive symptoms but discounts them because they make sense in the psychosocial context of the older patient (e.g., "Who would not be depressed in this situation?") or because he/she attributes them to comorbid physical problems.
    - Physician identifies depressive symptoms but does not make a diagnosis of depression because he/she does not want to offend the patient and the family.
    - Physician identifies depressive symptoms but does not make a diagnosis of depression because he or she believes that depression does not respond to treatment in older patients.

8. The advantages and disadvantages of using an inclusive vs exclusive approach when assessing depressive symptoms in older adults are summarized in the following table:

Approach	Advantages	Disadvantages
Inclusive	• False negative less likely (i.e., more sensitive) • More likely to identify depressive syndromes that are responsive to treatment	• False positives more likely (i.e., less specific) with higher likelihood of making a diagnosis of depression in patients whose symptoms are actually caused by a comorbid physical illness
Exclusive	• False positives less likely (i.e., more specific) with lower likelihood of making a diagnosis of depression in patients whose symptoms are actually caused by a comorbid physical illness	• False negative more likely (i.e., less sensitive) with higher likelihood of missing depression diagnosis in some patients whose depression would benefit from treatment

CASE DISCUSSION

1. In order to increase confidence in a diagnosis of a major depressive episode, consider:
   • The temporal course of his symptoms: if he has been diagnosed with depressive symptoms for several years but has developed anhedonia and a death wish over the last few weeks or months, the likelihood of a clinically treatable depression would increase.
   • The likelihood of a clinically treatable depression would be increased by the presence of other psychological symptoms (anxiety, worthlessness, hopelessness, helplessness).

2. Consider the following lab tests:
   • CBC to rule out anaemia that could explain the anergia
   • CT or a MRI to rule out brain metastases
   • TSH, calcium, phosphate, magnesium, albumin, B12, folates, electrolytes to rule out other medical conditions that could cause some of his depressive symptoms

3. In responding to the son's comment, consider:
   • It is true that many persons in similar circumstances could experience depressive symptoms; however, only 10–20% of patients with cancer have a clinical depression as severe as his father's (i.e., 80% do not).
   • Discuss the different presentation of depression in the elderly, the difficulties with diagnosis, the frequent comorbidities, the under-reporting of depressive symptoms by older patients, and the risk of suicide.
   • While the depression is perfectly understandable in this context, that does not mean it should not be treated or would not respond to treatment. One diagnoses and treats hip fractures even though they occur in the context of a fall and are perfectly understandable.
   • The patient may still live for several years and, while treating the depression will not take the cancer away, it should help the patient to feel better and to have a much better quality of life.

RECOMMENDED RESOURCES FOR REVIEW

Although these resources may not be specifically cited in the text, their approach informed the contents of the chapter, and they are recommended as useful further reading.

Blazer DG. Depression in late life: review and commentary. J Gerontol A Biol Sci Med Sci. 2003;58(3):M249–65. http://dx.doi.org/10.1093/gerona/58.3.M249. Medline:12634292

Butters MA, Young JB, Lopez O, et al. Pathways linking late-life depression to persistent cognitive impairment and dementia. Dialogues Clin Neurosci. 2008;10(3):345–57. Medline:18979948

REFERENCES

Beck AT, Kovacs M, Weissman A. Assessment of suicidal intention: the Scale for Suicide Ideation. J Consult Clin Psychol. 1979;47(2):343–52. http://dx.doi.org/10.1037/0022-006X.47.2.343. Medline:469082

Butters MA, Whyte EM, Nebes RD, et al. The nature and determinants of neuropsychological functioning in late-life depression. Arch Gen Psychiatry. 2004;61(6):587–95. http://dx.doi.org/10.1001/archpsyc.61.6.587. Medline:15184238

Davison TE, McCabe MP, Mellor D. An examination of the "gold standard" diagnosis of major depression in aged-care settings. Am J Geriatr Psychiatry. 2009;17(5):359–67. http://dx.doi.org/10.1097/JGP .0b013e318190b901. Medline:19390293

Drayer RA, Mulsant BH, Lenze EJ, et al. Somatic symptoms of depression in elderly patients with medical comorbidities. Int J Geriatr Psychiatry. 2005;20(10):973–82. http://dx.doi.org/10.1002/gps.1389. Medline:16163749

Harman JS, Schulberg HC, Mulsant BH, et al. The effect of patient and visit characteristics on diagnosis of depression in primary care. J Fam Pract. 2001;50(12):1068. Medline:11742610

Hegeman JM, Kok RM, van der Mast RC, et al. Phenomenology of depression in older compared with younger adults: meta-analysis. Br J Psychiatry. 2012;200(4):275–81. http://dx.doi.org/10.1192/bjp.bp.111.095950. Medline:22474233

Hendrie HC, Callahan CM, Levitt EE, et al. Prevalence rates of major depressive disorders: the effects of varying the diagnostic criteria in an older primary care population. Am J Geriatr Psychiatry. 1995;3(2):119–31. http://dx.doi.org/10.1097/00019442-199500320-00004

Koenig HG, George LK, Peterson BL, et al. Depression in medically ill hospitalized older adults: prevalence, characteristics, and course of symptoms according to six diagnostic schemes. Am J Psychiatry. 1997;154(10):1376–83. Medline:9326819

Kroenke K, Spitzer RL, Williams JB. The Patient Health Questionnaire-2: validity of a two-item depression screener. Med Care. 2003;41(11):1284–92. http://dx.doi.org/10.1097/01.MLR.0000093487.78664.3C. Medline:14583691

Mulsant BH, Ganguli M, Seaberg EC. The relationship between self-rated health and depressive symptoms in an epidemiological sample of community-dwelling older adults. J Am Geriatr Soc. 1997;45(8):954–8. http://dx.doi.org/10.1111/j.1532-5415.1997.tb02966.x. Medline:9256848

Schulberg HC, Mulsant B, Schulz R, et al. Characteristics and course of major depression in older primary care patients. Int J Psychiatry Med. 1998;28(4):421–36. http://dx.doi.org/10.2190/G23R-NGGN-K1P1-MQ8N. Medline:10207741

Szanto K, Gildengers A, Mulsant BH, et al. Identification of suicidal ideation and prevention of suicidal behaviour in the elderly. Drugs Aging. 2002;19(1):11–24. http://dx.doi.org/10.2165/00002512-200219010-00002. Medline:11929324

Whyte EM, Mulsant BH. Post stroke depression: epidemiology, pathophysiology, and biological treatment. Biol Psychiatry. 2002;52(3):253–64. http://dx.doi.org/10.1016/S0006-3223(02)01424-5. Medline:12182931

2.2 Bereavement in Older Adults

Cindy Grief, MD, MSc, FRCPC

INTRODUCTION

The topic of bereavement can be somewhat perplexing because of a multitude of terms and definitions, as well as controversial aspects of classification. Grappling with where to draw the line between the universal condition of bereavement and mental illness is a fundamental task for the geriatric psychiatrist, both philosophically and clinically. Dr Grief's chapter provides a helpful approach to understanding terminologies and controversies, as well as ideas to guide treatment.

CASE SCENARIO

Mrs T. is a 68-year-old woman who was widowed five months ago after her husband had a lengthy and painful death from cancer. She describes herself as very lonely, crying a lot, trying to go out with friends (but often cancelling), and finding her nights "terrible." Describe your approach to the treatment of bereavement in older adults.

OVERVIEW

1. Bereavement and the Diagnostic and Statistical Manual of Mental Disorders (DSM)

1.1 DSM-IV-TR Bereavement

- Symptoms of sadness, insomnia, poor appetite, weight loss, etc., are characteristic of a major depressive episode (MDE).
- Depressed mood is, however, considered "normal."
- Help is often sought for insomnia or anorexia.
- Cultural variation in expression is recognized.
- The diagnosis of MDE is generally not given within first 2 months after the loss.
- This is known as the bereavement exclusion (for an MDE).

1.2 Bereavement Exclusion

- In DSM-IV, an MDE was generally not diagnosed until 2 months after the loss in recognition of the overlap between acute grief and depression to avoid pathologizing normal grief.
- Depression could be diagnosed at any point after the loss if significant guilt, thoughts of death, feelings of worthlessness, marked psychomotor retardation, prolonged functional impairment, and/or psychosis were present.
- DSM-5 has eliminated the bereavement exclusion for the diagnosis of an MDE, suggesting an MDE be diagnosed even within the first 2 months after a loss if criteria met.
- This change has been met with controversy.

1.3 Controversy regarding the Elimination of the Bereavement Exclusion in DSM-5

1.3.1 "Con" Perspective: The Bereavement Exclusion Should Not Be Removed

- No validity, even for the 2 month cut-off post-loss, when an MDE is generally not diagnosed
- Exclusion should, in fact, be extended to 52 weeks.
- Depressive symptoms in the context of grief are fundamentally different in terms of course and prognosis (Wakefield, Schmitz, & Baer, 2011; Wakefield & First, 2012).

1.3.2 "Pro" Perspective: Agree with Removal of Bereavement Exclusion for Major Depression

- Bereavement-related depression (BRD) and major depressive disorder (MDD) are clinically similar with respect to nature of symptoms, severity, and duration (Kendler, Myers, & Zisook, et al., 2008).
- "No cardiologist in his or her right mind would write off angina in a grieving individual as bereavement rather than as a medical condition requiring further workup" (Zisook & Shuchter, 2001).

1.4 Bereavement and DSM-5

- In DSM-5, there is a note under MDE: "Responses to a significant loss (e.g., bereavement, financial ruin, losses from a natural disaster, a serious medical illness or disability) may include the feelings of intense sadness, rumination about the loss, insomnia, poor appetite, and weight loss noted in Criterion A, which may resemble a depressive episode. Although such symptoms may be understandable or considered appropriate to the loss, the presence of a major depressive episode in addition to the normal response to a significant loss should also be carefully considered."
    - In the bereavement literature, it is increasingly recognized that forced retirement, divorce, and other losses, as mentioned above, can trigger bereavement responses (Papa, Lancaster, & Kahler, 2014).
- Persistent complex bereavement disorder (PCBD) is listed as a condition for further study in DSM-5.
    - The bereavement literature uses both the term "complicated grief" (or "complicated grief disorder") and the term "prolonged grief disorder," which this condition parallels.
    - Refers to a problematic form of bereavement that is neither depression nor post-traumatic stress disorder (PTSD)

2. Bereavement and Normal Grief

2.1 Key Terms

- Bereavement is the death of someone close.
- Grief is the response.
- Mourning is the process set in motion by bereavement:
  - Acknowledging the finality of the loss
  - Re-envisioning life without the deceased
- Acute grief:
  - Neurovegetative symptoms, preoccupation with deceased
  - Early response, with intense affect, can be overwhelming.
  - Healing occurs with time.
- Integrated grief:
  - Permanent residual grief (Zisook & Shear, 2009)
  - Connection with deceased maintained, but feelings of distress are attenuated
  - Can access positive memories
  - Recalling deceased may evoke sadness and longing but not intense distress.
  - Adaptation to loss with capacity to engage in and derive pleasure from normal activities
  - Anniversary of the death, birthdays, and other milestones often trigger waves of grief.
- Complicated grief:
  - Lasting form of acute grief that does not heal and never recedes

2.2 How Does Healing Occur during the Course of Normal Grief?

- Kübler-Ross outlined the five-stage model of grief in her seminal 1969 book, *On Death and Dying*. Her work is highly respected, but more recent research offers alternative models.
- The Yale Bereavement Study (Maciejewski et al., 2007) tracked grief in older adults (mean age 62.9 years, 53.5% ≥ 65 years) 1 to 24 months following spousal loss with the Inventory of Complicated Grief (ICG).
  - Disbelief was not the first grief indicator; acceptance was dominant.
    - People can oscillate between stages; it is not necessarily a linear pattern.
- Dual process model of coping with bereavement
  - Often cited explanatory model (Stroebe & Schut, 1999)
  - In bereavement there are oscillations between loss-oriented coping and restoration-oriented coping:
    - Loss-oriented coping encompasses dealing with grief intrusion, avoidance, denial, and the need to break bonds with the deceased.
    - Restoration-oriented coping involves creating new roles and relationships.
- Attachment theory is also used to explain adaptation to normal grief (Shear et al., 2007; Kho et al., 2015).
  - Attachment relationships are key to adaptation in bereavement.
  - Internal working models have to be reconfigured after a loved one dies.

- – Humans resist separation and look for proximity.
- – Internalization of memories of deceased over time occurs.
- – It leads to acceptance of loss of physical connection.
- Normal grief and healing
  - – Resilience characterized 45.9% in Changing Lives of Older Couple data set (Bonnano et al., 2002)
  - – At 2 months post-loss, 49% of widowed classified as "no depression," n = 328, mean age 61 years (Zisook et al., 1997)
  - – Post-traumatic growth (Wagner, Forstmeier, & Maercker, 2007) can lead to positive changes in self-perception and relationships.

3. Outcomes of Bereavement

3.1 Medical Outcomes
(Cohen, Granger, & Fuller-Thomson, 2015; Hall et al., 1997; Martikainen & Valkonen, 1996; Mostofsky et al., 2012; Schleifer et al., 1983; Stahl & Schulz, 2014; Carey et al., 2014)

- Increased mortality
- Increased risk of myocardial infarction (MI)
  - – Within first 24 hours of bereavement, risk increased 21x
- Sleep disruption
- Impaired immune function (Hughes, Connor, & Harkin, 2016)
- Increased cancer rates

3.2 Mental Health Outcomes

- Increased rates of substance use
- Anxiety disorders, PTSD
- 10–20% develop complicated grief
- Suicide (Byrne & Raphael, 1997)
  - – 57 widowers aged 65+, assessed at 6 weeks and 13 months post-loss
    - ▪ 14% of widowers reported suicidal thoughts or actions at 6 weeks
    - ▪ 15.4% at 13 months (0% in married group)
    - ▪ Thoughts of suicide in older widowers at 13 months post-loss even without other depressive symptoms
  - – Increased risk of suicide around anniversaries of death
- Depression in bereavement
  - – Rates of MDD in widowhood cited in various studies (Clayton, 1990; Zisook & Shuchter, 1991; Zisook et al., 1994)
    - ▪ Approximately 25% at 2 to 7 months post-loss
    - ▪ 15% at 13 months (not assessed at one year to avoid effect of anniversary reaction) (Zisook & Shuchter, 1991; Zisook et al., 1994)
    - ▪ Subsyndromal depressive symptoms persist at higher rates
- Normal grief vs depression
  - – Thoughts/ruminations
    - ▪ Normal grief includes a preoccupation with thoughts and memories of deceased.

- In depression, thoughts are self-critical, pessimistic; thoughts about death may include wanting to join deceased because of feelings of worthlessness or inability to cope with distress.
  - Self-esteem
    - Preserved in grief
    - In depression, feelings of worthlessness and self-loathing (DSM-5)

4. Assessment

- Identifying data
  - Age, cultural background
- Narrative of death
  - Circumstances of death
  - Perception of expectedness
  - Relationship with deceased
  - Secondary losses
  - Caregiver burden
    - Caregivers may neglect their health.
    - Caregivers are vulnerable to BRD when it is a difficult, painful death.
    - Caregivers of persons with dementia may experience ambiguous loss – a series of losses that might not be recognized by others, also referred to as "disenfranchised grief," a term that refers to situations where individuals feel their grief goes unacknowledged. A spouse's loss of memory, functional impairment may not be noticed or marked by others. Other forms of ambiguous loss cited include the death of a pet, miscarriages (Zhang et al., 2008; Doka, 2006).
- Assessment
  - Explore anger, guilt
  - Early, intense grief-related distress, depressive symptoms (risk factors for later distress)
  - Suicidal ideation
  - Substance use
  - Cognitive status
  - Activities of daily living (ADLs) and instrumental ADLs (IADLs)
  - Past psychiatric history, especially for MDD
  - Past medical history
    - Cardiovascular risk factors, neglected health, nutrition, self-perceived poor health, physical limitations
  - Family history
  - Social/personal
    - Relationships, social support, socioeconomic status (SES)

5. Approach to Normal Grief

- Universal screening procedures appear to be of no benefit (Currier, Neimeyer, & Berman, 2008; meta-analysis of 61 controlled studies).

- Grief counselling is not effective and can cause iatrogenic worsening of problems (Neimeyer, 2000 – meta-analysis of 23 RCTs; note that this analysis was not specific to older adults).
- Explore rituals, anniversaries.
- Encourage exercise, balanced eating.
- In a study of n = 200 bereaved ≥ 50 years (mean 66.3 years)
  - Sleeping 6.5 to 9 hours per night in the months post-loss predicted better social and emotional health, greater energy.
  - Exercising ≥ 1 days per week significantly predicted better physical functioning (Chen, Gill, & Prigerson, 2005).
- Importance of social connections
  - Regular social activity decreased depressive symptomatology (Vanderwerker & Prigerson, 2004).

6. Management of Bereavement-Related Depression (BRD)

- Escitalopram: 12 week open-label for MDE, significant reduction in depressive symptoms, n = 30, mean 45.67 years (Hensley et al., 2009)
- Bupropion SR: 8 week open-label, n = 22, depressed widowed, significant reduction in depression (Zisook et al., 2001)
- Others: desipramine, nortriptyline
- Only 1 RCT for acute BRD pharmacotherapy (Reynolds et al., 1999)
  - n = 80 bereaved, ≥ 50 years
  - Nortriptyline + interpersonal psychotherapy (IPT); nortriptyline + medication clinic; placebo + IPT; placebo + medication clinic
  - Best outcome: nortriptyline and IPT
  - IPT alone no better than placebo for BRD

7. Complicated Grief (CG)

- Terminology is confusing in the literature.
  - Also referred to as complicated grief disorder (CGD) and prolonged grief disorder (PGD)
- Intense grief that persists > 6 months after the loss
- Traumatic distress
  - Sense of disbelief, anger, and bitterness
  - Distressing, intrusive thoughts related to the death
  - Avoidance of reminders of deceased
- Such distress also considered a key component of CGD and PGD
- PGD and CGD
  - PGD phenomenology distinct from anxiety, depression, and PTSD as shown by factor analytic studies on bereaved samples (Prigerson et al., 2009)
  - In DSM-5, prolonged grief disorder seems to be hinted at by persistent complex bereavement disorder, a condition for further study.
  - CGD discrete set of symptoms independent from BRD and PTSD but often comorbid (Golden & Dalgleish, 2010; Simon et al., 2007; Nakajima et al., 2012)
  - Rates of CGD nearly 10x higher among individuals with MDD (Sung et al, 2011; Simon et al., 2007; Nakajima et al. 2012)

- CGD/PGD linked to increased risk for hospitalizations, functional impairment, depression, suicidal thoughts
- Predicts medical and psychiatric morbidity, even when controlling for depressive symptoms (Shear, Ghesquiere, & Glickman, 2013; Simon, 2013)

7.1 Distinguishing CG from PTSD
(Shear et al., 2011)

Complicated grief	PTSD
• Trigger is loss	• Trigger is threat
• Yearning, sadness	• Fear
• Intrusive thoughts are person-related	• Intrusive thoughts are event-related
• Avoidance is loss-based	• Avoidance is fear-based
• Reminders pervasive	• Reminders linked to event

7.2 Some Risk Factors for Complicated Grief
(Simon, 2013)

- Childhood separation anxiety (Vanderwerker et al., 2006)
- Insecure attachment (Johnson et al., 2007)
- Dependent relationship with deceased
- Traumatic loss (Lobb et al., 2010)
- Close kinship relationship to the deceased (Lobb et al., 2010)

7.3 Cognitive Behavioural Principles behind CG
(Boelen, Van Den Hout, & Van Den Bout, 2006)

- Problems integrating the death of loved one into autobiographical memory
- Negative and self-blaming patterns of thinking that need to be challenged

8. Complicated Grief Treatment (CGT)
(Shear et al., 2005; Shear et al., 2014)

- CGT is a distinct therapy that incorporates both interpersonal psychotherapy (IPT) and cognitive behavioural therapy (CBT) techniques.
- CGT vs IPT, random assignment (Shear et al., 2005)
  - ICG score ≥ 30, 6 months post-death, medication for depression allowed
  - 95 men and women aged 18–85, 16 sessions
  - 3 phases, manualized
  - Outcome measures: treatment response of Clinical Global Improvement (CGI) score of 1 or 2, or as time to a 20-point or better improvement in self-report ICG
  - Improvement in complicated grief symptoms with both CGT and IPT
  - Response rate for CGT was higher (51%) than for IPT (28%; P = .02), and time to response was faster for complicated grief treatment (P = .02); number needed to treat was 4.3.
  - Authors concluded CGT superior treatment to IPT with higher response rates and faster time to response.

- Study expanded to include (n = 151) older adults >/ 50 years, mean age = 66.1 years (Shear et al., 2014)
    - Randomized to CGT or IPT for 16 weekly sessions
    - Response rate for CGT more than twice that for IPT

8.1 CG Treatment Phases

Sessions 1–3:
    - Psychoeducation
    - Story of death, relationship with deceased
    - Assessment of grief intensity
    - Focus on setting personal life goals
Sessions 4–10:
    - Address traumatic symptoms with imaginal revisiting exercises, in vivo exposure
    - Promote sense of connection with deceased
Sessions 11–16:
    - Termination phase

8.2 Key Elements of CG Treatment

- Goal-setting
    - Emphasis on life vs loss
    - Not about treatment goals, but lifetime goals
    - Encourage, facilitate, self-disclose
    - Reflect on progress
    - Revisit the death
        - Tell the story of the death and its aftermath, as though it's happening.
    - Ask them to report Subjective Units of Distress Scale (SUDS) rating
    - Create tapes for home use
    - Time in session left for debriefing and goal work
    - Loss-focused techniques
    - Imaginal conversations
        - Imagine your loved one can hear you and your questions or comments.
    - Use of pictures
    - Memory work
        - Ask them to record memories.
        - The goal is to be able to access both positive and negative memories.
- CGT with citalopram (Shear et al., 2016)
    - Placebo-controlled randomized clinical trial evaluated efficacy of citalopram combined with complicated grief therapy. Addition of citalopram helps depressive symptoms, but not complicated grief symptoms.

9. Final Points

- In the bereavement literature, the terms PGD and CG/CGD are all used and approximate similar clinical entities.
- There had been debate about the removal of the bereavement exclusion from DSM-5 and about the lack of inclusion of PGD.
- Persistent complex bereavement disorder, a condition for further study, is akin to complicated grief/prolonged grief disorder.
- The majority of older adults are resilient, yet bereavement is associated with adverse psychiatric and medical morbidity, including increased risk of mortality.
- Knowledge of risk factors for BRD and CGD can help guide assessment of the bereaved older adult.
- CGD and PGD can be distinguished from PTSD.
- Bereavement continues to be an area of active research, and there is much still to be learned about older adults.

QUESTIONS

1. List five negative medical outcomes associated with bereavement in the older adult.
2. What psychiatric conditions are associated with bereavement in the older adult?
3. What is the bereavement exclusion and why was it controversial?
4. Describe some symptoms associated with complicated grief and/or prolonged grief disorder.

ANSWERS

1. Negative medical outcomes with bereavement include:
   - Increased mortality from all causes
   - Increased cardiac events (especially increased risk of MI)
   - Hemodynamic changes with elevations in blood pressure observed
   - Impaired immune function
   - Increased cancer rates
   - Sleep dysfunction
   - Increased institutionalization and hospitalization
   - Negative health behaviours, e.g., alcohol and nicotine abuse
   - Self-neglect, e.g., not eating properly leading to nutritional deficiencies, not taking care of pre-existent health conditions

2. Psychiatric conditions associated with bereavement in later life include:
   - Major depressive disorder, as well as subsyndromal depression
   - Adjustment disorder
   - Anxiety disorders, including PTSD
   - Increased rates of substance use
   - Complicated/prolonged grief in 10–20%
   - Sleep disorders
   - Suicide, suicidal gestures
   - Worsening of pre-existing psychiatric and medical conditions

3. Regarding the DSM bereavement exclusion and its controversy:
   - In DSM-IV-TR, a major depression was generally not diagnosed until 2 months after the loss.
   - In DSM-IV-TR, therefore, the diagnosis of major depression had a bereavement exclusion.
   - This was in recognition of the overlap between acute grief and depression, and to avoid the pathologization of normal grief.
   - In DSM-5, the criteria for a major depressive episode no longer include a bereavement exclusion within the first 2 months post-loss.
   - Clinicians are encouraged to diagnose a major depression if criteria are met at any point during the course of grief.
   - Of note, even in DSM-IV-TR, criteria for an MDE might still be met before 2 months had elapsed if an individual presented with significant guilt, thoughts of death, feelings of worthlessness, marked psychomotor retardation, prolonged functional impairment, and/or psychosis.
   - Controversies:
     – There is evidence that bereavement-related depression and major depressive disorder are clinically similar with respect to nature of symptoms, severity, and duration (this is the majority opinion); however, some disagree and maintain that depressive symptoms in the context of grief are different in terms of course and prognosis.
     – Removal of the bereavement exclusion may increase the risk of overdiagnosing depression; to counter this, DSM-5 includes a footnote emphasizing that the normal and expected responses to a significant loss (not only due to death, but financial ruin, serious medical illness, etc.) include feelings of intense sadness and features that may resemble a depressive episode.
   - Of note, in DSM-5, an adjustment disorder may be diagnosed when symptoms do not represent normal bereavement, i.e., when "the intensity, quality, or persistence of grief reactions exceeds what normally might be expected," taking into account "cultural, religious, or age-appropriate norms."

4. Symptoms associated with complicated grief and/or prolonged grief disorder include:
   - Complicated grief
     – Acute grief that never becomes integrated
     – Attachment theory is central to understanding the construct.
     – Traumatic distress is a common feature (e.g., a sense of disbelief, anger, and bitterness; distressing, intrusive thoughts related to the death; avoidance of reminders of the deceased; separation distress).
   - Prolonged grief disorder was proposed for DSM-5 by Prigerson et al., 2009.
     – Features (with symptoms) include:
       ▪ Bereavement (loss of a significant other)
       ▪ Separation distress
       ▪ Cognitive, emotional, and behavioural symptoms: confusion about one's role in life or diminished sense of self; difficulty accepting the loss; avoidance of reminders of the reality of the loss; inability to trust others since the loss; bitterness or anger related to the loss; difficulty moving on with life; numbness since the loss; feeling that life is unfulfilling, empty,

or meaningless since the loss; feeling stunned, dazed, or shocked by the loss; feeling agitated, jumpy, or "on edge" since the loss

- – Diagnosis should not be made until at least 6 months after the loss.
- – Disturbance causes clinically significant impairment in social, occupational, or other important areas of functioning.
- • Note that in DSM-5 under other specified trauma and stressor-related disorder, persistent complex bereavement disorder can be diagnosed.
  - – This is a condition for further study and has its own set of proposed criteria, which are different from the above.
  - – It is most akin to complicated grief and PGD.
- • Whether you call it complicated/prolonged/persistent, or (formerly) traumatic grief, this construct is neither depression nor PTSD, but all these may be comorbid.

CASE DISCUSSION

A comprehensive assessment that includes obtaining a narrative of the circumstances of the death is warranted. One should ascertain whether the death was perceived as expected, relationship with the deceased, concurrent losses, presence of anger or guilt. It is also useful to ask about the anniversary of the death and other triggers.

Other considerations:

- • A good functional inquiry is important to elicit any depressive or anxiety symptoms, suicidal ideation, substance use, cognitive status, as well as symptoms of complicated/prolonged grief.
- • Past medical history should include cardiovascular risk factors.
- • Obtain family history and social history, including degree and quality of perceived social support, socioeconomic status, cultural and spiritual beliefs including mourning rituals, attachment history.
- • Perform a functional assessment, asking about ADL and IADLs.
- • Reassess if possible.
- • Be aware of anniversary reaction.
- • In follow-up, ask about suicidality (remember that early on, intense distress predicts later morbidity).
- • Complicated grief: consider CGT.
- • Bereavement/major depressive episode: choice of treatment depends on severity of depression.

RECOMMENDED RESOURCES FOR REVIEW

Although these resources may not be specifically cited in the text, their approach informed the contents of the chapter, and they are recommended as useful further reading.

Buckley T, Sunari D, Marshall A, et al. Physiological correlates of bereavement and the impact of bereavement interventions. Dialogues Clin Neurosci. 2012;14(2):129–39. PMID:22754285

Zhang B, El-Jawahri A, Prigerson HG. Update on bereavement research: evidence-based guidelines for the diagnosis and treatment of complicated bereavement. J Palliat Med. 2006;9(5):1188–203. http://dx.doi.org/10.1089/jpm.2006.9.1188. Medline:17040157

Zisook S, Corruble E, Duan N, et al. The bereavement exclusion and DSM-5. Depress Anxiety. 2012;29(5):425–43. http://dx.doi.org/10.1002/da.21927. Medline:22495967

Zisook S, Shear K. Grief and bereavement: what psychiatrists need to know. World Psychiatry. 2009;8(2):67–74. http://dx.doi.org/10.1002/j.2051-5545.2009.tb00217.x. Medline:19516922

REFERENCES

Boelen PA, Van Den Hout MA, Van Den Bout J. A cognitive-behavioral conceptualization of complicated grief. Clin Psychol Sci Pract. 2006;13(2):109–28. http://dx.doi.org/10.1111/j.1468-2850.2006.00013.x

Bonanno GA, Wortman CB, Lehman DR, et al. Resilience to loss and chronic grief: a prospective study fom preloss to 18-months postloss. J Pers SocPsychol. 2002;83(5):1150–64. Medline:12416919

Byrne GJ, Raphael B. The psychological symptoms of conjugal bereavement in elderly men over the first 13 months. Int J Geriatr Pyschiatry. 1997;12(2)241–51. Medline:9097218

Carey IM, Shah SM, DeWilde S, et al. Increased risk of acute cardiovascular events after partner bereavement: a matched cohort study. JAMA Intern Med. 2014;174(4):598–605. http://dx.doi.org/10.1001/jamainternmed.2013.14558. Medline:24566983

Chen JH, Gill TM, Prigerson HG. Health behaviors associated with better quality of life for older bereaved persons. J Palliat Med. 2005;8(1)96–106. http://dx.doi.org/10.1089/jpm.2005.8.96. PMID:15662178

Clayton P. Bereavement and depression. J Clin Psychiatry. 1990;51(Suppl):34–40. Medline:2195011

Cohen M, Granger S, Fuller-Thomson E. The association between bereavement and biomarkers of inflammation. Behav Med. 2015;41(2):49–59. Medline:24266503

Currier JM, Neimeyer RA, Berman JS. The effectiveness of psychotherapeutic interventions for bereaved persons: a comprehensive quantitative review. Psychol Bull. 2008;134(5):648–61. http://dx.doi.org/10.1037/0033-2909.134.5.648. Medline:18729566

Doka KJ. Grief: the constant companion of illness. Anesthesiol Clin. 2006;24(1):205–12. PMID:16487903

Golden AM, Dalgleish T. Is prolonged grief distinct from *bereavement*-related posttraumatic stress? Psychiatry Res. 2010;178(2):336–41. http://dx.doi.org/10.1016/j.psychres.2009.08.021. Medline:20493535

Hall M, Buysse DJ, Dew MA, et al. Intrusive thoughts and avoidance behaviors are associated with sleep disturbances in bereavement-related depression. Depress Anxiety. 1997;6(3):106–12. Medline:9442984

Hensley PL, Slonimski CK, Uhlenhuth EH, et al. Escitalopram: an open-label study of bereavement-related depression and grief. J Affect Disord. 2009;113(1–2):142–9. http://dx.doi.org/10.1016/j.jad.2008.05.016. Medline:18597854

Hughes MM, Connor TJ, Harkin A. Stress-related immune markers in depression: implications for treatment. Int J Neuropsychopharmacol. 2016;19(6):1–19. http://dx.doi.org/10.1093/ijnp/pyw001. Medline:26775294

Johnson JG, Zhang B, Greer JA, et al. Parental control, partner dependency, and complicated grief among widowed adults in the community. J Nerv Ment Dis. 2007;195(1):26–30. Medline:17220736

Kendler KS, Myers J, Zisook S. Does bereavement-related major depression differ from major depression associated with other stressful life events? Am J Psychiatry. 2008;165(11):1449–55. http://dx.doi.org/10.1176/appi.ajp.2008.07111757. Medline:18708488

Kho Y, Kane RT, Priddis L, et al. The nature of attachment relationships and grief responses in older adults: an attachment path model of grief. PLoS One. 2015;10(10):e0133703. http://dx.doi.org/10.1371/journal.pone.0133703. PMCID: PMC4603668

Lobb EA, Kristjanson LJ, Aoun SM, et al. Predictors of complicated grief: a systematic review of empirical studies. Death Stud. 2010;34(8):673–98. Medline:24482845

Maciejewski PK, Zhang B, Block SD, et al. An empirical examination of the stage theory of grief. JAMA. 2007;297(7):716–23. http://dx.doi.org/10.1001/jama.297.7.716. Medline:17312291

Martikainen P, Valkonen T. Mortality after the death of a spouse: rates and causes of death in a large Finnish cohort. Am J Public Health.1996;86:1097–93. Medline:8712266

Mostofsky E, Maclure M, Sherwood JB, et al. Risk of acute myocardial infarction after the death of a significant person in one's life: the Determinants of Myocardial Infarction Onset Study. Circulation. 2012;125(3):491–6. http://dx.doi.org/10.1161/CIRCULATIONAHA.111.061770. Medline:22230481

Nakajima S, Masaya I, Akemi S, et al. Complicated grief in those bereaved by violent death: the effects of post-traumatic stress disorder on complicated grief. Dialogues Clin Neurosci. 2012;14(2):210–14.

Neimeyer RA. Searching for the meaning of meaning: grief therapy and the process of reconstruction. Death Stud. 2000;24(6):541–58. Medline:11503667

Papa A, Lancaster NG, Kahler J. Commonalities in grief responding across bereavement and non-bereavement losses. J Affect Disord. 2014;161:136–43. http://dx.doi.org/10.1016/j.jad.2014.03.018. Medline:24751321

Prigerson HG, Horowitz MJ, Jacobs SC, et al. Prolonged grief disorder: psychometric validation of criteria proposed for *DSM-V* and *ICD-11*. PLoS Med. 2009;6(8):e1000121. http://dx.doi.org/10.1371/journal .pmed.1000121. Medline:19652695

Reynolds CF, Miller MD, Pasternak RE, et al. Treatment of bereavement-related major depressive episodes in later life: a controlled study of acute and continuation treatment with nortriptyline and interpersonal psychotherapy. Am J Physchiatry.1999;156(2):202–8. Medline:9989555

Schleifer SJ, Keller SE, Camerion M, et al. Suppression of lymphocyte stimulation following bereavement. JAMA. 1983;250(3):374–7. http://dx.doi.org/10.1001/jama.1983.03340030034024. Medline:6854901

Shear K, Frank E, Houck PR, et al. Treatment of complicated grief: a randomized controlled trial. JAMA. 2005;293(21):2601–8. http://dx.doi.org/10.1001/jama.293.21.2601. Medline:15928281

Shear MK, Ghesquiere A, Glickman K. Bereavement and complicated grief. Curr Psychiatry Rep. 2013;15(11):406. http://dx.doi.org/10.1007/s11920-013-0406-z. Medline:24068457

Shear MK, Monk T, Houck PR, et al. An attachment-based model of complicated grief including the role of avoidance. Eur Arch Psychiatry Clin Neurosci. 2007;257(8)453–61. http://dx.doi.org/10.1007/s00406-007-0745-z. Medline:17629727

Shear MK, Reynolds CF 3rd, Simon NM, et al. Optimizing treatment of complicated grief: a randomized clinical trial. JAMA Psychiatry. 2016. [epub ahead of print]. http://dx.doi.org/10.1001/jamapsychiatry .2016.0892. PMID:27276373

Shear MK, Simon N, Wall M, et al. Complicated grief and related bereavement issues for DSM-5. Depress Anxiety. 2011;28(2):103–17. http://dx.doi.org/10.1002/da.20780. Medline:21284063

Shear MK, Wang Y, Skritskaya N, et al. Treatment of complicated grief in elderly persons: a randomized clinical trial. JAMA Psychiatry. 2014;71(11):1287–95. http://dx.doi.org/10.1001/jamapsychiatry.2014.1242. Medline:25250737

Simon NM. Treating complicated grief. JAMA. 2013;310(4):416–23. http://dx.doi.org/10.1001/jama.2013.8614. Medline:23917292

Simon NM, Shear KM, Thompson EH, et al. The prevalence and correlates of psychiatric comorbidity in individuals with complicated grief. Compr Psychiatry. 2007;48:395–9. Medline:17707245

Stahl ST, Schulz R. Changes in routine health behaviors following late-life bereavement: a systematic review. J Behav Med. 2014;37(4):736–55. http://dx.doi.org/10.1007/s10865-013-9524-7. Medline:23881308

Stroebe M, Schut H. The dual process model of coping with bereavement rationale and description. Death Stud. 1999;23(3):197–224. Medline:10848151

Sung SC, Dryman MT, Marks E, et al. Complicated grief among individuals with major depression: prevalence, comorbidity, and associated features. J Affect Disord. 2011;134(1–3):453–8. http://dx.doi.org/10.1016/ j.jad.2011.05.017. Medline:21621849

Vanderwerker LC, Jacobs SC, Parkes CM, et al. An exploration of associations between separation anxiety in childhood and complicated grief in later life. J Nerv Ment Dis 2006;194:121–3. Medline:16477190

Vanderwerker L, Prigerson HG. Social support and technological connectedness as protective factors in bereavement. Journal of Loss and Trauma: International Perspectives on Stress & Coping. 2004;9(1):45–57. http://dx.doi.org/10.1080/15325020490255304

Wagner B, Forstmeier S, Maercker A. Posttraumatic growth as a cognitive process with behavioral components: a commentary on Hoboll et al.(2007). Appl Psychol. 2007;56(3):407–16. http://dx.doi.org/10.1111/ j.1464-0597.2007.00295.x

Wakefield JC, First MB. Validity of the bereavement exclusion to major depression: does the empirical evidence support the proposal to eliminate the exclusion in the DSM-5? World Psychiatry. 2012;11(1):3–10. Medline:22294996

Wakefield JC, Schmitz MF, Baer JC. Relation between duration and severity in bereavement-related depression. Acta Psychiatr Scand. 2011;124(6):487–94. http://dx.doi.org/10.1111/j.1600-0447.2011.01768.x. Medline:21950650

Zhang B, Mitchell SL, Bambauer KZ, et al. Depressive symptom trajectories and associated risks among bereaved Alzheimer disease caregivers. Am J Geriatr Psychiatry. 2008;16(2):145–55. http://dx.doi.org/ 10.1097/JGP.0b013e318157caec

Zisook S, Paulus M, Shuchter SR, et al. The many faces of depression following spousal bereavement. J Affect Disord. 1997;45(1–2):85–94. Medline:9268778

Zisook S, Shuchter SR. Depression through the first year after the death of a spouse. Am J Psychiatry. 1991;148(10):1346–52. Medline:1897615

Zisook S, Shuchter SR. Treatment of the depressions of bereavement. American Behavioral Scientist. 2001;44(5)782–97. http://dx.doi.org/10.1177/0002764201044005006

Zisook S, Shuchter SR, Pedrelli P, et al. Bupropion sustained release for bereavement: results of an open trial. J Clin Psychiatry. 2001;62(4):227–30. Medline:11379835

Zisook S, Shuchter SR, Sledge PA, et al. The spectrum of depressive phenomena after spousal bereavement. J Clin Psychiatry. 1994;55(Suppl):29–36. Medline:8077167

2.3 Pharmacotherapy of Depression in Older Adults

Benoit H. Mulsant, MD, MS, FRCPC

INTRODUCTION

Major depression remains a common syndrome in the elderly, and knowledge of pharmacological management of this illness is a mainstay for the practicing clinician. Dr Mulsant provides a masterful review of the limited evidence-base in geriatric psychiatry, as compared to adult-age psychiatry, in this challenging area. The use of a systematic approach is highlighted in order to maximize treatment response and to help determine when to alter treatment. He also reviews safety, including the recent warnings guiding our safe use of these medications.

CASE SCENARIO

A 72-year-old woman experiences a first-ever episode of depression, characterized by low mood, anhedonia, severe insomnia, a 15-pound weight loss, and difficulty concentrating. She is treated by her family physician with sertraline 50 mg/day for four weeks. She experiences only minimal improvement and is referred to you for clinical management.

1. What do you do first to approach this situation?
2. What do you do next?
3. Four weeks later, she has shown almost complete resolution of all her symptoms and she is asking you when she will be able to decrease the dose or stop her antidepressant. What do you tell her?

OVERVIEW

1. Fighting Therapeutic Nihilism

Late-life depression is one of the few medical conditions in which treatment can make a rapid and dramatic difference in an older adult's level of function.

2. Argument for a Systematic Approach

This section presents some of the evidence supporting the use of a systematic approach when treating a depression in older adults. This approach (also referred to as "protocolized treatment," "algorithmic treatment," "integrated clinical pathways," or "stepped care") is contrasted with an individualized approach under "usual care" conditions. The overall conclusion is that when treating depression pharmacologically, the way one uses medications is more important than the medications one uses (Mulsant et al., 2014).

2.1 Advantages of a Systematic Approach

- Informed by best available evidence and guidelines
- Clinical experience ends up being derived from treating large numbers of patients with the same medications.
- Keeping the course: clinicians are protected against their personal biases and pressure from patients or families.
- The focus is on the patient.

2.2 Disadvantages of Individualized Approach (Usual Care)

- Often based on fads ("treatment du jour")
- Little cumulative experience due to small numbers of patients receiving many different medications
- Ill-advised or ill-timed changes in treatment
- Focus is on the treatment; making decision is exhausting.

2.3 Poor Outcomes of Usual Care for Depressed Patients Treated by Well-Trained Psychiatrists

- Study of six psychiatric clinics in Westchester County (US) (Meyers et al., 2002)
    - 165 patients with major depression
    - 65% received an antidepressant
        - 45% treatment adequacy (adequate dose for 4+ weeks)
        - Academic vs non-academic sites: 53% vs 36%, p = 0.04
    - Remission rate after 3 months: 30%
    - Adequate treatment: threefold higher likelihood of remission (OR = 3.2; p = 0.04)

2.4 Superiority of Systematic Approach ("Clinical Protocol") over Individualized Approach ("Usual Care") for the Treatment of Depression in Late Life

- Two examples of randomized comparisons for late-life depression:
    1. IMPACT (Unützer et al., 2002)
    2. PROSPECT (Bruce et al., 2004; Alexopoulos et al., 2005; Alexopoulos et al., 2009)
- Meta-analyses of interventions for treatment-resistant depression in late-life (Cooper et al., 2011)

3. Possible Criteria for Choosing an Antidepressant for an Older Adult

- US guidelines (Alexopoulos et al., 2001)
- UK guidelines (Baldwin et al., 2002)
- Canadian guidelines (Buchanan et al., 2006; Canadian Coalition for Seniors' Mental Health, 2006)
- Evidence on efficacy (Kok, Nolen, & Heeren, 2012)
- Evidence on tolerability or safety (Mottram, Wilson, & Strobl, 2006)
- Cost

3.1 Guidelines

Why do we rely on expert opinion?
- Many antidepressants available
- Few good comparative trials in older adults
- Not clear how optimal dosages and side effects are different in older adults

An example: *Expert consensus guideline: pharmacotherapy of depressive disorders in older patients* (Alexopoulos et al., 2001)

2001 geriatric depression guideline selection of expert panel
- Experts held federal or other grants.
- Experts published influential papers on late-life depression.
- All invited experts (n = 50) agreed to participate.
- Experts were blind to the sponsors of the study.
- Selective serotonin reuptake inhibitors (SSRIs) were favoured regardless of severity of depression.

3.2 Evidence that Antidepressants Are Efficacious
(Pinquart, Duberstein, & Lyness, 2006)

- Meta-analysis of 62 placebo-controlled studies (n = 3921)
- Favourable outcomes: drugs: 66% vs placebo: 31%

> "Available treatments for depression work, with effect sizes that are moderate to large."
> (Pinquart, Duberstein, & Lyness, 2006)

3.3 What to Do with the Large Therapeutic Effects of Placebo when Treating Depression in Late Life

- Similar to effects seen in younger patients
- Placebo does not equal "no treatment" (Mulsant et al., 2014; Roose et al., 2004; Schatzberg & Roose, 2006). Patients treated with placebo receive:
  - Thorough baseline medical and psychological evaluation
  - Frequent and lengthy visits
- Process of care in research trials not representative of usual care

When considering that antidepressant medications seem to be more efficacious than placebos only for those with severe depression, "it is more accurate to state that patients with severe depression do not respond as well to placebo as patients with less severe depression rather than that patients with severe depression respond better to medication than patients with non-severe depression" (Roose et al., 2004).

In other words, the superiority of antidepressants over placebo is apparent only in those with severe depression who are hard to treat; those with mild or moderate depression do well, regardless of whether they are treated with an antidepressant or a placebo.

3.4 Potential Safety Concerns in Older Adults Treated with Antidepressants

- Drug-drug interactions (Mulsant & Pollock, 2015)
- Hyponatremia (Fabian et al., 2004)
- Falls and fractures (Joo et al., 2002)

- GI bleeds (Yuan, Tsoi, & Hunt, 2006)
- Cardiovascular effects (Johnson et al., 2006)
- Cognitive impairment (Mulsant & Pollock, 2015)
- Worsening of suicidality (Juurlink et al., 2006)
- Bone metabolism and osteoporosis (Shea et al., 2013; Gebara et al., 2014)

3.5 Cardiac Safety Concerns for Citalopram and Escitalopram in Older Adults

3.5.1 Similar US and Canadian Safety Warnings regarding Cardiac Effects of Citalopram in Older Adults

"The maximum recommended dose of citalopram is 20 mg per day for patients with hepatic impairment, patients who are older than 60 years of age, patients who are CYP 2C19 poor metabolizers, or patients who are taking concomitant cimetidine (Tagamet®) or another CYP2C19 inhibitor, because these factors lead to increased blood levels of citalopram, increasing the risk of QT interval prolongation and Torsade de Pointes."

> US Food and Drug Administration (FDA) Drug Safety Warning, August 2011
> (http://www.fda.gov/Drugs/DrugSafety/ucm297391.htm)

"A thorough QT study ... has shown that citalopram causes dose-dependent QT prolongation ... 20 mg per day is the maximum recommended dose for patients with hepatic impairment, patients who are 65 years of age or older, patients who are CYP2C19 poor metabolizers, or patients who are taking concomitant cimetidine or another CYP2C19 inhibitor ... ECG monitoring is recommended in patients with risk factors for Torsade de Pointes such as congestive heart failure, recent myocardial infarction, bradyarrhythmias."

> Health Canada Advisory, January 2012 (http://www.healthycanadians.gc.ca/
> recall-alert-rappel-avis/hc-sc/2012/14672a-eng.php)

3.5.2 Different US and Canadian Safety Warnings regarding Cardiac Effects of Escitalopram in Older Adults

"Although the antidepressant effects of the drugs are known to be limited to the S-isomer, the difference between the effects of citalopram racemate and escitalopram on the QT interval presumably means that the QT effects are not specific to the S-isomer ... [C]italopram causes dose-dependent QT interval prolongation that is clinically significant with the 60 mg daily dose ... Given that these findings were not observed with escitalopram, there are no changes planned for escitalopram at this time."

> US FDA Drug Safety Warning, March 2012 (http://www.fda.gov/
> Drugs/DrugSafety/ucm297391.htm)

"Cipralex can cause ... QT interval prolongation ... Use of Cipralex is **discouraged** in patients who are also taking drugs that prolong QT interval or that decrease electrolyte levels in the body. Examples ... include ... drugs used to treat heart rhythm problems, certain antipsychotics, certain antidepressants, opioid painkillers and certain drugs used to treat infections ... diuretics (water pills) and laxatives (including enemas) ... 10 mg per day is the maximum recommended dose for patients who are 65 years of age or older."

> Health Canada Warning, May 2012 (http://www.healthycanadians.gc.ca/
> recall-alert-rappel-avis/hc-sc/2012/13674a-eng.php)

4. A Systematic Approach to Treatment-Resistant Depression

Clinicians have struggled for a long time with how to interpret results of clinical trials:

> "All who drink of this remedy recover in a short time except those whom it does not help, who all die. Therefore, it is obvious that it fails only in incurable cases."
>
> Galen on clinical trials – 180 AD

When treating depression pharmacologically, clinicians need to select a few drugs (i.e., their "private" formulary) and use them in a systematic way. Each clinician needs to answer these questions:

- What is my first-line intervention?
- What is my second-line intervention?
- What is my third-line intervention?
- How long should each of these steps last?
- When do I switch medications? When do you I combine/augment medications?

4.1 Guideline Recommendations for the Pharmacotherapy of Major Depression
(Alexopoulos et al., 2001; Buchanan et al., 2006; CCSMH, 2006)

Table 2.3.1 outlines recommendations from the 2001 US expert consensus guidelines and the 2006 Canadian guidelines from the Canadian Coalition for Seniors' Mental Health.

4.1.1 Does It Matter Which Antidepressant One Uses?

Results of randomized placebo-controlled trials for the *acute treatment* of older patients with major depression have been published for citalopram, duloxetine, escitalopram, fluoxetine, paroxetine, sertraline, venlafaxine, and vortioxetine. There are no published placebo-controlled trials for desvenlafaxine, mirtazapine, levomilnacipran, or vilazodone.

Positive placebo-controlled trials exist for fluoxetine (1 of 3 published trials), paroxetine (1/1), sertraline (1/1), duloxetine (2/3), and vortioxetine (1/1), but not for citalopram (0/1), escitalopram (0/2), or venlafaxine (0/1). However, when experts select an antidepressant, they assume that all these drugs have similar efficacy and chose specific drugs based on pharmacologic profile (class, pharmacokinetics, potential for drug-drug interactions) and common adverse effects.

In the US and Canadian guidelines, published in 2001 and 2006 respectively (see Table 2.3.1), experts avoided fluoxetine (due to its long half-life and high potential for drug-drug interactions [DDIs]) and paroxetine (due to its uncomfortable symptoms upon discontinuation, high potential for DDIs, and potential anticholinergic effects). They favoured sertraline or citalopram, based on their tolerability and perceived safety. With the more recent concerns about citalopram cardiac effects (see section 3.5), one would suspect that experts would now avoid citalopram and favour escitalopram instead.

Unlike venlafaxine, the serotonin norepinephrine reuptake inhibitor (SNRI) duloxetine has been shown to be more efficacious than placebo in the acute treatment of older patients with major depressive disorder, but Canadian and US experts do not favour it over venlafaxine (Mulsant et al., 2014).

When experts were asked to pick a single first-line antidepressant to treat a generic older patient with depression (Mulsant et al., 2014), they avoided fluoxetine (long half-life, high potential for drug-drug interaction) and paroxetine (uncomfortable symptoms upon discontinuation, high potential for drug-drug interaction), and favoured sertraline or escitalopram based on the good tolerability and safety of these drugs.

Table 2.3.1: Canadian and US Guideline Recommendations for Pharmacotherapy
of Major Depression in Older Adults

	2001 US Expert Consensus Guidelines	**2006 Canadian Guidelines**
Preferred treatment	An antidepressant (selective serotonin reuptake inhibitor [SSRI] or venlafaxine XR preferred) plus psychotherapy	An antidepressant, psychotherapy, or a combination of both if the depression is of mild or moderate severity; a combination of an antidepressant and psychotherapy for a severe depression
Specific antidepressant	Citalopram and sertraline are preferred with paroxetine as another first-line option	Citalopram, sertraline, venlafaxine, bupropion, or mirtazapine
Starting dose	Begin with "somewhat lower doses" than in younger adults	Half of the dosage recommended for younger adults
Increases in doses	Wait 2–4 weeks before increasing a low dosage if there is little or no response, and 3–5 weeks if there is a partial response	Aim for "an average dose" within one month if the medication is well tolerated. In the absence of improvement after at least 2 weeks on "an average dose", increase dosage gradually (up to maximum recommended dosage) until clinical improvement or limiting side effects are observed
When to change treatment	After 3–6 weeks at a "therapeutic" or the maximum tolerated dose" if there is little or no response; after 4–7 weeks if there is a partial response	After at least 4 weeks at the maximum tolerated or recommended dosage if there is no or minimal response; after 4–8 weeks if there is some partial response
What to do in case of minimal or no response to initial antidepressant	Preferred option: switch to venlafaxine or bupropion. Alternative option: switch to nortriptyline, mirtazapine, or another SSRI	Consider "all reasonable treatment options" including ECT, combination of antidepressants or mood stabilizers, addition of psychotherapy
What to do in case of partial response to initial antidepressant	Combine or augment initial antidepressant with another agent	Switch to another antidepressant of the same or another class while considering the risk of losing the improvements made with the first treatment
Agents to consider for combination or augmentation	Bupropion, lithium, or nortriptyline	Mirtazapine, bupropion, or lithium

SSRI = selective serotonin reuptake inhibitor; ECT: electroconvulsive therapy
Adapted from Mulsant et al., 2014 with permission from Elsevier.

The issue of whether one should continue to use citalopram in older patients in view of the QTc warnings from the US FDA and Health Canada (see section 3.5) is an important one. Experts agree that we should avoid starting it in older patients. However, they would not automatically discontinue or decrease it in an older patient who has done well on it and is tolerating it (i.e., the electrocardiogram [ECG] shows a normal QTc). This becomes a medico-legal issue: the patient (or substitute decision maker [SDM]) should be informed of the risks of continuing citalopram (i.e., a low risk of sudden death) versus discontinuing it and switching to another antidepressant (i.e., a risk of recurrence of depression that could be severe and not respond to another antidepressant).

A related but different issue exists for escitalopram: while Health Canada urges caution when using it in older patients, the US FDA does not, concluding that the risk of QTc prolongation is solely due to R-citalopram.

4.1.2 Augmentation vs Switching?

There is evidence supporting the efficacy of either a switching strategy or an augmenting strategy in older adults who have failed to respond to first-line antidepressants (Cooper et al., 2011; Lenze et al., 2015). However, the switching strategy may be safer in older patients. For example, in one study comparing the tolerability and safety of augmenting/ combining vs switching antidepressants, the discontinuation rates due to adverse events were 51% with augmentation vs 8% with switching. The rates of falls were 42% with augmentation vs 24% with switching (Joo et al, 2002). Thus, guidelines (see Table 2.3.1) favour switching to augmenting unless patients have a partial response that they want to preserve while aiming for a full remission (a partial response would correspond to a relative decrease of at least 20% or 30% on a depression scale after 4 to 6 weeks of treatment with a therapeutic dosage of an antidepressant).

Psychosocial interventions can also be used to augment antidepressant pharmacotherapy. In older persons, interpersonal psychotherapy (IPT) is an attractive option given its focus on role transition and grief/losses (Reynolds et al., 2010). Problem-solving therapy (PST) also makes a lot of sense when treating older depressed patients who appear to be "stuck."

4.1.3 When Should One Do a Treatment Change?

Some studies suggest that older patients respond more slowly than younger patients, but these studies are not direct comparisons of patients in both age groups treated with the same drugs, using the same titration, and the same target dosage. There are very few studies in which younger and older patients are treated using the same treatment protocol. In these few studies, older and younger patients respond similarly (same rates of response, same time to response). Still, most physicians (and most studies) titrate antidepressant medications more slowly in older patients. This practice may be the reason why these older patients take a longer time to respond.

Comorbid physical disorders or anxiety may also require slower titration of antidepressants, also explaining some of the slower rates of response observed in these patients (Andreescu et al., 2007). Severe depression is harder to treat, but it is not clear that it takes a longer time to respond when it responds to treatment.

Data from studies in younger patients suggest that, in the absence of any improvement (or with minimal improvement), one should switch after as early as 2 weeks. However, in older patients, the data support that one should switch in the absence of response or with minimal response (corresponding to a relative decrease of less than 20% on a depression scale) after 4–5 weeks of treatment with a therapeutic dose of an antidepressant. The likelihood of full response within 5 to 6 weeks of a switch is about 40–50% vs the likelihood of full response if one continues the initial antidepressant for another 5 to 6 weeks (i.e., for a full 10–12 week trial), which is only 20–30% (Mulsant et al., 2006).

4.1.4 Do Not Give Up!

In older patients who appear not to be responding to pharmacotherapy, if one keeps trying after one year of treatment (3 to 6 different steps), the overall response rate for those who do not give up is around 90% (Kok, Nolen, & Heeren, 2009; Whyte et al., 2004). Unfortunately, after a couple of failed trials, many patients get discouraged and give up;

many physicians also get discouraged and stop trying. When older patients are not responding to a first-line intervention, it is very important to inform them that their depression is harder to treat than the typical depression (Tew et al., 2006), but that it is almost certain they will get better if they don't give up and if "we" (patient and clinician working as a team) keep trying. This type of information, support, and encouragement may be lifesaving: it may make the difference between a patient giving up and killing him- or herself and a patient recovering.

4.1.5 How Long Should Older Adults Take Their Antidepressant?

There is a paucity of continuation and maintenance studies in older patients who have responded acutely to an antidepressant and even fewer long-term maintenance studies (Kok, Heeren, & Nolen, 2011; Wilkinson & Izmeth, 2012). The benefits of long-term ("maintenance") antidepressant have been shown in randomized controlled trials for up to three years in older patients presenting with a recurrent depression (i.e., in those who have experienced several episodes of depression) and for two years in those presenting with a single depression (i.e., older patients experiencing their first episode of depression) (Kok, Heeren, & Nolen, 2011; Reynolds et al., 2006). If an older patient is in remission, is tolerating his or her antidepressant (i.e., experiencing no or minimal side effects), and is willing to stay on it, he or she should be encouraged to stay on it "forever." When older patients want to stop their antidepressant and the clinician is unable to convince them not to do so, they should be supported, the antidepressant dosage should be tapered down slowly (e.g., over at least 2 to 3 months, avoiding the winter or the anniversary of the death of a loved one), and the patient should be followed frequently.

4.2 What Is New since 2006?

- Is there a special role for newer antidepressants?
  - Escitalopram – no (Bose, Li, & Gandi, 2008; Kasper, de Swart, & Friis Andersen, 2005)
  - Desvenlafaxine – unknown (no relevant geriatric data)
  - Duloxetine – probably (Katona, Hanson, & Olsen, 2012; Raskin et al., 2007; Robinson et al., 2014)
  - Vortioxetine – maybe (Katona, Hanson, & Olsen, 2012)
  - Levomilnacipran – unknown (no relevant geriatric data)
  - Vilazodone – unknown (no relevant geriatric data)
- Is there a role in the treatment of geriatric (unipolar non-psychotic) depression for some atypical antipsychotics?
  - Quetiapine XR – maybe (Katila et al., 2013)
  - Aripiprazole – probably (Lenze et al., 2015 ; Sheffrin et al., 2009; Steffens et al., 2011)
  - Lurasidone – unknown (no relevant data)

4.3 A Comment on Electroconvulsive Therapy in Late-Life Depression

- Age is not a predictor of response/remission (Tew et al., 1999).
- Non-response to ECT predicted by:
  - Prior resistance to pharmacotherapy
  - Chronicity of episode (2 years or longer) (Dombrovski et al., 2005)

When clinicians are considering ECT because of a lack of response to several pharmacologic trials, clinicians should not wait more than 18 months before recommending ECT.

5. Conclusions

Late-life depression:
- Can be effectively treated
- Requires a systematic approach
- Success requires persistence
- Do not give up!

QUESTIONS

1. List two SSRIs and an SNRI that have been shown to be more efficacious than placebo in the acute treatment of older patients with major depressive disorder.
2. List one SSRI that has been associated with prolongation of the corrected QT (QTc) interval in at a recent (2014) placebo-controlled trial involving older patients.
3. List five safety concerns raised by the use of antidepressants in older persons.
4. List three possible pharmacologic strategies to manage an older depressed person who has failed to respond to a first-line antidepressant.
5. List two factors that have been associated with longer times to response or lower response rates when treating late-life depression pharmacologically.
6. Discuss some of the care issues associated with poor or incomplete response to pharmacotherapy in late-life depression.
7. Describe the advantages and disadvantages of switching vs augmenting antidepressants when an older patient has failed to improve sufficiently with a first-line antidepressant.

ANSWERS

1. Four SSRIs and one SNRI have been shown to be more efficacious than placebo in the acute treatment of older patients with major depressive disorder:
   - Sertraline
   - Fluoxetine
   - Paroxetine
   - Vortioxetine
   - Duloxetine

   This was a trick question! Many clinicians are surprised to hear that placebo-controlled trials do not favour the use of citalopram and escitalopram in older depressed patients, because the US 2001 guidelines and Canadian 2006 guidelines recommended citalopram as a first-line antidepressant for geriatric patients and experts are now recommending escitalopram. This is a reminder that expert opinion is informed by evidence but it is not necessarily evidence based. Results from one placebo-controlled trial of citalopram in the *acute* treatment of older patients with major depressive disorder (MDD) and two of escitalopram have been published. The findings from these three trials show no difference in efficacy between placebo and the active antidepressant.

   By contrast, both citalopram and escitalopram have one (of one) positive published placebo-controlled continuation/maintenance trial in older patients with MDD. However, it is easier to establish the superiority of an antidepressant over placebo in a continuation/maintenance treatment trial than in an acute treatment trial. More than half of placebo-controlled acute trials in younger and older adults with MDD fail, while there are almost no failed continuation/maintenance placebo-controlled antidepressant trials. This makes sense clinically: once a patient has responded to a medication, he or she is at high risk of relapse/recurrence if the medication is withdrawn.

2. Citalopram is the SSRI that has been associated with prolongation of the QTc interval in a recent (2014) placebo-controlled trial involving older patients with dementia (Drye et al., 2014).

3. Safety concerns raised by the use of antidepressants in older persons include:

- Drug-drug interactions
- Hyponatremia (usually asymptomatic and transient but it can be severe) due to syndrome of inappropriate antidiuretic hormone secretion (SIADH)
- Falls
- Hip fractures
- Gastrointestinal bleeding
- Cardiovascular effects (QTc prolongation) that can lead to death
- Cognitive impairment
- Worsening of suicidality (at initiation of antidepressant)
- Increase in bone metabolism leading to osteoporosis
- Increased blood pressure
- Orthostatic hypotension
- Blurred vision
- Sedation
- Serotonin syndrome

4. Possible pharmacologic strategies to manage an older depressed person who has failed to respond to a first-line SSRI antidepressant include:

- Optimizing dosage and duration (i.e., ensuring an adequate trial)
- Checking for proper adherence
- Switching to another SSRI (e.g., sertraline, escitalopram)
- Switching to an SNRI (e.g., venlafaxine, duloxetine)
- Switching to an antidepressant from another class (e.g., bupropion, mirtazapine)
- Switching to a tricyclic antidepressant (TCA; e.g., nortriptyline) or to quetiapine
- Augmenting with bupropion, lithium, or nortriptyline
- Augmenting with an atypical antipsychotic (e.g., aripiprazole, quetiapine)

5. Factors that have been associated with longer times to response or lower response rates when treating late-life depression pharmacologically include:

- Inadequate dose or duration of treatment
- Poor adherence
- Duration of depressive episode
- Severity of depressive episode
- Serotonin transporter genotype
- Failure to respond to previous antidepressant
- Comorbid anxiety
- Comorbid substance misuse
- Comorbid physical illness/frailty
- Executive dysfunction

6. Some care issues associated with poor or incomplete response to pharmacotherapy in late-life depression include:

- Not following a systematic approach, including selecting a medication associated with adverse effects and low adherence

- Keeping the medication dosage too low
- Changing medication too early or too late
- Giving up

7. This table summarizes the advantages and disadvantages of switching vs augmenting antidepressants when an older patient has failed to improve sufficiently with a first-line antidepressant.

	Advantages	**Disadvantages**
Switching	• Avoids polypharmacy and associated DDI, adverse effects, and costs • Better adherence	• Potential loss of partial response in patients who appeared not to respond to first antidepressant • Risk of adverse effects and delays associated with discontinuation • Titration of new antidepressant may take a long time, resulting in further delays
Augmenting	• Preserves partial response • Avoids adverse effects and delays associated with discontinuation	• Polypharmacy and associated DDI, adverse effects, and costs • Greater potential for non-adherence

DDI = drug-drug interaction

CASE DISCUSSION

1. As an approach to this situation, take the following steps:
   - Review the differential diagnosis: possibilities include major depressive disorder, dementia, and mood disorder due to a general medical condition (e.g., hypothyroidism, low B12, sleep apnea) or a substance-induced mood disorder (e.g., in the context of alcohol or opioid dependence).
   - Assess adherence to treatment.
   - Determine if suicidal thoughts are present, and address them if they are.
   - Consider non-pharmacological measures (e.g., exercise, sleep hygiene, socialization, psychotherapy, or other psychosocial interventions).

2. Next steps would include:
   - Review clinical factors that may be associated with a delay in response (e.g., comorbid anxiety).
   - Wait for 2 to 4 more weeks to see whether the patient responds (4 weeks is relatively short).
   - Consider an increase in dosage (e.g., to 100 mg/day).

3. Regarding continuing or stopping her antidepressant once she remits, consider the following:
   - The best evidence suggests that people who experience a major depressive episode in late life that remits with antidepressant treatment are protected against

relapses and recurrences if they continue their antidepressant at the dose to which they responded.

- While studies have shown benefits of long-term (maintenance) treatment for two to three years, experts recommend lifelong treatment (i.e., as long as it is tolerated).

RECOMMENDED RESOURCES FOR REVIEW

Although these resources may not be specifically cited in the text, their approach informed the contents of the chapter, and they are recommended as useful further reading.

Cooper C, Katona C, Lyketsos K, et al. A systematic review of treatments for refractory depression in older people. Am J Psychiatry. 2011;168(7):681–8. http://dx.doi.org/10.1176/appi.ajp.2011.10081165. Medline:21454919

Kok RM, Heeren TJ, Nolen WA. Continuing treatment of depression in the elderly: a systematic review and meta-analysis of double-blinded randomized controlled trials with antidepressants. Am J Geriatr Psychiatry. 2011;19(3):249–55. http://dx.doi.org/10.1097/JGP.0b013e3181ec8085. Medline:21425505

Kok RM, Nolen WA, Heeren TJ. Efficacy of treatment in older depressed patients: a systematic review and meta-analysis of double-blind randomized controlled trials with antidepressants. J Affect Disord. 2012;141(2–3):103–15. http://dx.doi.org/10.1016/j.jad.2012.02.036. Medline:22480823

Mulsant BH, Blumberger DM, Ismail Z, et al. A systematic approach to pharmacotherapy for geriatric major depression. Clin Geriatr Med. 2014;30(3):517–34. http://dx.doi.org/10.1016/j.cger.2014.05.002. Medline:25037293

REFERENCES

Alexopoulos GS, Katz IR, Bruce ML, et al. Remission in depressed geriatric primary care patients: a report from the PROSPECT study. Am J Psychiatry. 2005;162(4):718–24. Medline:15800144

Alexopoulos GS, Katz IR, Reynolds CF, et al. Pharmacotherapy of depression in older patients: a summary of the expert consensus guidelines. J Psychiatr Pract. 2001;7(6):361–76.

Alexopoulos GS, Reynolds CF, Bruce ML, et al. Reducing suicidal ideation and depression in older primary care patients: 24-month outcomes of the PROSPECT study. Am J Psychiatry. 2009;166(8):882–90. http://dx.doi.org/10.1176/appi.ajp.2009.08121779. Medline:19528195

Andreescu C, Lenze EJ, Dew MA, et al. Effect of comorbid anxiety on treatment response and relapse risk in late-life depression: controlled study. Br J Psychiatry. 2007;190(4):344–9. Medline:17401042

Baldwin RC, Chiu E, Katona C, et al. Guidelines on depression in older people: practicing the evidence. London: Martin Dunitz; 2002.

Bose A, Li D, Gandhi C. Escitalopram in the acute treatment of depressed patients aged 60 years or older. Am J Geriatr Psychiatry. 2008;16(1):14–20. http://dx.doi.org/10.1097/JGP.0b013e3181591c09. Medline:18165459

Bruce ML, Ten Have TR, Reynolds CF, et al. Reducing suicidal ideation and depressive symptoms in depressed older primary care patients: a randomized controlled trial. JAMA. 2004;291(9):1081–91. Medline:14996777

Buchanan D, Tourigny-Rivard MF, Cappeliez P, et al. National guidelines for seniors' mental health: the assessment and treatment of depression. Can J Geriatr. 2006;9(Suppl 2):S52–8.

Canadian Coalition for Seniors' Mental Health (CCSMH). National guidelines for seniors' mental health: the assessment and treatment of depression. Toronto: CCSMH; 2006. http://www.ccsmh.ca/en/projects/depression.cfm

Dombrovski AY, Mulsant BH, Haskett RF, et al. Predictors of remission after electroconvulsive therapy in unipolar major depression. J Clin Psychiatry. 2005;66(8):1043–9. Medline:16086621

Drye LT, Spragg D, Devanand DP, et al.; CitAD Research Group. Changes in QTc interval in the citalopram for agitation in Alzheimer's disease (CitAD) randomized trial. PLoS One. 2014;9(6):e98426. http://dx.doi.org/10.1371/journal.pone.0098426. Medline:24914549

Gebara MA, Shea ML, Lipsey KL, et al. Depression, antidepressants, and bone health in older adults: a systematic review. J Am Geriatr Soc. 2014;62(8):1434–41. http://dx.doi.org/10.1111/jgs.12945. Medline:25039259

Health Canada. Celexa (citalopram): association with abnormal heart rhythms – for health professionals. 25 January 2012. Accessed 28 May 2016. http://www.healthycanadians.gc.ca/recall-alert-rappel-avis/hc-sc/2012/14672a-eng.php

– Antidepressant Cipralex (escitalopram): updated information regarding dose-related heart risk. 7 May 2012. Accessed 28 May 2016. http://www.healthycanadians.gc.ca/recall-alert-rappel-avis/hc-sc/2012/13674a-eng.php

Fabian TJ, Amico JA, Kroboth PD, et al. Paroxetine-induced hyponatremia in older adults: a 12-week prospective study. Arch Intern Med. 2004;164(3):327–32. http://dx.doi.org/10.1001/archinte.164.3.327. Medline:14769630

Johnson EM, Whyte E, Mulsant BH, et al. Cardiovascular changes associated with venlafaxine in the treatment of late-life depression. Am J Geriatr Psychiatry. 2006;14(9):796–802. Medline:16943176

Joo JH, Lenze EJ, Mulsant BH, et al. Risk factors for falls during treatment of late-life depression. J Clin Psychiatry. 2002;63(10): 936–41. Medline:12416604

Juurlink DN, Mamdani MM, Kopp A, et al. The risk of suicide with selective serotonin reuptake inhibitors in the elderly. Am J Psychiatry. 2006;163(5):813–21. Medline:16648321

Kasper S, de Swart H, Fiirs Andersen H. Escitalopram in the treatment of depressed elderly patients. Am J Geriatr Psychiatry. 2005;13(10):884–91. Medline:16223967

Katila H, Mezhebovsky I, Mulroy A, et al. Randomized, double-blind study of the efficacy and tolerability of extended release quetiapine fumarate (quetiapine XR) monotherapy in elderly patients with major depressive disorder. Am J Geriatr Psychiatry. 2013;21(8):769–84. http://dx.doi.org/10.1016/j.jagp .2013.01.010. Medline:23567397

Katona C, Hansen T, Olsen CK. A randomized, double-blind, placebo-controlled, duloxetine-referenced, fixed-dose study comparing the efficacy and safety of Lu AA21004 in elderly patients with major depressive disorder. Int Clin Psychopharmacol. 2012;27(4):215–23. http://dx.doi.org/10.1097/YIC.0b013e3283542457. Medline:22572889

Kok RM, Nolen WA, Heeren TJ. Outcome of late-life depression after 3 years of sequential treatment. Acta Psychiatr Scand. 2009;119(4):274–81. http://dx.doi.org/10.1111/j.1600-0447.2008.01295.x. Medline:19053970

Lenze EJ, Mulsant BH, Blumberger DM, et al. Efficacy, safety, and tolerability of augmentation pharmacotherapy with aripiprazole for treatment-resistant depression in late life: a randomised, double-blind, placebo-controlled trial. Lancet. 2015;386(10011):2404–12. http://dx.doi.org/10.1016/S0140-6736(15)00308-6. Medline:26423182

Meyers BS, Sirey JA, Bruce M, et al. Predictors of early recovery from major depression among persons admitted to community-based clinics: an observational study. Arch Gen Psychiatry. 2002;59(8):729–35. Medline:12150649

Mottram, P., Wilson, K., Strobl, J. Antidepressants for depressed elderly. Cochrane Database Syst Rev. 2006;(1):CD003491. Medline:16437456

Mulsant BH, Houck PR, Gildengers AG, et al. What is the optimal duration of a short-term antidepressant trial when treating geriatric depression? J Clin Psychopharmacol. 2006;26(2):113–20. Medline:16633138

Mulsant BH, Pollock BG. Psychopharmacology. In: Blazer DG, Steffens DC, Thakur ME (editors). The American psychiatric publishing textbook of geriatric psychiatry. 5th ed. Arlington, VA: American Psychiatric Publishing; 2015. p. 527–87.

Pinquart M, Duberstein PR, Lyness JM. Treatments for later-life depressive conditions: a meta-analytic comparison of pharmacotherapy and psychotherapy. Am J Psychiatry. 2006;163(9):1493–501. Medline:16946172

Raskin J, Wiltse CG, Siegal A, et al. Efficacy of duloxetine on cognition, depression, and pain in elderly patients with major depressive disorder: an 8-week, double-blind, placebo-controlled trial. Am J Psychiatry. 2007;164(6):900–9. Medline:17541049

Reynolds CF, Dew MA, Martire LM, et al. Treating depression to remission in older adults: a controlled evaluation of combined escitalopram with interpersonal psychotherapy versus escitalopram with depression care management. Int J Geriatr Psychiatry. 2010;25(11):1134–41. http://dx.doi.org/10.1002/gps.2443. Medline:20957693

Reynolds CF, Dew MA, Pollock BG, et al. Maintenance treatment of major depression in old age. N Engl J Med. 2006;354(11):1130–8. http://dx.doi.org/10.1056/NEJMoa052619. Medline:16540613

Robinson M, Oakes TM, Raskin J, et al. Acute and long-term treatment of late-life major depressive disorder: duloxetine versus placebo. Am J Geriatr Psychiatry. 2014;22(1):34–45. http://dx.doi.org/10.1016/j.jagp .2013.01.019. Medline:24314888

Roose SP, Sackeim HA, Krishnan KR, et al.; Old-Old Depression Study Group. Antidepressant pharmacotherapy in the treatment of depression in the very old: a randomized, placebo-controlled trial. Am J Psychiatry. 2004;161(11):2050–9. http://dx.doi.org/10.1176/appi.ajp.161.11.2050. Medline:15514406

Schatzberg A, Roose S. A double-blind, placebo-controlled study of venlafaxine and fluoxetine in geriatric outpatients with major depression. Am J Geriatr Psychiatry. 2006;14(4):361–70. Medline:16582045

Shea ML, Garfield LD, Teitelbaum S, et al. Serotonin-norepinephrine reuptake inhibitor therapy in late-life depression is associated with increased marker of bone resorption. Osteoporos Int. 2013;24(5):1741–9. http://dx.doi.org/10.1007/s00198-012-2170-z. Medline:23358607

Sheffrin M, Driscoll HC, Lenze EJ, et al. Pilot study of augmentation with aripiprazole for incomplete response in late-life depression: getting to remission. J Clin Psychiatry. 2009;70(2):208–13. Medline:19210951

Steffens DC, Nelson JC, Eudicone JM, et al. Efficacy and safety of adjunctive aripiprazole in major depressive disorder in older patients: a pooled subpopulation analysis. Int J Geriatr Psychiatry. 2011;26(6):564–72. http://dx.doi.org/10.1002/gps.2564. Medline:20827794

Tew JD, Mulsant BH, Haskett RF, et al. Acute efficacy of ECT in the treatment of major depression in the old-old. Am J Psychiatry. 1999;156(12):1865–70. Medline:10588398

Tew JD, Mulsant BH, Houck PR, et al. Impact of prior treatment exposure on response to antidepressant treatment in late life. Am J Geriatr Psychiatry. 2006;14(11):957–65. Medline:17068318

Unützer J, Katon W, Callahan CM, et al. Collaborative care management of late-life depression in the primary care setting: a randomized controlled trial. JAMA. 2002;288(22):2836–45. Medline:12472325

US Food and Drug Administration. [Internet]. FDA drug safety communication: revised recommendations for Celexa (citalopram hydrobromide) related to a potential risk of abnormal heart rhythms with high doses. 24 August 2001. Accessed 28 May 2016. http://www.fda.gov/Drugs/DrugSafety/ucm297391.htm

Whyte EM, Basinski J, Frahi P, et al. Geriatric depression treatment in nonresponders to selective serotonin reuptake inhibitors. J Clin Psychiatry. 2004;65(12):1634–41. Medline:15641868

Wilkinson P, Izmeth Z. Continuation and maintenance treatments for depression in older people. Cochrane Database Syst Rev. 2012;11:CD006727. http://dx.doi:10.1002/14651858.CD006727.pub2

Yuan Y, Tsoi K, Hunt RH. Selective serotonin reuptake inhibitors and risk of upper GI bleeding: confusion or confounding? Am J Med. 2006;119(9):719–27. Medline:16945603

2.4 Bipolar Disorder in Older Adults

Kenneth Shulman, MD, FRCPC

INTRODUCTION

Bipolar disorder is a complex and challenging serious mental illness in younger adults, and with advanced age come additional considerations for geriatric psychiatrists. In this chapter Dr Shulman provides an overview of the epidemiology of bipolar disorder and how its presentation and epidemiology can differ in older adults when compared to younger adults. Some of the medical considerations that may influence the course of bipolar disorder or influence treatment are then reviewed.

CASE SCENARIO

An 84-year-old man has a history of bipolar II disorder and vascular disease. He was stable on maintenance lithium 450 mg QHS (0.8 mmol/L) for several years. Because of concerns about subtle cognitive changes and increased serum creatinine with decreased estimated glomerular filtration rate (eGFR), the patient decided to discontinue lithium, at the encouragement of his nephrologist. The patient refused other maintenance medications and then became mildly hypomanic for two years, with two brief mild depressive phases followed by a severe major depression.

1. What treatment options should a clinician now consider?
2. What are the risks and benefits the clinician must balance?
3. What other factors should be taken into account in ongoing management?

OVERVIEW

1. Bipolar Disorder in Older Adults: Unique Features

1.1 Epidemiology in Old Age
(Depp & Jeste, 2004; Kessler et al., 2005; Moorhead & Young, 2003; Leboyer et al., 2005)

- Lower prevalence in old age (1/3 of younger persons with bipolar disorder)
- Late onset (> 50) (5–10% of all bipolars)
- 6% of geriatric psychiatry outpatient visits
- 8–10% of geriatric psychiatry – inpatients
- 70% females

2. Clinical Features
(Sajatovic & Kessing, 2010; Tsai et al., 2002)

- Clinical presentation similar to mixed age samples
- Course of illness may be more heterogeneous
- Reduced risk of suicide vs young bipolars

3. Medical Comorbidities
(Gildengers et al., 2008)

- Cardiovascular + cerebrovascular
- Hypertension
- Diabetes and obesity
- Hyperlipidemia
- Atopic diseases (allergic rhinitis and asthma)

3.1 Cerebrovascular Risk and Bipolarity
(Subramaniam, Dennis, & Byrne, 2007; Cassidy & Carroll, 2002)

- Framingham Stroke Risk Score
- Higher in late-onset older bipolars
- Increased risk of stroke
- Lesions in right orbito-frontal cortex

3.2 Neuroimaging Correlates in Late Life
(Fujikawa, Yamawaki, & Touhouda, 1995; Beyer et al., 2004)

- Reduction of grey matter (late onset > early onset)
- Increase in deep white matter hyperintensities (DWMH) (cerebrovascular disease)
- Reduced size of caudate
- Silent cerebral infarctions (covert strokes)

4. Cognition and Bipolar Disorder (Euthymic State)
(Delaloye et al., 2009; Schouws et al., 2012; Martino, Strejilevich, & Manes, 2013)

- Late-onset bipolar disorder (> 50) – a distinct subtype
- Worsened cognition (executive dysfunction)
- Less genetic load
- Medical comorbidity (vascular risk factors)
- Is lifelong bipolar disorder neuroprogressive? – mixed evidence
- Is late-onset bipolar disorder a distinct subtype? – robust evidence

4.1 Cognition, Executive Function, and Bipolar Disorder
(Gildengers et al., 2013)

- Worsened response inhibition
- Worsened set shifting
- Worsened attention

- Increased disability
- No progression at 2 year follow-up

4.2 Neuroprogression in Bipolar Disorder
(Berk et al., 2011)

- Progression, acceleration, refractoriness
- ↑ dopamine ↑ glutamate
- Mitochondrial dysfunction → oxidative stress
- Reduced neurotrophins (brain-derived neurotrophic factor [BDNF])
- ↑ inflammation (C-reactive protein, interleukin 1B, tumour necrosis factor)
- Targets for mood stabilizers

4.3 Oxidative Stress + Mitochondrial Dysfunction
(Berk et al., 2011)

- ↑ pro-oxidants: anti-oxidants
- ↑ reactive oxygen species
- Damage to DNA, proteins
- Cognitive decline (aging)

5. Other Determinants of Mania in Older Adults

- Affective vulnerability
- Aging
- Heterogeneous cerebral pathology
- Lesion localization

6. Summary of Mania in Older Adults: Special Features
(Shulman et al., 1992)

- Late age of onset
- Neurologic comorbidity
- Medical comorbidity
- Cognitive impairment
- Increased mortality

7. Pharmacotherapy of Bipolar Disorder in Older Adults: A Focus on Lithium and Other Mood Stabilizers

7.1 Evidence-Based Treatment Guidelines
(Young, 2005)

- Lithium remains a first-line treatment (American Psychiatric Association [2002]; British Association for Pharmacology [Goodwin & Young, 2003]; Texas Medication Algorithm Project [Suppes et al., 2005]; Canadian Network for Mood and Anxiety Treatments [CANMAT; Yatham et al., 2006])
- No randomized controlled trials in old age: GERI-BD study results (lithium better than valproate – unpublished)

7.2 Other Mood Stabilizers in Older Adults

7.2.1 Acute Manic or Mixed States (Sajatovic et al., 2008)

- Monotherapy with lithium, quetiapine, or divalproex
- Combination for partial responders

7.2.2 Acute Bipolar Depression (Sajatovic et al., 2011)

- Lithium or quetiapine
- Add lamotrigine for partial responders
- Cautious use of antidepressants (SSRIs)
- Electroconvulsive therapy (ECT) for refractory depression or acute safety concerns

7.2.3 Maintenance Treatment

Secondary analyses, extrapolation from mixed age samples
- Lithium
- Divalproex
- Lamotrigine

8. Psychological Modalities

- Cognitive behavioural therapy (CBT), interpersonal psychotherapy (IPT), family-focused therapy (FFT), psychoeducation, psychosocial

9. Special Considerations for Lithium Carbonate in Older Adults
(Shulman, 2010)

- Altered pharmacokinetics/dynamics
- Therapeutic range (geriatric levels 0.3–0.8)
- Renal effects
- Drug interactions
- Toxicity/delirium
- Hypothyroidism
- Hyperparathyroidism
- Parkinsonism

9.1 Lithium and Renal Effects
(Rej, Herrmann, & Shulman, 2012)

- Nephrogenic diabetes insipidus (NDI)
- Acute renal failure
- Chronic renal failure

9.1.1 Lithium and NDI in Older Adults

- 1.8–85%
- Age, Li^+ duration, Li^+ level $\propto$ urine osmolality
- Not clinically significant

9.1.2 Acute Renal Failure in Older Adults Using Long-Term Lithium

- 10% decline in renal function per decade after age 40
- Lithium toxicity → acute renal failure (1.5%/year)
- $Li^+ > 1.5 = 5.4/100\ 000$/person year
- Few deaths

9.1.3 Chronic Renal Failure and Lithium in Chronic Users

- Prevalence (1.2–34%)
- Creatinine > 150 mmol/l (1.2%)
- End stage renal disease (0.5%)

9.1.4 Chronic Renal Failure and Lithium: Clinical Correlates

- Age > 70
- Li^+ level, duration
- Prior lithium intoxication
- Medical comorbidities (vascular)
- Relationship with lithium still unclear

9.1.5 Hospitalization for Lithium Toxicity and Use of Other Medications
(Juurlink et al., 2004)

- RR (95% CI) for thiazides 1.8 (1.0–3.3)
- RR (95% CI) for loop diuretics 3.4 (2.3–5.0)
- RR (95% CI) for angiotensin-converting enzyme (ACE) inhibitors 2.5 (1.8–3.5)
- RR (95% CI) for non-steroidal anti-inflammatory drugs (NSAIDs) 1.4 (1.0–1.9)

9.2 Incidence of Delirium with New Users of Lithium or Divalproex (Older Adults)
(Shulman et al., 2005b)

- Lithium no worse than divalproex
- HR for lithium 1.00 as reference drug vs HR for divalproex 1.36 (0.94–1.97)

9.3 Kaplan–Meier Curves Time to Thyroxine Treatment as Proxy for Hypothyroidism
(Shulman et al., 2005a)

- Thyroid replacement needed in 6% of lithium-treated older adults (twice general population)

9.4 Calcium and Parathyroid Levels (Meta-Analysis) Lithium vs Controls
(McKnight et al., 2012; Szalat, Mazeh, & Freund, 2009)

- ↑ calcium
- ↑ parathyroid hormone (PTH)
- ↑ 1° hyperparathyroidism (10% vs 0.1%)

9.5 Lithium and Parkinsonism

- Tremor is common
- Inappropriate Rx with dopaminergic drugs?
- Prescribing cascade if lithium effect is not recognized
- Pharmacoepidemiology as a research approach

10. Lithium and Neuroprotection: Glycogen Synthase Kinase (GSK)
(Tajes et al., 2008)

- Lithium - ↓GSK 3
- ↓GSK 3 - ↓β amyloid ↓tangles
- ↓GSK 3 -↓cell apoptosis

10.1 Bipolar Disorder, Lithium, and Neuroprotection vs Other Mood Stabilizers
(Hajek et al., 2012)

- Increased total grey matter
- Increased hippocampal volume
- ↓ white matter microstructural abnormalities
- Rate of dementia related to number of lithium prescriptions – protective effect of having prescriptions for lithium (HR < 1.0) (Kessing et al., 2008)

Disease modifying for amnestic mild cognitive impairment (MCI) (Forlenza et al., 2011)

10.2 Bipolar Disorder and Dementia

- Risk of dementia on re-admission (Kessing & Nilsson, 2003; Kessing et al., 2008; Kessing, Forman, & Andersen, 2010)
- Greatest for depression
- Mania risk for dementia may be mitigated by lithium use

11. BALANCE Study: Relapse Prevention Bipolar I
(The BALANCE Investigators and Collaborators, 2010)

- Randomized, open-label, 3 groups (valproate, lithium, combination)
- Up to 24 months follow-up
- Mean age 43
- 1° outcome – new intervention for emergent mood disorder
- Findings:
    - Lithium + valproate better than valproate
    - Lithium better than valproate

12. Risk of Psychiatric Admission: Valproate vs Lithium
(Kessing et al., 2011)

- The rate of hospital admissions was significantly increased for valproate as compared to lithium (HR of 1.33, 95% CI 1.18–1.48).

13. Increased Risk of Suicide Attempts and Death: Divalproex vs Lithium
(Goodwin et al., 2003)

Divalproex vs lithium
- RR (95%CI) for suicide attempts in emergency room 1.8 (1.4–2.2)
- RR (95%CI) for suicide attempts with hospitalization 1.7 (1.2–2.3)
- RR (95%CI) for suicide deaths 2.7 (1.1–6.3)

14. Old Age: Psychiatrists' Preferences
(Ephraim & Prettyman, 2009)

For acute mania – lithium 35.1% and valproate 28.2%
For prophylaxis – lithium 69.7% and valproate 13.3%

15. Trends in Lithium Use

Decreasing use of lithium and increased use of divalproex without adequate evidence throughout the 1990s and early 2000s (Shulman et al., 2003)
- Prevalence of lithium prescriptions increases from < 1/1000 in young adults to 4/1000 in the 65+ age group, but incidence of lithium prescriptions dramatically decrease in older adults (Bramness, Weitoft, & Hallas, 2009).

16. Summary of Evidence for Lithium in Older Adults
(Shulman, 2010)

- Good evidence for effectiveness of lithium
- Concerns regarding lithium treatment in older adults (toxicity, renal, thyroid, calcium, Parkinsonism)
- Need for geriatric-specific lithium levels (e.g., 0.3–0.8)?
- Dramatic change in prescription patterns without evidence
- Evidence for neuroprotection?

QUESTIONS

1. List five risk factors for mania in old age.
2. Describe a medical approach to the assessment of late-onset mania.
3. What is the role of neuroimaging in late-life bipolar disorder?
4. Describe the risks and benefits of lithium therapy in old age.
5. What is the role and significance of cognitive dysfunction in late-life bipolar disorder?
6. How is late-life mania a paradigm for a neuropsychiatric disorder?
7. Why might there be few early-onset bipolar patients in late life?

ANSWERS

1. Risk factors for mania in old age include:
   - Family history of mood disorder in first-degree relatives
   - Previous affective episodes (mania and/or depression) and/or affective vulnerability
   - Central nervous system (CNS) disorders, especially cerebrovascular disease affecting the right orbital frontal cortex
   - History of substance abuse

- Significant vascular risk factors, including diabetes
- Other brain lesions (e.g., traumatic brain injury [TBI], tumours)

2. In developing an approach to assessment of late-onset mania, consider:
   - Overall goals are to rule out secondary mood disorders (e.g., those due to general medical condition or to substances) and delirium
   - Thorough history: cardiovascular risk factors, history of cerebrovascular disease or other medical conditions that may influence selection of therapies, complete medication history, family psychiatric history
   - Obtain collateral history whenever possible
   - Thorough physical examination with a focus on the neurological examination
   - Cognitive screening test
   - Neuroimaging if there is a history of head injury or localizing signs of a cerebrovascular event, or if there is minimal family history of mood disorder
   - Lab investigations, including haematology, thyroid function, blood sugar, renal function, calcium, liver function, B12, and folate
   - Review of medications, especially recent changes (e.g., steroids, thyroxine, dopaminergic agents, antidepressants, β-2 agonists)

3. Regarding the role of neuroimaging in late-life bipolar disorder:
   - Identify possible underlying brain lesions that may have precipitated mania and may also be treatable or surgically correctable.
   - Identify the extent of cerebrovascular disease, including silent cerebral infarctions (may highlight the need for more aggressive treatment of vascular risk factors).
   - Establish a baseline for longitudinal follow-up.
   - Neuroimaging is more important in late-onset cases and sub-acute onset of mania.

4. The table below summarizes the risks and benefits of lithium in older adults with bipolar disorder.

Benefits	Risks
• One of the most effective mood stabilizers, recommended by all consensus guidelines and treatment algorithms	• Toxicity due to narrow therapeutic range; impaired renal function with age; drug interactions including commonly used drugs in old age (e.g., NSAID, diuretics [both loop and thiazide], ACE inhibitors)
• Potential for neuroprotection	• Hypothyroidism
• Inexpensive	• Hyperparathyroidism
• Reduces risk for suicide	• Possible renal damage (controversial)
• Decreased short-term mortality	• QT interval prolongation
• Treats all phases of bipolar disorder	• Need for careful monitoring
	• Increased sensitivity to neurological side effects due to increased permeability of the BBB
	• Diminished urine concentrating ability
	• Weight gain
	• Tremor
	• Possible skin/hair symptoms

ACE = angiotensin-converting enzyme; BBB = blood-brain barrier; NSAID = non-steroidal anti-inflammatory drug

5. Cognitive dysfunction is an important consideration in late-life bipolar disorder because:
   - Bipolarity is associated with frontal-executive dysfunction and language impairment, even in a euthymic state.
   - It may affect adherence.
   - It may reflect vascular CI and the need to address vascular risk factors.
   - Lithium treatment of bipolar disorder may be neuroprotective and prevent progression of dementia.
   - There is an increased risk of dementia in older adults with bipolar disorder.
   - Some medications used to treat bipolar disorder have adverse effects on cognition.

6. Late-life mania is a paradigm for a neuropsychiatric disorder in that:
   - It is a late-onset form of secondary mania associated with underlying brain pathology most commonly affecting the right orbital frontal cortex, often involving vascular lesions.
   - Late-life mania may be precipitated by CNS drugs such as steroids and dopaminergic agents.
   - It is associated with cognitive impairment.
   - Brain lesions or neurodegenerative changes may convert unipolar depression to bipolar disorder.
   - Multifactorial etiology includes genetics, developmental factors, and neurological lesions.

7. Potential reasons for fewer early-onset bipolar patients in late life include:
   - Increased mortality due to medical burden, including substance abuse
   - Increased mortality due to high-risk behaviours leading to accidental death
   - Increased mortality secondary to suicide
   - Burnout over time
   - In recent years we have seen better treatment for bipolar disorder and patients may have stabilized without recurrence.
   - Patient may have poor recall of earlier affective episodes.
   - Missed diagnosis
   - Patients with dementia may cease to have bipolar symptoms.

CASE DISCUSSION

1. Treatment options include:
   - Re-challenge with a lower dose of lithium and lower serum levels (0.4 to 0.6 mmol/L).
   - Consult with a nephrologist regarding renal function and monitor renal function carefully.
   - Consider alternative mood stabilizers such as lamotrigine.
   - Consider quetiapine monotherapy (but must balance against vascular risk factors).
   - Consider low dose of two mood stabilizers if necessary.
   - Consider ECT.
   - Clinician must balance the risk of mood instability against the side effects and toxicity associated with lithium therapy (see question #4).

- Balance risks associated with other mood stabilizers such as carbamazepine, lamotrigine, and atypical antipsychotic.
- Always consider the possible role of substance abuse.
- Consider psychotherapy/psychoeducation.
- Rule out other psychiatric comorbidities.
- Meet with caregiver(s) and family to increase adherence and permit rapid recognition of recurrence.
- Consider combination of mood stabilizer/atypical antipsychotic with a first-line antidepressant.

2. It will be important to balance:
- Benefits of treatment, including resolution of mood symptoms and improved quality of life (QOL)
- Risks of ongoing mood instability (e.g., cognitive impairment, morbidity, mortality, suicide)
- Risks of medications
  - Lithium (see question #4)
  - Quetiapine (metabolic side effects)

3. Other factors to consider in ongoing management include:
- Careful monitoring of serum lithium levels and renal function if lithium is restarted
- Monitoring for non-adherence, given lithium's narrow therapeutic range
- Suicide risk
- Ongoing cognitive impairment
- Kidney function
- Substance abuse
- Previous responses to other medications
- Suitability for ECT, and its acceptability for both patient and family

RECOMMENDED RESOURCES FOR REVIEW

Although these resources may not be specifically cited in the text, their approach informed the contents of the chapter, and they are recommended as useful further reading.

Forlenza OV, Diniz BS, Radanovic M, et al. Disease-modifying properties of long-term lithium treatment for amnestic mild cognitive impairment: randomized controlled trial. Br J Psychiatry. 2011;198(5):351–6. http://dx.doi.org/10.1192/bjp.bp.110.080044

Gildengers AG, Whyte EM, Drayer RA, et al. Medical burden in late-life bipolar and major depressive disorders. Am J Geriatr Psychiatry. 2008;16(3):194–200. http://dx.doi.org/10.1097/JGP.0b013e318157c5b1. Medline:18310550

Shulman KI. Lithium for older adults with bipolar disorder: should it still be considered a first-line agent? Drugs Aging. 2010;27(8):607–15. http://dx.doi.org/10.2165/11537700-000000000-00000. Medline:20658789

REFERENCES

American Psychiatric Association. Practice guidelines for the treatment of patients with bipolar disorder. Washington, DC: American Psychiatric Press; 2002.

BALANCE Investigators and Collaborators. Lithium plus valproate combination therapy versus monotherapy for relapse prevention in bipolar I disorder (BALANCE): a randomized open-label trial. Lancet. 2010;375(9712):385–95. http://dx.doi.org/10.1016/S0140-6736(09)61828-6. Medline:20092882

Berk M, Kapczinski F, Andreazza AC, et al. Pathways underlying neuroprogression in bipolar disorder: focus on inflammation, oxidative stress and neurotrophic factors. Neurosci Biobehav Rev. 2011;35(3):804–17. http://dx.doi.org/10.1016/j.neubiorev.2010.10.001. Medline:20934453

Beyer JL, Kuchibhatla M, Payne M, et al. Caudate volume measurement in older adults with bipolar disorder. Int J Geriatr Psychiatry. 2004;19(2):109–14. http://dx.doi.org/10.1002/gps.1030. Medline:14758576

Bramness JG, Weitoft GR, Hallas J. Use of lithium in the adult populations of Denmark, Norway and Sweden. J Affect Disord. 2009;118(1–3):224–8. http://dx.doi.org/10.1016/j.jad.2009.01.024. Medline:19249102Cassidy F, Carroll BJ. Vascular risk factors in late onset mania. Psychol Med. 2002;32(2):359–62. http://dx.doi.org/10.1017/S0033291701004718. Medline:11866328

Delaloye C, Moy G, Baudois S, et al. Cognitive features in euthymic bipolar patients in old age. Bipolar Disord. 2009;11(7):735–43. http://dx.doi.org/10.1111/j.1399-5618.2009.00741.x. Medline:19719786

Depp CA, Jeste DV. Bipolar disorder in older adults: a critical review. Bipolar Disord. 2004;6(5):343–67. http://dx.doi.org/10.1111/j.1399-5618.2004.00139.x. Medline:15383127

Ephraim E, Prettyman R. Attitudes of old age psychiatrists in England and Wales to the use of mood stabilizer drugs. Int Psychogeriatr. 2009;21(3):576–80. http://dx.doi.org/10.1017/S1041610209008667. Medline:19257918

Fujikawa T, Yamawaki S, Touhouda Y. Silent cerebral infarctions in patients with late-onset mania. Stroke. 1995;26(6):946–9. http://dx.doi.org/10.1161/01.STR.26.6.946. Medline:7762043

Gildengers AG, Chisholm D, Butters MA, et al. Two-year course of cognitive function and instrumental activities of daily living in older adults with bipolar disorder: evidence for neuroprogression? Psychol Med. 2013;43(4):801–11. http://dx.doi.org/10.1017/S0033291712001614. Medline:22846332

Goodwin FK, Fireman B, Simon GE, et al. Suicide risk in bipolar disorder during treatment with lithium and divalproex. JAMA. 2003;290(11):1467–73. http://dx.doi.org/10.1001/jama.290.11.1467. Medline:13129986

Goodwin GM, Young AH. The British Association for Psychopharmacology guidelines for treatment of bipolar disorder: a summary. J Psychopharmacol. 2003;17(4 Suppl):3–6. Medline:14964624

Hajek T, Kopecek M, Höschl C, et al. Smaller hippocampal volumes in patients with bipolar disorder are masked by exposure to lithium: a meta-analysis. J Psychiatry Neurosci. 2012;37(5):333–43. http://dx.doi.org/10.1503/jpn.110143. Medline:22498078

Juurlink DN, Mamdani MM, Kopp A, et al. Drug-induced lithium toxicity in the elderly: a population-based study. J Am Geriatr Soc. 2004;52(5):794–8. http://dx.doi.org/10.1111/j.1532-5415.2004.52221.x. Medline:15086664

Kessing LV, Forman JL, Andersen PK. Does lithium protect against dementia? Bipolar Disord. 2010;12(1):87–94. http://dx.doi.org/10.1111/j.1399-5618.2009.00788.x. Medline:20148870

Kessing LV, Hellmund G, Geddes JR, et al. Valproate v. lithium in the treatment of bipolar disorder in clinical practice: observational nationwide register-based cohort study. Br J Psychiatry. 2011;199(1):57–63. http://dx.doi.org/10.1192/bjp.bp.110.084822. Medline:21593515

Kessing LV, Nilsson FM. Increased risk of developing dementia in patients with major affective disorders compared to patients with other medical illnesses. J Affect Disord. 2003;73(3):261–9. http://dx.doi.org/10.1016/S0165-0327(02)00004-6. Medline:12547295

Kessing LV, Søndergård L, Forman JL, et al. Lithium treatment and risk of dementia. Arch Gen Psychiatry. 2008;65(11):1331–5. http://dx.doi.org/10.1001/archpsyc.65.11.1331. Medline:18981345

Kessler RC, Berglund P, Demler O, et al. Lifetime prevalence and age-of-onset distributions of DSM-IV disorders in the National Comorbidity Survey Replication. Arch Gen Psychiatry. 2005;62(6):593–602. http://dx.doi.org/10.1001/archpsyc.62.6.593. Medline:15939837Leboyer M, Henry C, Paillere-Martinot ML, et al. Age at onset in bipolar affective disorders: a review. Bipolar Disord. 2005;7(2):111–18. http://dx.doi.org/10.1111/j.1399-5618.2005.00181.x. Medline:15762851

Martino DJ, Strejilevich SA, Manes F. Neurocognitive functioning in early-onset and late-onset older patients with euthymic bipolar disorder. Int J Geriatr Psychiatry. 2013;28(2):142–8. http://dx.doi.org/10.1002/gps.3801. Medline:22451354

McKnight RF, Adida M, Budge K, et al. Lithium toxicity profile: a systematic review and meta-analysis. Lancet. 2012;379(9817):721–8. http://dx.doi.org/10.1016/S0140-6736(11)61516-X. Medline:22265699

Moorhead SR, Young AH. Evidence for a late onset bipolar-I disorder sub-group from 50 years. J Affect Disord. 2003;73(3):271–7. http://dx.doi.org/10.1016/S0165-0327(01)00476-1. Medline:12547296

Rej S, Herrmann N, Shulman K. The effects of lithium on renal function in older adults--a systematic review. J Geriatr Psychiatry Neurol. 2012;25(1):51–61. http://dx.doi.org/10.1177/0891988712436690. Medline:22467847

Sajatovic M, Calabrese JR, Mullen J. Quetiapine for the treatment of bipolar mania in older adults. Bipolar Disord. 2008;10(6):662–71. http://dx.doi.org/10.1111/j.1399-5618.2008.00614.x. Medline:18837860

Sajatovic M, Coconcea N, Ignacio RV, et al. Aripiprazole therapy in 20 older adults with bipolar disorder: a 12-week, open-label trial. J Clin Psychiatry. 2008;69(1):41–6. http://dx.doi.org/10.4088/JCP.v69n0106. Medline:18312036

Sajatovic M, Gildengers A, Al Jurdi RK, et al. Multisite, open-label, prospective trial of lamotrigine for geriatric bipolar depression: a preliminary report. Bipolar Disord. 2011;13(3):294–302. http://dx.doi.org/10.1111/j.1399-5618.2011.00923.x. Medline:21676132

Sajatovic M, Kessing LV. Bipolar disorder in the elderly. In: Yatham LN, Maj M, editors. Bipolar disorder: clinical and neurobiological foundations. Singapore: Markono Print Media; 2010. http://dx.doi.org/10.1002/9780470661277.ch38

Schouws SN, Stek ML, Comijs HC, et al. Cognitive decline in elderly bipolar disorder patients: a follow-up study. Bipolar Disord. 2012;14(7):749–55. http://dx.doi.org/10.1111/bdi.12000. Medline:22998105

Shulman KI, Rochon P, Sykora K, et al. Changing prescription patterns for lithium and valproic acid in old age: shifting practice without evidence. BMJ. 2003;326(7396):960–1. http://dx.doi.org/10.1136/bmj.326.7396.960. Medline:12727769

Shulman KI, Sykora K, Gill S, Mamdani M, Anderson G, et al. New thyroxine treatment in older adults beginning lithium therapy: implications for clinical practice. Am J Geriatr Psychiatry. 2005a;13(4):299–304. http://dx.doi.org/10.1097/00019442-200504000-00005. Medline:15845755

Shulman KI, Sykora K, Gill S, Mamdani M, Bronskill S, et al. Incidence of delirium in older adults newly prescribed lithium or valproate: a population-based cohort study. J Clin Psychiatry. 2005b;66(4):424–7. http://dx.doi.org/10.4088/JCP.v66n0403. Medline:15816783

Shulman KI, Tohen M, Satlin A, et al. Mania compared with unipolar depression in old age. Am J Psychiatry. 1992;149(3):341–5. http://dx.doi.org/10.1176/ajp.149.3.341. Medline:1536272

Subramaniam H, Dennis MS, Byrne EJ. The role of vascular risk factors in late onset bipolar disorder. Int J Geriatr Psychiatry. 2007;22(8):733–7. http://dx.doi.org/10.1002/gps.1730. Medline:17146839

Suppes T, Dennehy EB, Hirschfeld RM, et al.; Texas Consensus Conference Panel on Medication Treatment of Bipolar Disorder. The Texas implementation of medication algorithms: update to the algorithms for treatment of bipolar I disorder. J Clin Psychiatry. 2005;66(7):870–86. http://dx.doi.org/10.4088/JCP.v66n0710. Medline:16013903

Szalat A, Mazeh H, Freund HR. Lithium-associated hyperparathyroidism: report of four cases and review of the literature. Eur J Endocrinol. 2009;160(2):317–23. http://dx.doi.org/10.1530/EJE-08-0620. Medline:19001061

Tajes M, Gutierrez-Cuesta J, Folch J, et al. Lithium treatment decreases activities of tau kinases in a murine model of senescence. J Neuropathol Exp Neurol. 2008;67(6):612–23. http://dx.doi.org/10.1097/NEN.0b013e3181776293. Medline:18520779

Tsai SY, Kuo CJ, Chen CC, et al. Risk factors for completed suicide in bipolar disorder. J Clin Psychiatry. 2002;63(6):469–76. http://dx.doi.org/10.4088/JCP.v63n0602. Medline:12088157

Yatham LN, Kennedy SH, O'Donovan C, et al.; Guidelines Group, CANMAT. Canadian Network for Mood and Anxiety Treatments (CANMAT) guidelines for the management of patients with bipolar disorder: update 2007. Bipolar Disord. 2006;8(6):721–39. http://dx.doi.org/10.1111/j.1399-5618.2006.00432.x. Medline:17156158

Young RC. Evidence-based pharmacological treatment of geriatric bipolar disorder. Psychiatr Clin North Am. 2005;28(4):837–69, viii. http://dx.doi.org/10.1016/j.psc.2005.09.011. Medline:16325732

2.5 Anxiety Disorders in Older Adults

Laura Gage, MD, FRCPC

INTRODUCTION

Anxiety disorders are among the most common mental disorders encountered in older adults, and symptoms of anxiety also frequently occur with other mental health conditions such as depression and dementia. While anxiety disorders are common in geriatric psychiatry clinical environments, they have not received as much attention as other common mental health conditions. Anxiety disorders in older adults can represent either the new onset of anxiety disorders late in life or aging with anxiety disorders that developed earlier. In this chapter Dr Gage has provided an overview of the epidemiology of anxiety disorders, highlighting some of the unique features in older adults along with a review of evidence-based treatments for anxiety disorders.

CASE SCENARIO

Mrs P. is a 77-year-old woman who lives on her own. She has a longstanding history of generalized anxiety disorder (GAD). She is referred to you from her family physician for a consultation due to worsening symptoms of her anxiety disorder. She has increased worries around her physical health following several falls, and now visits her family physician frequently due to complaints of dizziness and shakiness. Her family doctor feels that she is medically stable. Her sleep has recently deteriorated, and she now has decreased appetite with some mild weight loss. Her medical history includes chronic obstructive pulmonary disease (COPD), diabetes mellitus, and hypothyroidism.

Her medications include levothyroxine 0.1 mg po od, metformin 500 mg po bid, albuterol 2 puffs 4 h prn, citalopram 30 mg po od, and zopiclone 5 mg po hs. Her citalopram was increased from 20 mg, and the zopiclone was added one week ago by the family doctor with no effect to date.

1. What is your approach to assessing contributions to the patient's symptomatology?
2. What should be considered in assisting the family doctor with developing a preliminary management plan?

OVERVIEW

1. Epidemiology

1.1 Trends in Epidemiology
(Bland et al., 1988; Regier et al., 1988; Streiner, Cairney, & Veldhuizen, 2006; Gum, King-Kallimanis, & Kohn, 2009; Beekman et al., 1998; Préville et al., 2010)

- Wide variation in epidemiological data in anxiety disorders in older adults
- Anxiety disorders among the most common late-life psychiatric diagnoses, but less common than in younger age groups
- GAD and phobic disorders most common among the anxiety disorders
- More common in women than in men

1.2 Limitations to Epidemiological Data
(Streiner et al., 2009; Corna et al., 2010; Smith, Ingram, & Brighton, 2009)

- Challenges in the epidemiology and diagnosis of anxiety disorders in the older adults include the following:
  - Screening tools are usually developed for younger people.
  - Older adults tend to minimize symptoms.
    - May use different language to describe anxiety
    - Tend to attribute symptoms to physical symptoms/illnesses
    - May have difficulty remembering symptoms
  - Subsyndromal but clinically relevant symptoms would not be captured.

1.3 Age of Onset
(Kessler et al., 2005; Le Roux, Gatz, & Wetherell, 2005)

- Anxiety disorders usually have an early age of onset.
- Late-onset anxiety disorders are more often associated with depression or dysthymia.
- It is important to consider medical causes with late-onset anxiety.
- Panic disorder has a particularly low late-life incidence.
- In contrast, late-onset agoraphobia is *more* commonly seen.

2. Risk Factors for Anxiety Disorders in Older Adults
(Smith, Ingram, & Brighton, 2009; Wolitzky-Taylor et al., 2010; Lenze & Wetherell, 2011)

- Physical illness, psychosocial stress, depression, cognitive impairment, female gender, advanced age, lower educational or professional levels, external locus of control, family history of anxiety disorder, alcohol or drug use; others mentioned in the literature include being unmarried, poor self-rated health, adverse events in childhood, neuroticism, being childless, and functional limitations.
- Age-related protective factors may include social support, religiosity, physical activity, cognitive stimulation, and effective coping skills.

3. Course

3.1 Anxiety Disorders Are Persistent in Older Adults
(Schuurmans et al., 2005; Lenze et al., 2005a)

- Anxiety disorders are among the most persistent mental health syndromes.
- Average duration of 20+ years

3.2 Symptom Expression

- Overall, quite similar to younger population with only minor differences (which will be reviewed for each disorder)

4. Relationship between Anxiety and Cognitive Impairment

4.1 Evidence Is Limited, but Supports That Anxiety Is Associated with Accelerated Cognitive Decline
(Beaudreau & O'Hara, 2008; Sinoff & Werner, 2003; Lenze & Wetherell, 2011)

- Older brains are less able to downregulate hypothalamic-pituitary-adrenal (HPA) axis.
- Chronic anxiety activates HPA axis leading to elevated cortisol, and this is thought to damage hippocampus and alter N-methyl-D-aspartate (NMDA) receptor activity.
- Another proposed mechanism is an increase in β-amyloid 42 peptide and tau hyperphosphorylation due to excessive HPA activation.
- There may also be accelerated aging at a cellular level with telomere shrinkage associated with chronic anxiety.
- Some of these changes may be reversible with treatment.

5. Generalized Anxiety Disorder

5.1 Presentation in Older Adults
(Diefenbach, Stanley, & Beck, 2001; Wolitzky-Taylor et al., 2010; Schoevers et al., 2005)

- Most common anxiety disorder in older adults (along with phobias)
- Less severe symptom presentation compared to younger age group
- Higher percentage of health worries and worries about the well-being of the family compared to younger age group
- Can be challenging to determine when anxiety is excessive in the older adults

5.2 High Medical Comorbidity
(Sable & Jeste, 2001; Smith, Ingram, & Brighton, 2009)

- There is a bidirectional relationship between medical illness and anxiety.
  - Comorbid anxiety is often associated with increased mortality in medically unwell patients.
  - Anxiety often manifests somatically, which can be mistaken as having a medical etiology.
  - Alternatively, many medical conditions can mimic symptoms of anxiety.
  - Symptoms from medical issues can be frightening, in turn causing anxiety.

– Medication side effects can include anxiety symptoms.

– Disability/lifestyle changes from having medical illness can cause anxiety.

5.3 High Comorbidity with Depression
(Flint, 1994)

• Comorbid anxiety with depression is associated with increased suicidality, decreased treatment responsiveness, and increased severity of symptoms (Hopko et al., 2000; Flint & Rifat, 1997; Lenze et al., 2000).

• Longitudinally, anxiety symptoms appear to lead to depressive symptoms, more likely than vice versa (Wetherell, Gatz, & Pedersen, 2001).

5.4 Controlled Pharmacological Trials of GAD in Older Adults

• Escitalopram (Lenze et al., 2009)
  – Randomized controlled trial (RCT), non-industry funded
  – Low-medium treatment response
  – Fatigue most common adverse drug reaction
• Citalopram (Lenze et al., 2005b)
  – Small RCT, partially industry funded
  – 65% treatment vs 24% placebo response rate
• Sertraline (Schuurmans et al., 2006)
  – RCT, sertraline vs cognitive behavioural therapy (CBT) vs waitlist
  – Non-industry funded
  – Sertraline and CBT equally effective, modest effect size
• Serotonin norepinephrine reuptake inhibitors (SNRIs) (e.g., duloxetine, venlafaxine) (Davidson et al., 2008; Katz et al., 2002)
  – Retrospective pooled analysis of industry funded trials of 65+ population
  – Similar effect sizes and side effects to younger population
  – No prospective trials in older adults specifically
• Quetiapine XR (Mezhebovsky et al., 2013)
  – RCT, industry funded
  – Similar remission rates as reported in younger populations
  – Risk/benefit ratio must be considered in the context of other available treatment options
• Pregabalin (Montgomery et al., 2008)
  – RCT, industry funded
  – Modest efficacy
  – Well tolerated
• Buspirone (2 trials)
  – Open trial, industry funded, 605 patients 65+ (Robinson, Napoliello, & Schenk, 1988)
    ▪ Modest effect size and favourable side-effect profile
  – Small single-blind RCT, non-industry funded (Mokhber et al., 2010)
    ▪ Buspirone vs sertraline equally effective

5.5 Cognitive Behavioural Therapy

- In terms of psychotherapy for anxiety disorders in older adults, CBT for GAD has had the most extensive controlled research trials.
- Meta-analysis shows moderate effect sizes (Hendriks et al., 2008).
- Some studies suggest that the most effective part of CBT for anxiety disorders in older adults may be the relaxation training, which can be fairly easily incorporated into regular practice (Thorp et al., 2009).

6. Panic Disorder

6.1 Presentation in the Elderly
(Lindesay, 1991; Eaton et al., 1989)

- Lower prevalence rates than in younger age groups; not known why less frequent in late life; possibilities include:
  - Age bias in diagnostic criteria
  - Age-related changes in cognitive style
  - Age-related changes in neurotransmitters (i.e., maintenance of γ-aminobutyric acid [GABA], decrease in noradrenergic activity, decrease in cholecystokinin)
  - Disorder-associated mortality
  - Cohort effect
- Late-onset is uncommon. When late onset is seen, carefully search for depression, medical causes.
- Fewer panic symptoms and higher level of functioning compared to younger population; however, agoraphobic avoidance does not decline with age.
- Bidirectional relationship with medical comorbidity is similar to that reviewed in section 5.2 in this chapter.

6.2 Pharmacotherapy Trials of Panic Disorder in Older Adults

- Paroxetine vs CBT vs waitlist (Hendriks et al., 2010)
- RCT, industry funded
- Paroxetine and CBT equally effective, reduction of panic attack rate by about 75%

7. Agoraphobia

7.1 Presentation in Older Adults
(Corna et al., 2007; Ritchie et al., 2013; McCabe et al., 2006)

- Agoraphobia in older adults often late onset
- Less often associated with panic disorder as compared to younger adults
- Onset may be related to change in health status, falls
- More common in women and those widowed/divorced
- Often preceded by depression

7.2 Pharmacotherapy Trials in Older Adults

- No controlled pharmacotherapy trials in older adults for agoraphobia without panic disorder

- One positive RCT trial (paroxetine = CBT) of panic disorder with concurrent agoraphobia (Hendriks et al., 2009)

8. Social Anxiety Disorder

8.1 Presentation in Older Adults
(Flint, 2005; Cairney et al. 2007)

- Few epidemiological studies are available.
- Limited data suggests the prevalence to be lower than in younger adults.
- Severity may decrease with age and then increase again after 80.
- Older adults are more likely to have greater anxiety over a greater number of situations relative to younger adults.

8.2 Pharmacotherapy Trials in Older Adults

- No controlled pharmacotherapy trials of social anxiety disorder in older adults to date

9. Post-traumatic Stress Disorder

(Note: in the DSM-5 post-traumatic stress disorder [PTSD] has been moved out of the anxiety disorders section.)

9.1 Presentation in Older Adults
(Acierno et al., 2006; Creamer & Parslow, 2008; Böttche, Kuwert, & Knaevelsrud, 2012)

- Lower prevalence rate in older adults than in younger population
- Older adults may develop PTSD less frequently after traumatic events than younger adults do.
    - Early life traumas result in higher rates of PTSD than late-life traumas.
    - Unclear if this is related to a cohort effect or autonomic reactivity/brain changes with age
- Re-experiencing symptoms decline with age but avoidance increases.
- Delayed-onset PTSD is fairly rare, but reactivation more frequent.
    - Reactivation may be related to analogous historical events or triggered by age-related losses (i.e., retirement, deaths).

9.2 Pharmacological Trials in Older Adults

- Prazosin (Raskind et al., 2007)
    - Mixed ages, but included some geriatric population
    - RCT, non-industry funded
    - Decreased trauma nightmares, sleep disturbance, and global clinical status improved

10. Obsessive-Compulsive Disorder

(Note: in the DSM-5 obsessive-compulsive disorder [OCD] has been moved out of the anxiety disorders section.)

10.1 Presentation in Older Adults
(Regier et al., 1988; Kohn et al., 1997)

- Low prevalence rates (0.8% 12-month prevalence)
- Fewer symmetry and counting rituals
- Increased handwashing rituals and fears of sinning obsessions

10.2 Hoarding
(Ayers et al., 2010; Grisham & Norberg, 2010)

- Hoarding occurs more often and more severely in elderly.
- Often involves single, unmarried, older women
- In elderly, hoarding symptoms may be secondary to dementia, stroke, alcoholism, severe depression, among other etiologies.

(Note: in the DSM-5, hoarding is recognized as a distinct disorder [part of the OCD and related conditions section] and has been removed from the anxiety disorders section.)

10.3 Pharmacotherapy Trials in Older Adults

- No controlled pharmacotherapy trials of OCD in older adults to date

11. Benzodiazepines in Anxiety Disorders

11.1 Controlled Trials of Benzodiazepines in Older Adults for Anxiety Disorders Are Rare

- Only one RCT of benzodiazepines for anxiety in older adults (Koepke et al., 1982)
- Oxazepam efficacious over placebo, but only had voluntary reporting of side effects

11.2 Age-Related Pharmacokinetic and Pharmacodynamic Changes Increase the Potential for Benzodiazepine Side Effects in Older Adults
(Madhusoodanan & Bogunovic, 2004)

- Side effects include the following:
    - Falls
    - Impaired driving skills
    - Cognitive impairment
    - Respiratory function affected
    - Potential to cause disinhibition
    - Risk of dependence
    - Rebound anxiety
    - Sedation

11.3 Guidelines Caution to Use Benzodiazepines Judiciously in Older Adults
(Madhusoodanan & Bogunovic, 2004; Canadian Psychiatric Association, 2006; National Collaborating Centre for Mental Health [NICE], 2011)

- Benzodiazepines should be avoided or used only for short periods if possible.
- If used, conjugated benzodiazepines (e.g., lorazepam, oxazepam, temazepam) are recommended (over oxidatively metabolized benzodiazepines), as they have no active metabolites and clearance is relatively unaffected by age.

12. Final Points

- Anxiety disorders are relatively common in late life.
- High rates of comorbidity with depression

- Bidirectional, complex interactions with medical illness
- Late-onset anxiety is less common, and one must consider comorbid medical causes or depression.
- Recent years have seen a significant increase in RCTs for CBT and pharmacotherapy for GAD, but the remainder of the anxiety disorders remain poorly studied.

QUESTIONS

1. List the risk factors and protective factors associated with anxiety disorders in older adults.
2. Present some explanations as to why GAD is relatively more common in older adults and panic disorder is less common in older adults.
3. Discuss some potential adaptations of CBT for anxiety to older adults.
4. Summarize the difference in the presentation of various anxiety disorders in older adults as compared to the younger population.
5. Why is it of particular importance to consider your differential in late-onset anxiety? List five alternative causes other than a primary anxiety disorder.
6. Using a patient with COPD and panic disorder as an example, discuss the interplay between medical and anxiety disorders in older adults.
7. Does chronic anxiety cause cognitive decline? Explain the association between anxiety disorders and cognitive decline in older adults.

ANSWERS

1. This table provides a summary of the risk factors and protective factors associated with anxiety disorders in older adults.

Risk Factors	Protective Factors
• Female gender	• Social support
• Depression	• Religiosity
• Cognitive impairment	• Physical activity
• Advanced age	• Cognitive stimulation
• Physical illness	• Effective coping skills
• Poor self-rated health	• Converse of any of the other risk factors
• Neuroticism	
• Childless	
• Psychosocial stress	
• Adverse events in childhood	
• Lower education or professional level	
• External locus of control	
• Being unmarried	
• Alcohol use or drug use	
• Family history of anxiety disorder	
• Functional limitations	

2. Proposed explanations for why panic disorders are less common in older adults include the following:
   - Lower levels of panic disorder in older adults may be due to age-related changes in brain structure and function, or peripheral physiology that decrease autonomic responses and therefore decrease panic attack symptomatology, leading to relatively lower levels of panic disorder in the older population.
   - Some changes that have been hypothesized are decreased norepinephrine and cholecystokinin activity with maintenance of GABA activity.
   - Increase in adaptive behaviours that regulate emotions, leading to less panic, may play a role.

   Proposed explanations for GAD being more common in older adults include:
   - With GAD, age-related executive dysfunction decreases ability to inhibit worry, leading to relatively higher levels of GAD.
   - Functional connectivity changes between the amygdala and frontal lobe may play a role.
   - Increased medical comorbidity and/or functional impairment with aging may play a role.
   - GAD is more prevalent throughout the lifespan than panic disorder, and this pattern continues in late life.
   - Increased exposure to biomedical and psychosocial stressors (e.g., cognitive impairment, functional limitation, poor social supports, etc.), changes, and losses may play a role.
   - Many medications can produce anxiety-like symptoms.

3. Adaptations of CBT for anxiety in older adults include:
   - Emphasis on psychoeducation
   - Use of relaxation
   - Slower pace
   - Increased repetition and review of concepts
   - Increased focus on behavioural approach
   - Engagement of family
   - Fewer abstract concepts
   - Audiotape sessions for review between appointments
   - Include religion (for those with religious beliefs)
   - Reminder phone calls between sessions
   - More focus on medical concerns
   - Written summary of sessions for patients with cognitive decline

   (See also chapter 2.7)

4. Differences in presentations of anxiety disorders in older adults, compared to the younger population include:
   - *GAD*: more worry about health-related vs work-related issues; anxiety may manifest somatically in late life
   - *OCD*: fewer symmetry concerns/counting rituals; greater fear of having sinned; increased hand washing; increased compulsive hoarding
   - *PTSD*: fewer "re-experiencing" symptoms but increased avoidance symptomatology

- *Specific phobias*: more environmental phobias (e.g., fear of lightning and heights); fear of falling quite common
- *Social phobia*: severity declines until age 80 and then increases again; elderly endorse greater anxiety for a number of situations when compared to younger adults
- *Agoraphobia*: less likely to have comorbid panic disorder; more likely to be triggered by change in health status or fall; late onset is more common than among the other disorders
- *Panic disorder*: decreased panic symptoms; less anxiety and arousal; higher level of functioning

5. With the exception of agoraphobia, it is less likely for anxiety disorders to begin in late life. Other potential causes include:
   - Depression
   - Physical illness (e.g., supraventricular tachycardia, hypoglycemia, hyperthyroidism, Parkinson's, temporal lobe seizures, hypocalcemia, COPD)
   - Medication toxicity (particularly sympathomimetics, salbutamol, theophylline, thyroxine, caffeine, amphetamines)
   - Withdrawal from alcohol or benzodiazepines
   - Dementia
   - Delirium

6. Regarding the interplay between anxiety disorders and COPD (and other medical comorbidities) in older adults:
   - In older patients with medical comorbidities, there is more functional impairment, morbidity, and mortality in the presence of anxiety.
   - Anxiety is associated with increased risk of developing physical illness (especially cardiovascular).
   - Between 18% and 50% of COPD patients report anxiety symptoms (GAD and panic disorder more frequent).
   - COPD symptoms can mimic physiological symptoms of anxiety and can produce fearful bodily sensations, in turn provoking increased anxiety.
   - Pharmacological treatment of COPD can cause anxiety symptoms.
   - COPD patients can develop anxiety about their physical symptoms or in response to the disability and lifestyle changes imposed by the medical disease.
   - Older adults tend to attribute anxiety symptoms to the physical disease and consequently anxiety disorders may be underdiagnosed.

7. Regarding anxiety and cognitive decline in older adults:
   - There is an association between anxiety and cognitive decline, although the exact nature of this relationship has not yet been determined (may be bidirectional).
   - The predominant proposed mechanism is that chronic anxiety activates the HPA axis with increased release of corticotropin-releasing factor (CRF), leading to increased release of cortisol; cortisol desensitizes central glucocorticoid receptors and alters NMDA receptor activity with synaptic and morphological change of the hippocampus and prefrontal cortex.

- Another proposed mechanism is an increase in β-amyloid 42 peptide and tau hyperphosphorylation due to excessive HPA activation.
- There may also be accelerated aging at a cellular level with telomere shrinkage associated with chronic anxiety.

CASE DISCUSSION

1. Assessment of the contributions would include the following:
   - Evaluation of medical conditions/issues
     - In terms of medical contribution, her diabetic control, thyroid function, COPD/respiratory status should be reviewed as they could be contributing.
     - She should also be evaluated for any newly developed medical conditions and for any change in her cognition.
     - Rule out urinary tract infection (UTI).
     - Assess for evidence of COPD exacerbation or chest infection.
     - Consider a CT head to rule out silent vascular disease or infarct.
   - Assessment of cognitive and functional status
   - Review of her medications
     - Evaluate the effect of the increased citalopram (above maximum recommended dosing), which could contribute to falls or cause akathisia and agitation.
     - Please see chapter 2.3 regarding citalopram and QTc prolongation.
     - Addition of zopiclone may contribute to falls.
     - Albuterol can cause similar side effects and may be contributing.
     - As well, ensure that there are no other changes in medications, new over-the-counter medications; her ability to manage her medications independently should be reviewed.
   - A reassessment of her psychiatric diagnosis should occur, particularly reviewing for comorbid depression and alcohol use.
2. An approach to management would include the following considerations:
   - A multimodal plan should be based on a more in-depth assessment.
   - Possible pharmacological changes
     - Lower dosage of citalopram and possibly switch to mirtazapine as second line (may also help with sleep).
     - Discontinue zopiclone, as it has been ineffective and may be contributing to falls.
   - Possible nonpharmacological interventions should focus on her psychiatric symptoms.
     - Education
     - Sleep behaviour management
     - Relaxation training
     - Increasing social supports

RECOMMENDED RESOURCES FOR REVIEW

Although these resources may not be specifically cited in the text, their approach informed the contents of the chapter, and they are recommended as useful further reading.

Beaudreau SA, O'Hara R. Late-life anxiety and cognitive impairment: a review. Am J Geriatr Psychiatry. 2008;16(10):790–803. http://dx.doi.org/10.1097/ JGP.0b013e31817945c3. Medline:18827225

Gonçalves DC, Byrne GJ. Interventions for generalized anxiety disorder in older adults: systematic review and meta-analysis. J Anxiety Disord. 2012;26(1):1–11. http://dx.doi .org/10.1016/j.janxdis.2011.08.010. Medline:21907538

Lenze EJ, Wetherell JL. A lifespan view of anxiety disorders. Dialogues Clin Neurosci. 2011;13(4):381–99. Medline:22275845

Wolitzky-Taylor KB, Castriotta N, Lenze EJ, et al. Anxiety disorders in older adults: a comprehensive review. Depress Anxiety. 2010;27(2):190–211. http://dx.doi.org/ 10.1002/da.20653. Medline:20099273

REFERENCES

Acierno R, Ruggiero KJ, Kilpatrick DG, et al. Risk and protective factors for psychopathology among older versus younger adults after the 2004 Florida hurricanes. Am J Geriatr Psychiatry. 2006;14(12):1051–9. http://dx.doi.org/10.1097/01.JGP.0000221327.97904.b0. Medline:17035356

Ayers CR, Saxena S, Golshan S, et al. Age at onset and clinical features of late life compulsive hoarding. Int J Geriatr Psychiatry. 2010;25(2):142–9. http://dx.doi.org/10.1002/gps.2310. Medline:19548272

Beekman AT, Bremmer MA, Deeg DJ, et al. Anxiety disorders in later life: a report from the Longitudinal Aging Study Amsterdam. Int J Geriatr Psychiatry. 1998;13(10):717–26. http://dx.doi.org/10.1002/(SICI)1099-1166(1998100)13:10<717::AID-GPS857>3.0.CO;2-M. Medline:9818308

Bland RC, Stebelsky G, Orn H, et al. Psychiatric disorders and unemployment in Edmonton. Acta Psychiatr Scand Suppl. 1988;77(S338):72–80. http://dx.doi.org/10.1111/j.1600-0447.1988.tb08550.x. Medline:3165598

Böttche M, Kuwert P, Knaevelsrud C. Posttraumatic stress disorder in older adults: an overview of characteristics and treatment approaches. Int J Geriatr Psychiatry. 2012;27(3):230–9. http://dx.doi.org/10.1002/gps.2725. Medline:21538540

Cairney J, McCabe L, Veldhuizen S, et al. Epidemiology of social phobia in later life. Am J Geriatr Psychiatry. 2007;15(3):224–33. PMID: 17213375

Canadian Psychiatric Association. Clinical practice guidelines. Management of anxiety disorders. [Erratum in: Can J Psychiatry. 2006;51(10):623]. Can J Psychiatry. 2006;51(8 Suppl 2):9S–91S. Medline:16933543

Corna LM, Cairney J, Herrmann N, et al. Panic disorder in later life: results from a national survey of Canadians. Int Psychogeriatr. 2007;19(6):1084–96. http://dx.doi.org/10.1017/S1041610207004978. Medline:17367554

Corna LM, Gage L, Cairney J, et al. Psychiatric disorder in later life: a Canadian perspective. In: Cairney J, Streiner DL, editors. Mental disorders in Canada: an epidemiologic perspective. Toronto: University of Toronto Press; 2010. p. 227–57. http://www.utppublishing.com/Mental-Disorder-in-Canada-An-Epidemiological-Perspective.html

Creamer M, Parslow R. Trauma exposure and posttraumatic stress disorder in the elderly: a community prevalence study. Am J Geriatr Psychiatry. 2008;16(10):853–6. http://dx.doi.org/10.1097/01.JGP.0000310785.36837.85. Medline:18474685

Davidson J, Allgulander C, Pollack MH, et al. Efficacy and tolerability of duloxetine in elderly patients with generalized anxiety disorder: a pooled analysis of four randomized, double-blind, placebo-controlled studies. Hum Psychopharmacol. 2008;23(6):519–26. http://dx.doi.org/10.1002/hup.949. Medline:18478624

Diefenbach GJ, Stanley MA, Beck JG. Worry content reported by older adults with and without generalized anxiety disorder. Aging Ment Health. 2001;5(3):269–74. http://dx.doi.org/10.1080/13607860120065069. Medline:11575066

Eaton WW, Kramer M, Anthony JC, et al. The incidence of specific DIS/DSM-III mental disorders: data from the NIMH Epidemiologic Catchment Area Program. Acta Psychiatr Scand. 1989;79(2):163–78. PMID: 2784251

Flint AJ. Epidemiology and comorbidity of anxiety disorders in the elderly. Am J Psychiatry. 1994;151(5):640–9. http://dx.doi.org/10.1176/ajp.151.5.640. Medline:8166303

– Anxiety and its disorders in late life: moving the field forward. Am J Geriatr Psychiatry. 2005;13(1):3–6. http://dx.doi.org/10.1097/00019442-200501000-00002. Medline:15653934

Flint AJ, Rifat SL. Anxious depression in elderly patients. Response to antidepressant treatment. Am J Geriatr Psychiatry. 1997;5(2):107–15. Medline:9106374

Grisham JR, Norberg MM. Compulsive hoarding: current controversies and new directions. Dialogues Clin Neurosci. 2010;12(2):233–40. Medline:20623927

Gum AM, King-Kallimanis B, Kohn R. Prevalence of mood, anxiety, and substance-abuse disorders for older Americans in the national comorbidity survey-replication. Am J Geriatr Psychiatry. 2009;17(9):769–81. http://dx.doi.org/10.1097/JGP.0b013e3181ad4f5a. Medline:19700949

Hendriks GJ, Keijsers GP, Kampman M, et al. A randomized controlled study of paroxetine and cognitive-behavioural therapy for late-life panic disorder. Acta Psychiatr Scand. 2010;122(1):11–9. http://dx.doi.org/10.1111/j.1600-0447.2009.01517.x. Medline:19958308

Hendriks GJ, Oude Voshaar RC, Keijsers GP, et al. Cognitive-behavioural therapy for late-life anxiety disorders: a systematic review and meta-analysis. Acta Psychiatr Scand. 2008;117(6):403–11. http://dx.doi.org/10.1111/j.1600-0447.2008.01190.x. Medline:18479316

Hopko DR, Bourland SL, Stanley MA, et al. Generalized anxiety disorder in older adults: examining the relation between clinician severity ratings and patient self-report measures. Depress Anxiety. 2000;12(4):217–25. http://dx.doi.org/10.1002/1520-6394(2000)12:4<217::AID-DA5>3.0.CO;2-6. Medline:11195758

Katz IR, Reynolds CF III, Alexopoulos GS, et al. Venlafaxine ER as a treatment for generalized anxiety disorder in older adults: pooled analysis of five randomized placebo-controlled clinical trials. J Am Geriatr Soc. 2002;50(1):18–25. http://dx.doi.org/10.1046/j.1532-5415.2002.50003.x. Medline:12028242

Kessler RC, Berglund P, Demler O, et al. Lifetime prevalence and age-of-onset distributions of DSM-IV disorders in the National Comorbidity Survey Replication. [Erratum in: Arch Gen Psychiatry. 2005 Jul;62(7):768] Arch Gen Psychiatry. 2005;62(6):593–602. http://dx.doi.org/10.1001/archpsyc.62.6.593. Medline:15939837

Koepke HH, Gold RL, Linden ME, et al. Multicenter controlled study of oxazepam in anxious elderly outpatients. Psychosomatics. 1982;23(6):641–5. PMID: 6750675

Kohn R, Westlake RJ, Rasmussen SA, et al. Clinical features of obsessive-compulsive disorder in elderly patients. Am J Geriatr Psychiatry. 1997;5(3):211–5. http://dx.doi.org/10.1097/00019442-199700530-00004. Medline:9209562

Lenze EJ, Mulsant BH, Mohlman J, et al. Generalized anxiety disorder in late life: lifetime course and comorbidity with major depressive disorder. Am J Geriatr Psychiatry. 2005a;13(1):77–80. http://dx.doi.org/10.1097/00019442-200501000-00011. Medline:15653943

Lenze EJ, Mulsant BH, Shear MK, Dew MA, et al. Efficacy and tolerability of citalopram in the treatment of late-life anxiety disorders: results from an 8-week randomized, placebo-controlled trial. Am J Psychiatry. 2005b;162(1):146–50. http://dx.doi.org/10.1176/appi.ajp.162.1.146. Medline:15625213

Lenze EJ, Mulsant BH, Shear MK, Schulberg HC, et al. Comorbid anxiety disorders in depressed elderly patients. Am J Psychiatry. 2000;157(5):722–8. http://dx.doi.org/10.1176/appi.ajp.157.5.722. Medline:10784464

Lenze EJ, Rollman BL, Shear MK, et al. Escitalopram for older adults with generalized anxiety disorder: a randomized controlled trial. JAMA. 2009;301(3):295–303. http://dx.doi.org/10.1001/jama.2008.977. Medline:19155456

Le Roux H, Gatz M, Wetherell JL. Age at onset of generalized anxiety disorder in older adults. Am J Geriatr Psychiatry. 2005;13(1):23–30. http://dx.doi.org/10.1097/00019442-200501000-00005. Medline:15653937

Lindesay J. Phobic disorders in the elderly. Br J Psychiatry. 1991;159:531–41. PMID: 1751864

Madhusoodanan S, Bogunovic OJ. Safety of benzodiazepines in the geriatric population. Expert Opin Drug Saf. 2004 Sep;3(5):485–93. http://dx.doi.org/10.1517/14740338.3.5.485. Medline:15335303

McCabe L, Cairney J, Veldhuizen S, et al. Prevalence and correlates of agoraphobia in older adults. Am J Geriatr Psychiatry. 2006;14(6):515–22. http://dx.doi.org/10.1097/01.JGP.0000203177.54242.14. Medline:16731720

Mezhebovsky I, Mägi K, She F, et al. Double-blind, randomized study of extended release quetiapine fumarate (quetiapine XR) monotherapy in older patients with generalized anxiety disorder. Int J Geriatr Psychiatry. 2013;28(6):615–25. http://dx.doi.org/10.1002/gps.3867. Medline:23070803

Mokhber N, Azarpazhooh MR, Khajehdaluee M, et al. Randomized, single-blind, trial of sertraline and buspirone for treatment of elderly patients with generalized anxiety disorder. Psychiatry Clin Neurosci. 2010;64(2):128–33. http://dx.doi.org/10.1111/j.1440-1819.2009.02055.x. Medline:20132529

Montgomery S, Chatamra K, Pauer L, et al. Efficacy and safety of pregabalin in elderly people with generalised anxiety disorder. Br J Psychiatry. 2008;193(5):389–94. http://dx.doi.org/10.1192/bjp.bp.107.037788. Medline:18978320

National Collaborating Centre for Mental Health (UK). Generalised anxiety disorder in adults: management in primary, secondary and community care. NICE Clinical Guidelines, no. 113. Leicester (UK): British Psychological Society; 2011. PMID: 22536620

Préville M, Boyer R, Vasiliadis HM, et al.; Scientific Committee of the ESA Study. Persistence and remission of psychiatric disorders in the Quebec older adult population. Can J Psychiatry. 2010;55(8):514–22. Medline:20723279

Raskind MA, Peskind ER, Hoff DJ, et al. A parallel group placebo controlled study of prazosin for trauma nightmares and sleep disturbance in combat veterans with post-traumatic stress disorder. Biol Psychiatry. 2007;61(8):928–34. http://dx.doi.org/10.1016/j.biopsych.2006.06.032. Medline:17069768

Regier DA, Boyd JH, Burke JD Jr, et al. One-month prevalence of mental disorders in the United States. Based on five epidemiologic catchment area sites. Arch Gen Psychiatry. 1988;45(11):977–86. http://dx.doi.org/10.1001/archpsyc.1988.01800350011002. Medline:3263101

Ritchie K, Norton J, Mann A, et al. Late-onset agoraphobia: general population incidence and evidence for a clinical subtype. Am J Psychiatry. 2013;170(7):790–8. http://dx.doi.org/10.1176/appi.ajp.2013.12091235. Medline:23820832

Robinson D, Napoliello MJ, Schenk J. The safety and usefulness of buspirone as an anxiolytic drug in elderly versus young patients. Clin Ther. 1988;10(6):740–6. Medline:3219687

Sable JA, Jeste DV. Anxiety disorders in older adults. Curr Psychiatry Rep. 2001;3(4):302–7. http://dx.doi.org/10.1007/s11920-001-0023-0. Medline:11470037

Schoevers RA, Deeg DJ, van Tilburg W, et al. Depression and generalized anxiety disorder: co-occurrence and longitudinal patterns in elderly patients. Am J Geriatr Psychiatry. 2005;13(1):31–9. http://dx.doi.org/10.1097/00019442-200501000-00006. Medline:15653938

Schuurmans J, Comijs HC, Beekman AT, et al. The outcome of anxiety disorders in older people at 6-year follow-up: results from the Longitudinal Aging Study Amsterdam. Acta Psychiatr Scand. 2005;111(6):420–8. PMID: 15877708

Schuurmans J, Comijs H, Emmelkamp PM, et al. A randomized, controlled trial of the effectiveness of cognitive-behavioral therapy and sertraline versus a waitlist control group for anxiety disorders in older adults. Am J Geriatr Psychiatry. 2006;14(3):255–63. http://dx.doi.org/10.1097/01.JGP.0000196629.19634.00. Medline:16505130

Sinoff G, Werner P. Anxiety disorder and accompanying subjective memory loss in the elderly as a predictor of future cognitive decline. Int J Geriatr Psychiatry. 2003;18(10):951–9. http://dx.doi.org/10.1002/gps.1004. Medline:14533128

Smith M, Ingram T, Brighton V. Detection and assessment of late-life anxiety. J Gerontol Nurs. 2009;35(7):9–15. http://dx.doi.org/10.3928/00989134-20090527-02. Medline:19650618

Streiner DL, Cairney J, Veldhuizen S. The epidemiology of psychological problems in the elderly. Can J Psychiatry. 2006;51(3):185–91. Medline:16618010

Streiner DL, Patten SB, Anthony JC, et al. Has 'lifetime prevalence' reached the end of its life? An examination of the concept. Int J Methods Psychiatr Res. 2009;18(4):221–8. http://dx.doi.org/10.1002/mpr.296. Medline:20052690

Thorp SR, Ayers CR, Nuevo R, et al. Meta-analysis comparing different behavioral treatments for late-life anxiety. Am J Geriatr Psychiatry. 2009;17(2):105–15. http://dx.doi.org/10.1097/JGP.0b013e31818b3f7e. Medline:19155744

Wetherell JL, Gatz M, Pedersen NL. A longitudinal analysis of anxiety and depressive symptoms. Psychol Aging. 2001;16(2):187–95. http://dx.doi.org/10.1037/0882-7974.16.2.187. Medline:11405307

2.6 Electroconvulsive Therapy in Older Adults

Daniel M. Blumberger, MD, MSc, FRCPC
Peter Chan, MD, FRCPC

INTRODUCTION

Electroconvulsive therapy (ECT) is one of the oldest psychiatric treatments, yet remains the most effective for severe depression. Geriatric psychiatrists must have a good foundation in knowledge of this procedure, even if only to be able to explain its use and rationale to patients and their caregivers. Drs Blumberger and Chan provide an in-depth overview, summarizing current knowledge as it applies to the use of ECT in the elderly patients.

CASE SCENARIO

Ms B. is a 66-year-old divorced, socially isolated, moderately obese woman, who retired early from teaching due to bipolar I disorder. She has had "mood swings" since delivering her first child at age 31, and was eventually diagnosed at age 52 after a psychotic manic episode. The manic/hypomanic episodes eventually stabilized with lithium 1200 mg/d and lamotrigine 200 mg/d over the last eight years. She has had bipolar depressive episodes since, with multiple trials of antidepressants for functionally disabling symptoms of anergia and hypersomnia, associated with her low mood. An inpatient course of bilateral ECT x6 was successful four years ago, but she complained of lingering cognitive impairment for months afterwards. She is currently on bupropion-XL 300 mg/d, dextroamphetamine 10 mg/d, and aripiprazole 5 mg/d, along with the mood stabilizers. Other conditions include type II diabetes and hypertension, for which she take metformin and ramipril. She is being seen as an outpatient, living alone, and has two supportive children, but they live in different cities. GDS-15 = 11; MoCA = 22/30.

1. What brain stimulation therapies can be offered?
2. What are the benefits, risks, and barriers for each therapeutic measure?
3. What additional conditions can there be that may influence outcome with brain stimulation?
4. How should her medications be managed during the course of brain stimulation treatment?
5. Should consideration be given for an ECT course as an outpatient?
6. What are the logistical barriers for outpatient maintenance ECT in her situation?

OVERVIEW

1. Overall Framework

- ECT is safe, and can be effective in elderly patients for mood disorders and some psychotic disorders, with or without concurrent dementia.
- There is a paucity of studies in geriatric patients, particularly those over age 80.
- Older adults with major depressive disorder respond to ECT better than younger adults, warranting consideration in the elderly, especially with psychotic depression, catatonia, intense suicidal ideas, or severe physical deterioration due to their mental illness.
- There is no standardized technique regarding ECT for the elderly, so stimulus dosing above seizure threshold, brief or ultrabrief pulse width parameters, and electrode placement should be guided by clinical parameters such as need for speed of response, cognitive impairment risk, and refractoriness to previous ECT stimulus/placement parameters.

2. Physiological Effects and Risks of ECT

2.1 Electric Stimulus

Parasympathetic (vagal) stimulation
- Risk of bradycardia and bradyarrhythmias
- Risk of asystole

Direct stimulation of muscles for jaw contraction
- Jaw clenching despite neuromuscular blockade
- Risk of dental, oral, jaw injuries

2.2 Seizure Induction

- Sympathetic discharge
  - Tachycardia
  - Hypertension
    - 2 to 4x increase in rate-pressure product
    - Risk of myocardial ischemia
    - Risk of abdominal aortic aneurysm rupture
    - Risk of stroke but no conclusive cases reported
  - May need pre-ECT beta blockers to attenuate
- Atrial or ventricular tachyarrhythmias – usually self-limiting
- Risk if severe aortic stenosis
- Increased cerebral blood flow/oxygen extraction/glucose metabolism
- Increased intracranial pressure – risk if brain tumour with midline shift
- More permeable blood-brain barrier
- Increased intraocular pressure – risk if closed angle glaucoma or recent retinal detachment
- Increased intragastric pressure – risk of reflux/aspiration

2.3 Indications

(American Psychiatric Association, 2001)

- Primary indications: general axis I (DSM-IV-TR) conditions for which ECT indicated
  - Depression
  - Mania and related conditions
  - Schizophrenia and related conditions
- Primary features for which ECT more likely to be prescribed: mood disorders
  - Acute suicidality with high risk of acting out suicidal thoughts
  - Psychotic features
  - Rapidly deteriorating physical status due to complications from the depression, such as poor oral intake
  - History of poor response to medications
  - History of good response to ECT
  - Patient preference
  - Risks of standard antidepressant treatment outweigh the risks of ECT, particularly in medically frail or elderly patients
  - Catatonic features
- Primary indications: mania
  - Primary features as reflected above
  - Extreme agitation
  - "Manic delirium"
- Primary indications: schizophrenia and related disorders
  - Positive symptoms with abrupt or recent onset
  - Catatonia
  - History of good response to ECT
  - Affective component of schizoaffective disorder
  - Refractory psychosis +/– clozapine
- Secondary indications
  - Catatonia unrelated to mood or psychotic disorder
  - Parkinson's disease and motor symptoms
  - Neuroleptic malignant syndrome
  - Mood disorder secondary to a physical condition
  - Refractory delirium
  - Intractable status epilepticus

3. Technique

3.1 Determinants of Beneficial Effects vs Cognitive Side Effects

- Waveform
  - Square pulse wave devices are now standard (Figure 2.6.1)
  - Older generation sine wave devices should not be used due to a much greater risk for cognitive impairment

Figure 2.6.1: Ultrabrief, Brief, and Sine Wave Pulses

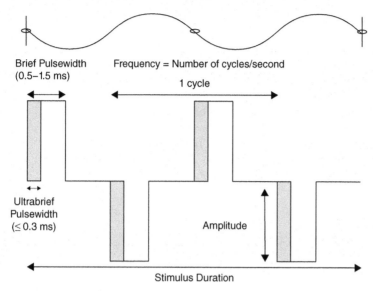

Source: Loo et al., 2012.

- Dosing
  - Incremental stimulus dosing to find seizure threshold is the best way to find seizure threshold (ST)
  - Right unilateral (RUL) ECT: aim for 4–6x ST; bitemporal (BT)/bifrontal (BF) ECT: aim for 1.5–2.5x ST
  - Stimulus dosing below this range increases the chance for lack of response
  - Stimulus dosing above this range increases the chances of cognitive dysfunction
- Placement: BT, RUL, BF
- Pulse width: standard/brief pulse width (SBPW) vs ultrabrief pulse width (UBPW)
  - Placement vs pulse width (see Table 2.6.1)
    - Brief pulse width, bitemporal ECT still considered the gold standard

Table 2.6.1: Differential Effects in Relation to Placement and Pulse Width

Placement	Therapeutic Range	Response	Cognitive Side Effects	Seizure Expression
RUL UBPW	4–6X ST	++	+	+
RUL SBPW	4–6X ST	++	+ (++)	++
BF UBPW	1.5–2.5X ST	++?	++	+ (++)
BF SBPW	1.5–2.5X ST	++	++	++
BT*	1.5–2.5X ST	++ (+++)	++ (+++)	++ (+++)

BF = bifrontal; BT = bitemporal7; RUL = right unilateral; SBPW = standard/brief pulse width (.5–1.5 ms); ST = seizure threshold; UBPW = ultrabrief pulse width (< 0.5 ms)

*Bitemporal SB PW: conflicting evidence for BT UBPW ECT (Sackeim, 2008); BT more rapid response compared to UL ECT

4. Seizure Threshold Determinants (Increased Threshold)

- Age: older > younger
- Male > female
- BF placement > BT placement > RUL placement
- Concurrent medications (e.g., benzodiazepines)
- Anaesthetic dosage
- Certain anaesthetic agents (esp. propofol) over others

5. ECT Response Rates vs Remission in Older Adults

5.1 General Response in Treating Major Depressive Disorder

- Generally: 75–85%
- Elderly: 80–90%
- Med-resistant (non-elderly): 60–70%

5.2 Speed of Response and Remission
(Husain et al., 2004)

- Multicentre, prospective randomized controlled trial (RCT); numerous subsequent publications from the CORE (Consortium of Researchers for ECT) group
- Mean age 56.2 years (range = 19–85 years), 30% psychotic depressed
- N = 253 major depressive disorder (MDD), 1.5T bitemporal ECT index series
- 86% completers, 80% response overall
- Treatment-resistant depression was not a predictor of response.
- Psychotic depressed cohort remitted faster compared to non-psychotic depressed cohort.
- Figure 2.6.2 shows the ECT number at which this cohort initially achieved responder status, sustained responder status, and remitter status.

Figure 2.6.2: Response and Remission during Index ECT: CORE Trial

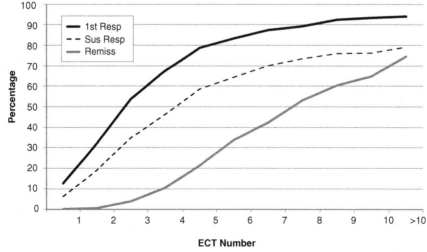

Source: Hussain et al., 2004.

- Prolonged Remission in Depressed Elderly (PRIDE) trial: recently completed RCT from the CORE group (Kellner et al., 2016)
  - Age 60 and over, unipolar depressed, 240 patients
  - RUL-UB pulse width ECT augmented with venlafaxine (phase 1); then remitters randomized to 6 months of continuation ECT plus venlafaxine and lithium, or continuation lithium and venlafaxine without ECT (phase 2)
  - Phase 1 index series showed 61.7% remitters, 28.3% dropout; it supports the efficacy of this form of ECT in the elderly. Phase 2 showed that the ECT plus medication group had statistically lower HAM-D scores than the medication alone group.

6. ECT for Late-Onset Depression

- Right unilateral and bilateral ECT placement can be effective.
- Possible cognitive improvement when Mini Mental State Examination (MMSE) < 24, as depressive symptoms remit, though less improvement seen with bilateral ECT (Tielkes et al., 2008).
- Dementia of depression (previously called "pseudodementia") can respond well to ECT (Wagner et al., 2011; Rapinesi et al., 2013).
- Late-onset geriatric depression is a predictor for developing dementia later (Barnes et al., 2012; Byers & Yaffe, 2011) as 2–4X risk, so monitor cognition longitudinally.

7. ECT for Depression in Dementia

- Cornell Scale for Depression in Dementia (CSDD) may help differentiate; Geriatric Depression Scale (GDS) validated for use in those with mild-moderate dementia with caregiver assistance in completing the scale.
- Mood disorders complicating dementia can respond well to ECT (Weintraub & Lippmann, 2001; Rao & Lyketsos, 2000), BUT:
  - Non-specific effects of ECT on agitation
  - Higher risk for post-ECT delirium and lingering cognitive disturbance – consider discussing during consent
  - Only five prospective trials (Oudman, 2012)
  - Open label case series or reports of effectiveness of ECT for refractory behavioural and psychological symptoms of dementia (BPSD) not necessarily related to depression (Ujkaj et al., 2012)

8. Consent
(American Psychiatric Association, 2001)

- Patients should be reviewed for ability to consent for, or refuse, ECT even if they have been deemed incapable of consenting to pharmacotherapy.
- Assent ≠ consent
- Depressed patients can be highly ambivalent and unable to make a decision, even though they may seem to understand and repeat the information given.
- Some may understand the information, but may still be deemed not capable to consent if they fail to appreciate the consequences or how it applies to their situation (Appelbaum, 2007).

- Severely depressed elderly patients can give consent, particularly with standardized ECT information (Lapid et al., 2004).
- Some patients with dementia may be capable of consenting to ECT; consistency in response when presented with the same information is a better gauge than ability to retain information from one day to the next.
- Figure 2.6.3 shows the percentage of Canadian ECT responding sites that endorsed discussing these six key elements for ECT consent.

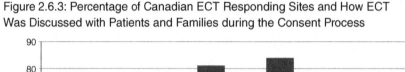

Figure 2.6.3: Percentage of Canadian ECT Responding Sites and How ECT Was Discussed with Patients and Families during the Consent Process

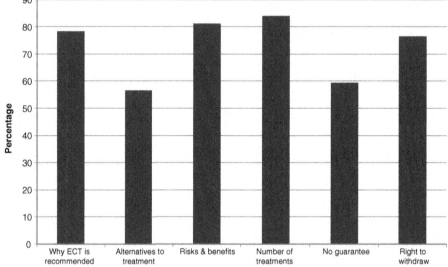

Reprinted with permission from Chan et al., 2012.

- Figure 2.6.4 shows the method (%) used by Canadian ECT responding sites to discuss ECT with patients and families during the consent process.
- ECT information video from the British Columbia ECT guidelines (British Columbia Ministry of Health Services & Mheccu, 2002) now available free:
  - http://www.canects.org/patients.php (English)
  - http://www.canects.org/french/accueil.php (French)
  - About 20 minutes long and shows a real-life ECT performed
  - Video available in English, French, Cantonese, Punjabi

9. Concurrent Psychotropic Medications

- Generally pharmacotherapy can be safely combined with ECT.
- Most patients on maintenance ECT are concurrently on maintenance pharmacotherapy, but maintenance ECT alone has been prescribed successfully.
- Despite theoretical concerns of bradycardia, prolonged seizure, or prolonged apnea with succinylcholine, cholinesterase inhibitors (ChEIs) can often be given safely and uneventfully during ECT. ChEIs should be continued in most instances, as there may

Figure 2.6.4: Methods of Providing ECT Information to Patients and Families

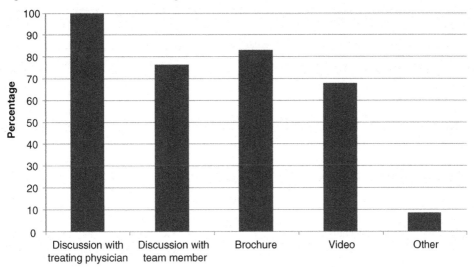

Reprinted with permission from Chan et al., 2012.

also be some risk for cognitive worsening if held during the ECT course (Hausner et al., 2011). Studies evaluating starting a ChEI in order to prevent or treat ECT-related cognitive dysfunction have been generally disappointing, and not recommended forroutine use at this time.

- For benzodiazepines, anticonvulsants (for use in bipolar disorder), or lithium, if unable to taper, then hold dose the night before the ECT and the morning of ECT prior to the treatment.

- If benzodiazepine dependent, especially at higher doses, do not taper abruptly prior to ECT due to risk of prolonged ECT-induced seizure. Elderly may have high seizure thresholds during the course of ECT, which will trigger a re-examination of any medications with anticonvulsant effect.

- Geriatric serum lithium level therapeutic range = 0.3–0.8 mEq/L. Theoretical risks of excessive cognitive disturbance, prolonged apnea, and spontaneous seizures with the combination, but it can be combined safely (Dolenc & Rasmussen, 2005).

- Emerging evidence that adding nortriptyline or venlafaxine prescribed early in an index ECT course can increase response rates (Sackeim et al., 2009).

- Most antidepressants can be safely given, but consider switch to another class during ECT if the patient already relapsed on the current medication regime.

- Bupropion and clozapine can significantly lower the seizure threshold, so warrant caution.

- See Table 2.6.2 for a comparison of recommendations on concomitant pharmacotherapy during ECT.

10. Tolerability

10.1 Overall Very Safe and Rapid-Acting Treatment

- One of the lowest risk procedures involving anaesthesia
- Major issues related to public misconceptions and acceptability of the procedure

Table 2.6.2: Comparison of Recommendations on Concomitant Pharmacotherapy during ECT

Medication	APA	UK	Haskett*	BC
Benzodiazepines	Taper if feasible	Avoid if possible	–	Taper or switch
Antipsychotics	OK	OK, caution with clozapine	More evidence	OK
MAOIs	Not usually d/c	OK	–	OK
Other antidepressants	OK	OK, caution with TCAs and venlafaxine	Augment	OK, avoid bupropion
Lithium	d/c or low level	d/c or low level	d/c	Low level OK
Anticonvulsant	d/c if for psych	OK to continue	–	OK
Zopiclone	OK if needed	OK to use	–	–
ChEIs	–	OK to use	–	–

d/c = discontinue; ECT = electroconvulsive therapy; MAOI = monoamine oxidase inhibitor; TCA = tricyclic antidepressant

*Adjunctive psychotropic medications during electroconvulsive therapy in the treatment of depression, mania, and schizophrenia (Haskett & Loo, 2010)

Adapted from American Psychiatric Association (APA), 2001; Waite & Easton, 2013; Hasket & Loo, 2010; British Columbia Ministry of Health Services/Mheccu, 2002.

10.2 Anaesthesia-Related Common Side Effects
(American Psychiatric Association, 2001; Datto, 2000)

- Burning on administration (methohexital, propofol)
- Muscle aches and pains (succinylcholine)
- Nausea
- Emergence paralysis

10.3 ECT-Related Common Side Effects
(American Psychiatric Association, 2001; Datto, 2000; Tess & Smetana, 2009)

- Bradycardia, transient asystole
- Cardiac ectopy (18% over 85), changes to ST segment
- Transient hypertension (67% over 85)
- Jaw pain
- Dental injury, orobuccal lacerations
- Headache
- Nausea and vomiting
- Postictal confusion
- Falls (36% in over 80, 14% in 65 to 80)

10.4 Measures to Manage ECT-Related Common Side Effects

- Atropine and glycopyrrolate to prevent bradycardia and asystole during titration
- Bite block every time to prevent dental injury
- Oral non-steroidal anti-inflammatory drugs (NSAIDs) pre- or post- treatment, ketorolac IV pre-treatment, intranasal sumatriptan for headaches
- Labetalol or esmolol for hypertension; should not use routinely due to reduction in seizure length and quality. Aggressive medical management is preferred. Don't hold antihypertensives before treatment.
- IV anti-emetic such as granisetron or ondansetron for nausea

10.5 Poor Quality (Poor Coherence, Amplitude, Regularity, and Postictal Suppression) or Missed Seizures

- Ensure vigorous pre-oxygenation.
- If patient on benzo consider flumazenil.
- Increase stimulus intensity.
- Consider switching electrode position; and/or
- Consider switching pulse width.
- Consider switching anaesthesia meds: methohexital less anticonvulsant than propofol; can reduce propofol and methohexital by combining with remifentanil.
- Consider ketamine if unable to achieve seizures; give midazolam post-seizure to prevent dissociation.

11. Cognitive Side Effects

11.1 Categories of Cognitive Impairment

- Postictal confusion disorientation lasting 15 to 60 minutes
- Postictal delirium (rare)
- Anterograde amnesia
- Retrograde amnesia
- Autobiographical memory impairment

11.2 Assessment of Cognitive Side Effects

(American Psychiatric Association, 2001; Greenberg & Kellner, 2005; Kumar et al., 2016)

- Formal vs informal
- Subjective vs objective
- Baseline assessment: Montreal Cognitive Assessment (MoCA), Columbia Autobiographical Memory Interview – Short Form (CAMI-SF), Modified Mini Mental State Examination (3MSE)
- Global cognition improves with remission of depression, but recall worsens
- Older age associated with more objective impairment of retrograde amnesia
- Patients with neurologic illness/dementia at higher risk of postictal delirium

11.3 Determinants of Cognitive Side Effects

- Electrode position (no difference between bifrontal and bitemporal); fewer cognitive side effects with RUL compared to bitemporal and bifrontal (Kellner et al., 2010)
- Pulse width: fewer side effects with ultrabrief (0.3 −0.37msec) compared to brief pulse (0.5 to 1.5 msec) (Sackeim et al., 2008)
- Concomitant medications: lithium associated with greater cognitive side effects (American Psychiatric Association, 2001)
- Anaesthetic doses/stimulus intensity: higher dose anaesthesia leads to higher stimulus intensity and thus greater cognitive side effects and worse outcomes (Bundy et al., 2010)
- Frequency of treatment (2x/week vs 3x/week): fewer cognitive side effects with twice weekly treatment compared to thrice weekly (Shapira et al., 1998)

12. Adverse Effects

12.1 Rare and Serious Side Effects
(American Psychiatric Association, 2001; Tess & Smetana, 2009; Datto, 2000)

- Deaths: 1/10 000 patients or 1/80 000 to 1/100 000 treatments (same as risk of general anaesthesia alone)
- Cardiovascular disease is high risk
- Over 80 are at higher risk
- Cardiovascular event
- Aspiration
- Allergic reaction or malignant hyperthermia

12.2 Other Rare Side Effects
(American Psychiatric Association, 2001; Tess & Smetana, 2009; Datto, 2000)

- Prolonged seizure (180 sec vs 120 sec) associated with greater postictal confusion; seizures can be terminated with double dose of induction agent, or 2 mg midazolam IV
- Spontaneous seizure
- Postictal delirium/agitation
- Prolonged apnea
- Mania or hypomania (stop treatment vs continue treatment until mood stabilizes)
- Ischemic stroke

13. Relative Contraindications

- Intracranial lesion with mass effect
- Recent stroke less than 1 month
- Recent myocardial infarction (MI) less than 1 month
- Unstable aneurysm or vascular malformation

QUESTIONS

1. List the three commonly applied electrode placements for ECT and the advantages vs disadvantages of each. How does this change with doing ultrabrief pulse width rather than brief pulse width ECT?
2. Discuss four strategies to lower seizure threshold prior to ECT or during the ECT session.
3. What are the theoretical concerns surrounding the use of cholinesterase inhibitors during ECT?
4. What are the theoretical concerns surrounding the use of lithium and ECT?
5. Your patient suffers from major depression and is at the moderate stage of Alzheimer's disease. You are the ECT consultant and practitioner. Outline the steps you would take, starting from initial contact to the end of the index course of ECT, and how it might differ from managing those without dementia. Would your approach differ if this person has severe dementia with BPSD?

ANSWERS

1. The table below summarizes the advantages and disadvantages of three commonly applied electrode placements.

ECT Type	Advantages	Disadvantages
BT	• Faster response than RUL • Considered gold standard • Good for patients who need rapid response	• More cognitive side effects compared to RUL
BF	• Faster response than RUL • Possibly fewer cognitive side effects compared to BT in elderly patients	• More cognitive impairment than RUL
RUL	• Response rates comparable to BT and BF • Ultrabrief pulse width ECT has good evidence for benefit • Fewer cognitive side effects • Good for patients with cognitive impairment while receiving bilateral ECT, or a history of cognitive side effects with bilateral ECT	• Need higher dosages (4–6x threshold), so may not be able to deliver therapeutic dose for elderly with high seizure thresholds • Slower response than with bilateral placement

BF = bifrontal; BT = bitemporal; ECT = electroconvulsive therapy; RUL = right unilateral

- Regarding ultrabrief pulse width:
  - Less cognitive risk associated with unilateral ECT, and possibly also with bilateral ECT (evidence still mounting)
  - Effective for RUL, but mixed results in bilateral ECT
  - Smaller dose delivered, resulting in more missed seizures and longer time to response and remission for some patients

2. Strategies to lower seizure threshold prior to ECT or during the ECT session include:
   - Hyperventilation and adequate pre-oxygenation prior to the ECT stimulus
   - Discontinue or taper anticonvulsants and benzodiazepines.
   - Consider intraoperative IV flumazenil for counteracting the effect of benzodiazepines.
   - Give medications to lower seizure threshold (e.g., chlorpromazine, bupropion).
   - Choice of anaesthetic agent (e.g., ketamine and etomidate lower threshold, propofol increases it)
   - May lower propofol or barbiturate dose by combining with remifentanil
   - Ensure adequate hydration (especially in elderly).
   - Switch to RUL ECT.
   - Note: caffeine and theophylline will lengthen seizure duration, but not necessarily change seizure threshold.

3. The theoretical concerns surrounding the use of cholinesterase inhibitors during ECT include:
   - Acetylcholine and succinylcholine broken down by pseudocholinesterase, so theoretically can lead to prolongation of succinylcholine effects (e.g., prolonged paralysis)
   - May enhance bradycardic response during ECT, so theoretically increases risk of asystole or prolonged seizures
   - Practically, can be given safely and often not discontinued prior to ECT (no clear evidence for positive cognitive outcomes during or post-ECT)

4. The theoretical concerns surrounding the use of lithium during ECT include:
   - Increased risk of postictal delirium, cardiac arrhythmias, and prolonged seizures
   - Worsening of cognition
   - Increased permeability of lithium into the brain during ECT ictal response
   - Decision is to continue at same dose, taper, or discontinue (geriatric therapeutic range is 0.3–0.8 usually); can hold dose the night before, and not give dose until after ECT session completed.

5. The issue of capacity and substitute decision maker is important, given the patient's moderate dementia and superimposed major depression; also, given the high rates of delirium, the patient could become incapable, even if he/she were capable prior to treatment. Additional considerations include:
   - Optimize the patient medically, minimize modifiable risk factors for delirium, and discuss the risk of delirium.
   - Consider administering ECT less frequently to begin, anticipating that there may be cognitive difficulties between sessions, although there may be no differences between patients with dementia, mild cognitive impairment (MCI), and normal cognition; cognitive function (measured by MMSE scores) may actually improve in patients with dementia following ECT, but this effect may be due to improvement in depression.
   - Differentiating depression from severe BPSD may be extremely difficult; some case reports and case series have shown that ECT has some effectiveness for BPSD, but this finding warrants further research consideration; one may use the Cornell Scale for Depression in Dementia to try to differentiate BPSD from symptoms of depression.
   - For dementia patients who benefit from ECT, deciding when to stop ECT may be difficult, especially as the dementia progresses further to a more "palliative" phase; however, there is no evidence to show that modified ECT (weekly or less frequently) is harmful at this stage of dementia.
   - Patients with dementia may have prolonged periods of confusion after ECT, though this is infrequent.

CASE DISCUSSION

1. ECT is preferable. Repetitive transcranial magnetic stimulation (rTMS) is an option, but clinics may not accept referrals for bipolar I disorder (risk of switching) and elderly (less response compared to younger adults using conventional rTMS).

2. The table below summarizes the benefits, risks, and barriers of ECT and rTMS
in this case.

Modality	Benefits	Risks/Barriers
ECT	• History of benefit (perhaps try RUL or BF first to lessen cognitive risk)	• Risk of switching to mania • Higher cognitive risk compared to rTMS • General anaesthesia required
rTMS	• Overall, risk of seizure low • Less cognitive risk compared to ECT • No anaesthetic required • Generally well tolerated • Less invasive	• Lower response rate for depression • Not readily available • Unproven for bipolar depression • Risk of seizure can be increased with use of bupropion or psychostimulants • Risk of switching to mania

BF = bifrontal; ECT = electroconvulsive therapy; rTMS = repetitive transcranial magnetic stimulation; RUL = right unilateral

3. It is important to consider other conditions that may influence the outcome with brain stimulation in this case:
   • Consider presence of obstructive sleep apnea with ECT and general anaesthesia.
   • Rule out hypothyroidism and hypercalcemia (while on lithium).
   • Rule out B12 deficiency (metformin, elderly, possible decreased intake).
   • Possible MCI or even (vascular) dementia (increases risk of cognitive side effects)
   • Possible substance abuse
   • Possible comorbid axis II disorder

4. The following considerations may be prudent in managing her medications during a course of brain stimulation treatment:
   • Consider holding bupropion due to risk for prolonged seizure.
   • Consider discontinuing or holding the morning dose of dextroamphetamine prior to ECT/rTMS due to increased risk of sympathomimetic effects with ECT stimulus, or slightly increased seizure risk with rTMS.
   • Likely safe to take aripiprazole just prior to ECT/rTMS
   • Use of lithium in ECT (see question # 6 above)
   • Discontinue, taper, or hold lamotrigine night before and morning of ECT due to higher seizure thresholds in the elderly, which may also climb during a course of ECT.
   • Take ramipril and other antihypertensives on the morning of ECT.
   • Hold metformin on the morning of ECT due to risk of hypoglycemia with fasting.
   • Take blood sugars before and after ECT.

5. Would not begin outpatient ECT, due to many comorbidities and lack of supervision at home. Obesity and possible obstructive sleep apnea are additional safety issues for anaesthesia.

6. Logistical barriers to address include transportation and supervision post-ECT, as well as cognitive dysfunction hampering adherence to fasting, attending appointments, and medications.

RECOMMENDED RESOURCES FOR REVIEW

Although these resources may not be specifically cited in the text, their approach informed the contents of the chapter, and they are recommended as useful further reading.

Kellner CH, Greenberg RM, Murrough JW, et al. ECT in treatment-resistant depression. Am J Psychiatry. 2012;169(12):1238–44. http://dx.doi.org/10.1176/appi.ajp.2012.12050648. Medline:23212054

Kerner N, Prudic J. Current electroconvulsive therapy practice and research in the geriatric population. Neuropsychiatry (London). 2014;4(1):33–54. http://dx.doi.org/10.2217/npy.14.3. PMID:24778709

Oudman E. Is electroconvulsive therapy (ECT) effective and safe for treatment of depression in dementia? A short review. J ECT. 2012;28(1):34–8. http://dx.doi.org/10.1097/YCT.0b013e31823a0f5a. Medline:22330702

Tess AV, Smetana GW. Medical evaluation of patients undergoing electroconvulsive therapy. N Engl J Med. 2009;360(14):1437–44. http://dx.doi.org/10.1056/NEJMra0707755. Medline:19339723

REFERENCES

American Psychiatric Association, Committee on Electroconvulsive Therapy. The practice of electroconvulsive therapy: recommendations for treatment, training, and privileging (A task force report of the American Psychiatric Association). 2nd ed. Washington, DC: American Psychiatric Association; 2001.

Appelbaum PS. Clinical practice. Assessment of patients' competence to consent to treatment. N Engl J Med. 2007;357(18):1834–40. http://dx.doi.org/10.1056/NEJMcp074045. Medline:17978292

Barnes DE, Yaffe K, Byers AL, et al. Midlife vs late-life depressive symptoms and risk of dementia: differential effects for Alzheimer disease and vascular dementia. Arch Gen Psychiatry. 2012;69(5):493–8. http://dx.doi.org/10.1001/archgenpsychiatry.2011.1481. Medline:22566581

Boylan LS, Haskett RF, Mulsant BH, et al. Determinants of seizure threshold in ECT: benzodiazepine use, anesthetic dosage, and other factors. J ECT. 2000;16(1):3–18. http://dx.doi.org/10.1097/00124509-200003000-00002. Medline:10735327

British Columbia Ministry of Health Services; Mental Health Evaluation & Community Consultation Unit (Mheccu). Electroconvulsive therapy: guidelines for health authorities in British Columbia. Vancouver, BC: British Columbia Ministry of Health; 2002. http://www.health.gov.bc.ca/library/publications/year/2002/MHA_ect_guidelines.pdf

Bundy BD, Hewer W, Andres FJ, et al. Influence of anesthetic drugs and concurrent psychiatric medication on seizure adequacy during electroconvulsive therapy. J Clin Psychiatry. 2010;71(6):775–7. http://dx.doi.org/10.4088/JCP.08m04971gre. Medline:20051218

Byers AL, Yaffe K. Depression and risk of developing dementia. Nat Rev Neurol. 2011;7(6):323–31. http://dx.doi.org/10.1038/nrneurol.2011.60. Medline:21537355

Chan P, Graf P, Enns M, et al. The Canadian Survey of Standards of Electroconvulsive Therapy Practice: a call for accreditation. Can J Psychiatry. 2012;57(10):634–42. Medline:23072955

Datto CJ. Side effects of electroconvulsive therapy. Depress Anxiety. 2000;12(3):130–4. http://dx.doi.org/10.1002/1520-6394(2000)12:3<130::AID-DA4>3.0.CO;2-C. Medline:11126187

Dolenc TJ, Rasmussen KG. The safety of electroconvulsive therapy and lithium in combination: a case series and review of the literature. J ECT. 2005;21(3):165–70. http://dx.doi.org/10.1097/01.yct.0000174383.96517.77. Medline:16127306

Dunne RA, McLoughlin DM. Systematic review and meta-analysis of bifrontal electroconvulsive therapy versus bilateral and unilateral electroconvulsive therapy in depression. World J Biol Psychiatry. 2012;13(4):248–58. http://dx.doi.org/10.3109/15622975.2011.615863. Medline:22098115

Enns MW, Reiss JP, Chan P. Electroconvulsive therapy: a position paper of the Canadian Psychiatric Association. Can J Psychiatry. 2010;55(6):insert 1–11.

Gosselin C, Graf P, Milev R, et al. Delivery of electroconvulsive therapy in Canada: a first national survey report on devices and technique. J ECT. 2013;29(3):225–30. http://dx.doi.org/10.1097/YCT.0b013e31827f135b. Medline:23519223

Greenberg RM, Kellner CH. Electroconvulsive therapy: a selected review. Am J Geriatr Psychiatry. 2005;13(4):268–81. Medline:15845752

Haskett RF, Loo C. Adjunctive psychotropic medications during electroconvulsive therapy in the treatment of depression, mania, and schizophrenia. J ECT. 2010;26(3):196–201. http://dx.doi.org/10.1097/YCT .0b013e3181eee13f. Medline:20805728

Hausner L, Damian M, Sartorius A, et al. Efficacy and cognitive side effects of electroconvulsive therapy (ECT) in depressed elderly inpatients with coexisting mild cognitive impairment or dementia. J Clin Psychiatry. 2011;72(1):91–7. http://dx.doi.org/10.4088/JCP.10m05973gry. Medline:21208587

Husain MM, Rush AJ, Fink M, et al. Speed of response and remission in major depressive disorder with acute electroconvulsive therapy (ECT): a Consortium for Research in ECT (CORE) report. J Clin Psychiatry. 2004;65(4):485–91. http://dx.doi.org/10.4088/JCP.v65n0406. Medline:15119910

Kellner CH, Husain MM, Knapp RG, et al. Right unilateral ultrabrief pulse ECT in geriatric depression: phase 1 of the PRIDE study. Am J Psychiatry. 2016; July 15 (epub ahead of print).

– A novel strategy for continuation ECT in geriatric depression: phase 2 of the PRIDE study. Am J Psychiatry. 2016; July 15 (epub ahead of print).

Kellner CH, Knapp R, Husain MM, et al. Bifrontal, bitemporal and right unilateral electrode placement in ECT: randomised trial. Br J Psychiatry. 2010;196(3):226–34. http://dx.doi.org/10.1192/bjp.bp.109.066183. Medline:20194546

Kumar S, Mulsant BH, Liu AY, et al. Systematic review of cognitive effects of electroconvulsive therapy in late-life depression. Am J Geriatr Psychiatry. 2016;24(7):547–65. [Epub ahead of print, 8 March 2016]. http://dx.doi.org/10.1016/j.jagp.2016.02.053. PMID:27067067

Lapid MI, Rummans TA, Pankratz VS, et al. Decisional capacity of depressed elderly to consent to electroconvulsive therapy. J Geriatr Psychiatry Neurol. 2004;17(1):42–6. http://dx.doi.org/10.1177/ 0891988703261996. Medline:15018698

Loo CK, Katalinic N, Martin D, et al. A review of ultrabrief pulse width electroconvulsive therapy. Ther Adv Chronic Dis. 2012;3(2):69–85. http://dx.doi.org/10.1177/ 2040622311432493. Medline:23251770

Rao V, Lyketsos CG. The benefits and risks of ECT for patients with primary dementia who also suffer from depression. Int J Geriatr Psychiatry. 2000;15(8):729–35. http://dx.doi.org/10.1002/1099-1166(200008) 15:8<729 ::AID-GPS193>3.0.CO;2-A. Medline:10960885

Rapinesi C, Serata D, Del Casale A, et al. Depressive pseudodementia in the elderly: effectiveness of electro-convulsive therapy. Int J Geriatr Psychiatry. 2013;28(4):435–8. http://dx.doi.org/10.1002/gps.3877. Medline:23468198

Sackeim HA, Dillingham EM, Prudic J, et al. Effect of concomitant pharmacotherapy on electroconvulsive therapy outcomes: short-term efficacy and adverse effects. Arch Gen Psychiatry. 2009;66(7):729–37. http:// dx.doi.org/10.1001/archgen psychiatry.2009.75. Medline:19581564

Sackeim HA, Prudic J, Devanand DP, et al. The impact of medication resistance and continuation pharmaco-therapy on relapse following response to electroconvulsive therapy in major depression. J Clin Psychopharma-col. 1990;10(2):96–104. http://dx.doi.org/10.1097/00004714-199004000-00004. Medline:2341598

Sackeim HA, Prudic J, Nobler MS, et al. Effects of pulse width and electrode placement on the efficacy and cognitive effects of electroconvulsive therapy. Brain Stimul. 2008;1(2):71–83. http://dx.doi.org/10.1016/ j.brs.2008.03.001. Medline:19756236

Shapira B, Tubi N, Drexler H, et al. Cost and benefit in the choice of ECT schedule. Twice versus three times weekly ECT. Br J Psychiatry. 1998;172(1):44–8. http://dx.doi.org/10.1192/bjp.172.1.44. Medline:9534831

Sienaert P, Peuskens J. Anticonvulsants during electroconvulsive therapy: review and recommendations. J ECT. 2007;23(2):120–3. http://dx.doi.org/10.1097/YCT.0b013e3180330059. Medline:17548985

Tielkes CE, Comijs HC, Verwijk E, et al. The effects of ECT on cognitive functioning in the elderly: a review. Int J Geriatr Psychiatry. 2008;23(8):789–95. http://dx.doi .org/10.1002/gps.1989. Medline:18311845

Ujkaj M, Davidoff DA, Seiner SJ, et al. Safety and efficacy of electroconvulsive therapy for the treatment of agitation and aggression in patients with dementia. Am J Geriatr Psychiatry. 2012;20(1):61–72. http:// dx.doi.org/10.1097/JGP.0b013e3182051bbc. Medline:22143072

van Schaik AM, Comijs HC, Sonnenberg CM, et al. Efficacy and safety of continuation and maintenance electroconvulsive therapy in depressed elderly patients: a systematic review. Am J Geriatr Psychiatry. 2012;20(1):5–17. http://dx.doi.org/ 10.1097/JGP.0b013e31820dcbf9. Medline:22183009

Wagner GS, McClintock SM, Rosenquist PB, et al. Major depressive disorder with psychotic features may lead to misdiagnosis of dementia: a case report and review of the literature. J Psychiatr Pract. 2011;17(6):432–8. http://dx.doi.org/10.1097/01 .pra.0000407968.57475.ab. Medline:22108402

Waite J, Easton A, editors; Royal College of Psychiatrists. The ECT handbook. 3rd ed. Fourth report of the Royal College of Psychiatrists' Special Committee on ECT (College Report CR176). London: Royal College of Psychiatrists; 2013.

Weintraub D, Lippmann SB. ECT for major depression and mania with advanced dementia. J ECT. 2001;17(1):65–7. http://dx.doi.org/10.1097/00124509-200103000-00014. Medline:11281520

2.7 Psychotherapy in Older Adults

Keri-Leigh Cassidy, MD, FRCPC
Lesley Wiesenfeld, MD, FRCPC
Janya Freer, MD, FRCPC

INTRODUCTION

An increasing number of recent treatment studies demonstrate the effectiveness of psychotherapy in the patients seen by geriatric psychiatrists. With some modifications in the focus and technique, we can use similar treatments as those used with younger patients. Drs Cassidy, Freer, and Wiesenfeld provide an evidence-based review of the field with examples from different types of psychotherapeutic interventions as well as specifics that apply to an older population.

CASE SCENARIO

Mrs C. is an active 67-year-old accountant who retired this year. After her retirement, she developed a major depressive episode (e.g., irritable with husband, tearful, loss of interest/socializing, insomnia, loss of appetite). She had hoped in her retirement to have more time with grandchildren and travel with her husband, but is now wondering what there is to look forward to after all. You are considering a course of interpersonal psychotherapy (IPT).

1. Choose an interpersonal problem area.
2. What are some useful questions to ask for the interpersonal problem area?
3. What are some of Mrs C.'s tasks in the chosen problem area?

OVERVIEW

1. Major Themes

- Relevance of using psychotherapy as a treatment in senior patients
- Overview of the evidence base for psychotherapy in late life
- Indications for the use of psychotherapy in older adults (cognitive behavioural therapy, interpersonal psychotherapy, psychodynamic psychotherapy, and reminiscence and group psychotherapies)
- Overview of models and core techniques used; differences among treatment approaches (cognitive behavioural therapy, interpersonal psychotherapy, psychodynamic, reminiscence, and group psychotherapies)
- Considerations and modifications of psychotherapy for older adults

2. History and Relevance

2.1 History of Psychotherapy for Older Adults

- The evidence base for psychotherapy for older adults lags compared to psycho-therapeutic treatments for depression/anxiety in younger adults, and compared to evidence for biological therapies.
- Psychotherapy for seniors is often not considered by clinicians.
- Resources remain scarce, and access to psychotherapy for older adults is limited.
- The field of psychiatry and psychotherapy has a historical negative bias towards older adults – due to ageism, clinicians may employ therapeutic nihilism and view older adults as "untreatable" with psychotherapy.

2.2 Medical Relevance: Arguments for Using Psychotherapy as a Treatment in Older Adults

(Walker & Clarke, 2001; de Beurs et al., 1999; Alexopoulos, 2005; Blazer, 1989; Kiosses, Leon, & Areán, 2011; Beekman et al., 1995)

- Anxiety and depressive disorders common in this age group – associated high morbidity/mortality.
- Older adults have heterogeneous response to medication.
    - Only 1/4 to 1/3 respond robustly to medications at 1–3 years follow-up.
    - Older adults are prone to relapse/recurrence.
        - Risk factors for relapse are older age at index, poor self-rated health, medical illness, social isolation, baseline anxiety, personality pathology.
- Medications' adverse effects: benzodiazepines – confusion, incontinence, falls (OR 1.5–2.0); SSRIs – hyponatremia, arrhythmias, falls (OR 1.5)

2.3 Psychological Relevance: Age-Related Vulnerabilities Suited to Psychotherapy

"The mark of a noble society is found … not in how it protects the powerful but in how it de-fends the vulnerable."

(Osei Darkwa, 1997)

- Physical change, chronic illness
- Loss/grief/bereavement – actual, anticipated
- Cognitive decline
- Role changes, e.g., retirement, parenting, spousal
- Productivity/creativity
- Abandonment – institutionalization
- Forced dependency
- Societal devaluation – shame, humiliation
- Loss of control, influence, vitality, leadership, and authority
- Economic losses
- Displacement by youth
- Sexual decline/concerns about attractiveness
- Facing regrets
- Relinquishing fantasies
- Facing foreshortened future
- Eriksonian stage of integrity vs despair impacting on a wish for a coherent narrative
- Facing and preparing for death

2.4 Practical Relevance: Older Adults Can Be Very Good Psychotherapy Candidates!

- Compliance/attendance
- Maturity
- Motivation

2.5 CBT's Social Relevance: Longevity, Resiliency, and the "Positive Psychiatry" Movement

(MacCourt et al., 2011; Alzheimer Society, 2010; Levy et al., 2002; Jeste et al., 2013; Poon et al., 2010)

- Longevity research indicates "outlook" is more important than life events or physical health factors.
- Centenarians share attributes of optimism, adaptability, positive attitudes towards aging.
- Older age is associated with higher self-rated successful aging.
- Additional years of life (7.5 years) is associated with positive vs negative self-perceptions of aging.
- There has been a national call for increased mental health promotion for older adults:
  - Mental Health Commission of Canada Guidelines for Older Adults
  - Alzheimer Society Rising Tide document
- International call for a "positive psychiatry" movement to actively promote resiliency in late life
- "The Fountain of Health Initiative for Optimal Aging" is a Canadian "positive psychiatry of aging" initiative. The Fountain of Health translates the science of healthy aging and resilience to the public and healthcare providers to help shift the disease paradigm of aging. Informed by cognitive behavioural therapy principles, Fountain of Health clinical tools can be used in the office to challenge negative age stereotypes, and help patients set and reach health behaviour change goals. See http://fountainofhealth.ca
- Cognitive behavioural therapy (CBT) holds particular relevance to identify and shift cognitions, such as attitudes about aging.
- More research is needed!

3. Evidence: Does Psychotherapy Work for Older Adults?

3.1 Summary of Evidence: General Overview

- Most of the existing evidence is regarding the treatment of depression
- Most commonly applied are:
  - Cognitive behavioural therapy (CBT)
  - Interpersonal psychotherapy (IPT)
  - Psychodynamic psychotherapy (PP)
- Best evidence for CBT
- Less evidence supporting IPT, but looks promising
- Some evidence to support problem-solving therapy (PST)
- Group therapy = individual treatment; small evidence base for short-term

- Psychodynamic psychotherapy (PP) – efficacy compared to medication has not been established
- Reminiscence psychotherapy (RP) research quality remains poor overall.
  - RP might improve depression, life satisfaction, self-esteem in older adults.
  - Modest psychosocial benefits of RP in older adults with dementia

3.2 Strongest Evidence Is for CBT

- Numerous meta-analyses support the efficacy of CBT in treating depression and anxiety in younger adults.
- Some published randomized controlled trials (RCTs) support CBT in late-life depression or anxiety.
- Newer meta-analyses also support use of CBT in late life (Table 2.7.1; further details provided in sections 3.2.1 to 3.2.4).

Table 2.7.1: Meta-Analyses Supporting the Use of CBT in Older Adults

Meta-analysis: Authors, Year	Number of Studies
Scogin & McElreath, 1994	17 studies
Koder, Brodaty, & Anstey, 1996	7 studies
Engels & Verney, 1997	17 studies
Gerson et al., 1999	45 studies
*Pinquart & Sörensen, 2001	122 studies
Pinquart, Duberstein, & Lyness, 2006	89 studies
*Wilson, Mottram, & Vassilas, 2008	Cochrane Review: 9 studies
* Kiosses, Leon, & Areán, 2011	144 studies

* = most key studies

3.2.1 Evidence for CBT in Older Adults with Depression

- RCT (Thompson et al., 2001)
  - Mild-moderate depressed older outpatients, n = 102
    - CBT plus desipramine > CBT alone > desipramine alone
- Meta-analysis (Pinquart & Sörensen, 2001)
  - Self-rated depression, n = 646
    - CBT vs psychoeducation, d: 0.64 (medium effect size) vs 0.29 (small effect size)
  - Clinician-rated depression, n = 342
    - CBT vs supportive, d: 1.18 (very large effect size) vs 0.61 (medium effect size)
- Meta-analysis (Kiosses, Leon, & Areán, 2011)
  - 6/404 studies included
  - Conclusion: "CBT probably efficacious, pending replication"

3.2.2 Evidence for CBT in Older Adults with Anxiety

- RCTs (generalized anxiety):
  - Barrowclough et al., 2001: n = 55; CBT; 71% (response rate at 12 mo. follow-up) vs support only 39% (response rate at 12 mo. follow-up)
  - Wetherell, Gatz, & Craske, 2003: n = 75; CBT; d = 0.79 (large effect size) vs discussion d = 0.36 (medium effect size) vs wait list d = 0.05 (small effect size)
  - Stanley et al., 2003: n = 85; CBT 45% (responders) vs control 8% (responders)

3.2.3 Cochrane Review: "Psychotherapy Treatments for Older Depressed People"
(Wilson et al., 2008)

- Meta-analysis
- 12 trials eligible for review
- 9 trials with data used in meta-analysis
- All examined CBT or psychodynamic therapies
- 7 trials with data for CBT vs. controls
- IPT data was insufficient for inclusion
- Conclusions:
  - CBT more effective than wait-list controls (weighted mean difference [WMD] -9.85, 95% CI -11.97 to -7.73) (5 trials)
  - Psychodynamic therapy = CBT (no sig diff) (3 trials)
  - CBT superior to active controls on Hamilton Rating Scale for Depression (HAM-D), but equivalent to active interventions on Geriatric Depression Scale (GDS) (3 trials)
  - Few high quality RCTs addressing psychotherapy for late-life depression
  - Small number and heterogeneity of trials/patients eligible for inclusion (the largest study of CBT vs wait-list controls was not included)
  - "CBT is efficacious in older people compared to wait-list controls."

3.2.4 "Enhanced" CBT for Older Adults
(Mohlman et al., 2003)

- Two pilot studies compared:
  - Pilot 1: standard CBT (n = 14) vs wait list (n = 13)
  - Pilot 2: "enhanced" CBT (n = 8) vs wait list (n = 7)
- "Enhanced" learning and memory aids:
  - Homework reminder
  - Troubleshooting calls
  - Weekly review of all concepts and techniques
- Conclusion: larger effect sizes for enhanced CBT vs standard CBT in older adults

3.3 Evidence for Interpersonal Psychotherapy in Older Adults
(Weissman et al., 1979; Miller, 2008)

- Efficacy established for younger adults in two initial studies
- Lack of RCTs and adequately powered studies in geriatric population for interpersonal psychotherapy (IPT)
- IPT in older adults most supported in the maintenance phase

- Ongoing controlled studies, IPT being adapted for depressed older adults with cognitive impairment
- Conclusion from Cochrane Review: "Insufficient evidence for inclusion in meta-analysis"

3.4 Problem-Solving Therapy (PST)

(Kiosses, Leon, & Areán, 2011)

- PST model: a form of CBT focusing on actions/goal setting
- Targets depression
- Systematically teaches patients skills to improve coping with *specific* everyday problems/life crises
- Techniques:
    - Identify problems
    - Brainstorm solutions
    - Create action plans
    - Evaluate effectiveness of plans in finding solutions

3.4.1 Evidence for Problem-Solving Therapy

- Two randomized control trials:
    - Areán & Cook, 2002: PST vs supportive therapy in 221 older subjects with major depressive disorder (MDD) and executive dysfunction
        - Greater reduction in depression (HAM-D) than supportive therapy participants at weeks 9 and 12
    - Alexopoulos 2005: PST vs reminiscence therapy
        - Greater reduction in depression for PST than reminiscence therapy or wait-list controls
- Conclusion from meta-analysis (Kiosses, Leon, & Areán, 2011): "PST is probably efficacious in reducing depression and disability in the elderly."

3.5 Treatment Initiation and Participation (TIP) Therapy

- TIP model: based on "theory of reasoned actions"
- Used in primary care in conjunction with medication
- Focus on thoughts/behaviours interfering with medication compliance
- Technique: uses CBT to improve adherence to pharmacological treatment (addresses stigma, fear)
- Brief intervention (3 sessions of 30 min each, and 2 follow-up phone calls)
- Identifies barriers to adherence to meds

3.5.1 Evidence for TIP Therapy (Sirey, Bruce, & Alexopoulos, 2005)

- RCT: 52 older adults with MDD
- Conclusion: greater reduction in depression at 12 weeks compared to treatment as usual (82% adhered to medication vs 43% controls)

3.6 Evidence for Dynamic Therapy
(Garner, 2002; Mackin & Areán, 2005)

- Brief dynamic psychotherapy has small evidence base for late-life depression
- Efficacy vs medication not yet established

3.7. Evidence for Reminiscence Therapy
(Webster, Bohlmeijer, & Westerhof, 2010; Mackin & Areán, 2005)

- Reminiscence therapy techniques target depression, self-esteem in elderly
- Modest psychosocial benefits in dementia
- Quality of literature varied
- Limitations: lack of conceptual clarity with respect to technique, target outcomes, poor experimental design

3.8 Evidence for Group Therapy
(Barlow et al., 2000; Leszcz, 2009; Pinquart & Sörensen, 2001; Payne & Marcus, 2008)

- Meta-analyses regarding effectiveness: greater improvement in group treatment vs controls
    - Significantly superior to no treatment for geriatric depression
- Evidence mixed with respect to group vs individual treatment:
    - "Rationally employed and conceptually sound groups" equally effective as individual treatment
    - Individual = group for self-rated depression
    - Greater improvements individual vs group for clinician-rated depression and self-rated well-being
    - Individual = group (effect sizes may be smaller than reported with younger adults)

4. Indications for Various Psychotherapies in Older Adults

Table 2.7.2 describes the indication and other suitability factors associated with the discussed psychotherapies.

5. Models and Techniques of Psychotherapy in Older Adults: Cognitive Behavioural Therapy

5.1 CBT Techniques: Phases (and Tasks) of Treatment

- Initial phase – weeks 1–4 (tasks: introduce model, set goals, introduce tools/materials)
- Intermediate phase – weeks 5–16 (tasks: use of automatic thought records, identifying hot thoughts/conditional assumptions, making cognitive shifts, behavioural experiments)
- Termination – weeks 16–20 (tasks: review of goals, identifying effective tools, work remaining, plans to address post-therapy period)

Table 2.7.2: Psychotherapies in Older Adults and Respective Indications

Modality	Indications/Suitability Factors
Cognitive behavioural therapy	• Geriatric depression, anxiety, insomnia • Relapse prevention • Patient able to identify automatic thoughts • Patient able to identify a here and now focus • Seeking symptoms resolution • Can be adapted successfully in mildly cognitively impaired patient
Interpersonal psycho-therapy	• Focus on grief, interpersonal disputes, and role transitions • Indicated for geriatric depression and relapse prevention • Addresses psychosocial triggers not addressed by medication treatment
Dynamic psychotherapy	• Focus on connections between past relationships, unresolved conflicts, defenses, and current functioning • Mechanism of change is insight • Requires sufficient psychological mindedness to participate and benefit from dynamic interpretations
Reminiscence psychotherapy	• For treatment of mild depressive symptoms • Can be adapted for support of patients with mild cognitive symptoms
Group psychotherapy	• For social isolation, interpersonal skills

5.2 The Cognitive Model: CBT "Triangles"

The following diagram, or triangle, demonstrates the relationship between thoughts, feelings, and behaviours, and is a useful model for understanding cognitive behavioural therapies (Figure 2.7.1).

• Dynamic, inter-relationship among thoughts, feelings, and behaviours
• Premise: all thoughts not created equally; some thoughts more helpful than others
• Methods: identify distorted/unhelpful thoughts (Figure 2.7.2) and change to more accurate/helpful thoughts
• Outcomes: helpful thoughts can improve moods and promote more adaptive behaviours

Figure 2.7.1: The Cognitive Triangle

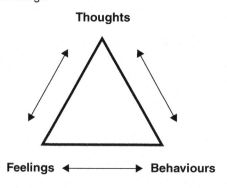

Figure 2.7.2: Cognitive Schema of Depression

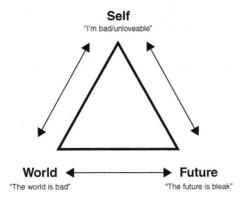

Self
"I'm bad/unloveable"

World
"The world is bad"

Future
"The future is bleak"

5.2.1 CBT Model: The Three Different Levels of Conscious Thought

- Automatic thoughts: "self-talk"; situation-specific
- Conditional assumptions
- Core beliefs: unconditional beliefs about self
  - Basic views of self, crosses all situations
  - Two main themes:
    - Sociotropic (interpersonal, relationships; example: "I'm unlovable")
    - Autonomous (work, performance; example: "I'm incompetent")

5.2.2 CBT: What Are Distortions?

- Distortions are patterns or types of thoughts that maintain negative thinking.
- Naming them allows for objectifying the thought patterns and questioning their validity.
- Examples of distortions:
  - *All or nothing**: sees things in black or white
    Example: "My vision is poor so I can never go anywhere."
  - *Overgeneralization*: sees a single negative event as a never ending pattern
    Example: "This antidepressant medication hasn't worked for me; I will never find one that does."
  - *Mind reading**: arbitrarily concludes someone is reacting negatively (without checking it out)
    Example: "She missed our lunch date because she doesn't like me anymore."
  - *Catastrophizing**: attributes extreme and horrible consequences of events (worst case scenario).
    Example: "I am sure this pain in my chest means I am having a heart attack."
  - *Disqualifying the positive**: rejects positive experiences; insists they "don't count"
    Example: "Just because I managed to make dinner for the whole family doesn't mean I'm capable in the kitchen – I just got lucky this time."
  - *Emotional reasoning*: assumes negative emotions reflect the way things are
    Example: "I feel hurt; therefore she intended to hurt my feelings."

– *Should statements**: motivates with guilt
    Example: "I *should* write my Christmas cards."
– *Labelling*: uses extreme overgeneralization, emotionally loaded language
    Example: "I am just an old 'has-been."
– *Personalization*: sees self as cause, responsible for negative outcomes
* = particularly common among depressed/anxious older adults

5.3 Common CBT Techniques

• *Socratic questions*: open-ended questions the patient has the knowledge to answer
    Example: "What are some other possible reasons your friend hasn't called lately?"
• *Guided discovery*: questions that bring information to the patient's attention
    Example: "How might you be able to apply this experience to other situations in the future?"
• *Collaborative empiricism*: patient and therapist work together to form hypotheses about patient's thoughts and behaviours
    Example: "Your homework last week was to phone your son, but you haven't been able to yet. Let's work together to try to better understand what might be getting in your way of achieving this goal."
• *Downward arrow technique*: therapist's method of questioning automatic thoughts to uncover core beliefs
    Example: "If that were true, then what would that mean about you?"

5.3.1 Ways to Untwist Thinking

• *Labelling distortions*: have patient identify which distortions he or she uses
    Example: "When you said 'The evening was a disaster,' what kind of distortion were you using?"
• *Cognitive continuum*: "thinking in shades of grey"
    Example: "You said you think you are a bad mother. How would you define the very worst mother? Or the very best mother? Now where would you put yourself on this scale?"
• *Automatic thought records*: weighing the evidence
    Example: "Using this thought record, what evidence is there for and against the accuracy of this thought?"
• *Double-standard technique*: judging the self more harshly than others
    Example, "If your good friend Mary was in this same situation, what would you say to her? How does compare to what you said to yourself?"
• *Pros and cons*: weighing risks to benefits
    Example: "What are possible advantages of attending a walking club? What are the disadvantages?"
• *Be a scientist*: check it out.
    Example: "Consider giving your friend a call, then record and examine your thoughts and mood after the phone call. Would you be willing to try and just see what happens?"

6. Models and Techniques of Psychotherapy in Older Adults: Interpersonal Psychotherapy

6.1 IPT: Model

- Manualized, time-limited, weekly outpatient treatment for depression
- Goals: relieve symptoms, address here and now (current not past)
- Methods:
    - Combines psychodynamics (exploration, clarification of affect) and CBT (behaviour change, reality checking)
    - Connection between depression onset and current interpersonal problems used as treatment focus
    - Symptoms/dysfunction secondary to depression and external relations to others are *not* considered an enduring aspect of personality or internal conflict.

6.2 Four IPT Problem Areas

- *Role dispute*: spouse, other family member (adult child), friend, other supports
- *Role transition*: relationship, health change, move, retirement, loss of ideal
- *Grief*: most commonly spouse or sibling, but may include parent, adult child, or significant caregiver; or loss of pet, health, home and/or other symbolic losses
- *Interpersonal deficits*: lack of social skills, ie. skills to negotiate changes of old-age, or initiating and maintaining relationships or supports

6.3 IPT Techniques: Three Phases of Treatment

- *Initial* (sessions 1–3): diagnostic evaluation and psychiatric history, explaining depression and IPT, and identifying the major problem area
- *Intermediate* (sessions 4–9): focus on the major problem area
- *Termination* (sessions 10–12): like a "graduation," this phase highlights a person's sense of competence, independence, and achievement in the therapy; the nature of depression and risk of recurrence reviewed

7. Psychodynamic Psychotherapy in Late Life

Two main schools of thought:
- Persistence of instinctual drives/wishes throughout life
- Second half of life is fundamentally different: "psychology of life's morning and a psychology of its afternoon" (Jung, 1929)

7.1 Tasks of Psychodynamic Psychotherapy
(Hildebrand, 1982)

- Hildebrand described several developmental tasks and difficulties of later life that might be amenable to psychodynamic techniques:
    - Fear of diminution
    - Threat of redundancy in roles
    - Need to reconsider/remake marital relationship after children have left
    - Awareness of aging, illness, and dependence

- – Awareness of limitations of what one can now achieve with the remainder of life
- – Feelings of failure in roles already executed (parenting, work, etc.)
- – Loss of partner/intimacy
- – Anticipatory narcissistic injury of mortality
- Psychotherapy undertaken with elderly adults, particularly very elderly adults, might be impacted by geriatric-specific features such as:
  - – Frailty or medical illness interfering with psychotherapeutic frame (transportation to appointments, sitting for appointments, frequency of appointments)
  - – Age difference between patient and therapist impacting transference and countertransference
  - – The impact of comorbid cognitive impairment on using psychodynamic techniques
  - – The role of the patient's family in patient's life and therapeutic undertaking

8. Reminiscence Psychotherapy
(Webster, Bohlmeijer, & Westerof, 2010)

- Defined as "remembering as a form of therapy"
- Introduced by Dr Robert Butler (geriatrician) in 1960s who coined term "life review"
- Type of narrative or biographically oriented psychotherapeutic technique
- Influenced by Eriksonian stage: integrity vs despair as developmentally important
- Encourages reflection on life narrative, with goal of incorporating a cohesive, positive sense of accomplishment and legacy
- Typical topics and foci are relationships, family, achievements, and adaptations
- Structured process of re-evaluation, resolution of conflicts, and integration of a coherent narrative of self
- Two main target populations: elderly adults with depressive symptoms and those with cognitive symptoms
- Dignity therapy developed for palliative population incorporates some reminiscence elements

9. Group Therapy: Model Misconceptions

- "Cheaper" or diluted psychotherapy
- Not as "worthwhile" as individual work
- Fears about group:
  - – Reveal and confess
  - – "Letting it all hang out"/loss of control
  - – Mental "contagion": get sicker by being with other patients; stigma of mental illness
  - – Shame
  - – Hostile strangers
- Buy-in to groups a challenge for depressed (withdrawn) and anxious (avoidant) patients
- Can be a challenge to engage older adults in groups!

9.1 Overcoming Obstacles to Group Attendance

- Make a personal connection
- Knowing the therapist; first-name basis helps
- Psychoeducation/address misconceptions
- Instil hope
- Outreach/home visit might be initially needed
- Address transportation to group
- Consider other barriers: hearing, vision, mobility
- Avoid interpretation of absences; accept that attendance may vary due to illness, transportation
- Consider therapist between-session phone calls to support attendance

9.2 Group Therapy Model: Yalom's 11 Therapeutic Factors
(Yalom & Leszcz, 2005)

- Instillation of hope*
- Universality*
- Imparting information
- Altruism
- Corrective recapitulation of the primary family group*
- Development of socializing techniques*
- Imitative behaviour*
- Interpersonal learning and feedback*
- Group cohesiveness*
- Catharsis
- Existential factors

* = specific advantages of group therapy > individual therapy

9.3 Generic Group Techniques

- Preparation: pre-group assessments, room set-up, supplies
- Phases of group:
    - Introductory: rationale for attending, demystification, rule and boundary setting
    - Transitional: tolerate differences, find commonality
    - Working: cohesive group, behaviour change
    - Termination: goodbyes, post-treatment planning

9.4 Specific Group Techniques

Outpatient cognitive behaviour group
- Structured, time-limited, closed membership
    - Substances, depression or anxiety
    - *Tasks*: focus on discrete changes in behaviour, decrease symptoms, alleviate suffering
    - *Techniques*:
        - Set concrete/realistic goals
        - Here and now focus
        - Follow an agenda
        - Assign and review homework aimed at goals

- Outpatient interpersonal
  - Not structured, time-unlimited, closed membership
  - *Tasks*: strive to better understand unconscious motivations and interpersonal interactions
  - *Techniques*:
    - Clarify, interpret the "here and now"
    - Intervene when there are strong emotions
    - Step in, summarize the data, and ask members for their interpretations
    - Example of here and now technique: "I'm not sure what's happening today in the group, but I notice _____ and _____ are looking at their watches, and _____ is exchanging glances with _____ whenever _____ is talking."

10. Current Issues

"The debate is not whether ... (psycho)therapy is applicable to the elderly ... but rather how to modify existing (treatments) so that they incorporate differences in thinking styles and age-related adjustment."

Koder, Brodaty, & Anstey (1996)

10.1 Sadavoy's "5 C's" of Psychogeriatrics
(Sadavoy, 2009)

- Chronicity
- Complexity
- Comorbidity
- Context
- Continuity: vulnerabilities held throughout life but expressed for the first time in late life
  - Can be difficult for therapist to understand
  - Move beyond the "mask of aging"
  - Therapist challenged to mobilize an authentic empathic response
  - Resonate empathically with both younger and older elements of patient

10.2 Practical Challenges of Psychotherapy with Older Adults: Suggested Modifications

- Frailty/poor physical health (e.g., transportation, immobility, arthritis in hands) → address transportation barriers, wheelchair accessible space; reduce writing requirements
- Sensory impairment (e.g., poor vision/hearing) → use large print materials, flipchart; speak clearly/one at a time in group; reduce background noise
- Cognitive changes/mild memory impairment→ build concepts weekly; use repetition; teach in multiple modalities (written, verbal); use mnemonics, symbols/images
- Age-specific themes/patient beliefs (e.g., loss and transition points, stigma of mental illness, attitudes to aging/ageism, health anxiety, being "too old to change," prejudice against younger therapist) → therapist can intentionally raise age-specific themes for exploration; draw from patient/group members experiences and attitudes
- Therapist beliefs (e.g., ageist assumptions, therapeutic nihilism) → therapist can be aware of, intentionally address thoughts/beliefs; seek supervision for support, discussion

10.3 Making CBT Work for Depressed and Anxious Older Adults
(Mohlman et al., 2003)

Strategies to overcome challenges and to increase compliance, learning: "enhanced" CBT

10.3.1 "Enhanced" Learning Techniques

- Simplified concepts and worksheets: large print, fewer columns
- Break down parts/build each week
- Repetition of major concepts and practices
- Teach in multiple modalities: flip chart, verbal, manuals
- Use mnemonics
- Support homework completion: mid-week phone call/coaching

10.3.2 Enhanced Group CBT Study
(Ursuliak et al., 2008)

- Criteria for referral to CBT: 65+ years old
- DSM-IV-TR diagnosis: depressive or anxiety disorder
- Criteria for exclusion from CBT:
    - Cognitive impairment (MMSE < 25)
    - Active psychotic illness
    - Significant medical condition
- Design: retrospective analysis of quality assurance data
    - Missing data collected by chart review
- Results:
    - N = 30
    - Total of 14 hours of CBT (7 weeks x 2 hours each)
    - N = 23 completers, 76.7%
    - 19/23 complete all 5 measures
    - 2/23 self-report measures only
    - Good retention (76.7%) and attendance rates (90.0%)
    - See also Table 2.7.3
- Depressive symptoms: severe → moderate-mild (large to very large effect size)
- Anxiety symptoms:
    - Clinician-rated: mild → remission (large effect size)
    - Self-report: mod → mild (small effect size)
- Quality of life:
    - ~1 pt. improvement (moderate effect size)

Enhanced group CBT: take home messages:
    - Statistically and clinically significant effects
    - Impressive outcome for a brief psychological intervention
    - Cost effective in group format
    - May be best option for some, avoids medications
    - More research needed

Table 2.7.3: Changes in Depression, Anxiety, and Quality of Life Scores in Enhanced Group CBT for Seniors Study

Average Pre-scores	Average Post-scores
BDI: 36 (severe)	BDI: 23 (moderate)
HAM-D: 35 (severe)	HAM-D: 9 (mild)
BAI: 37 (moderate)	BAI: 21 (mild)
HAM-A: 20 (mild)	HAM-A: 7 (remission)
PQoL: 3.74	PQoL: 4.8 (n = 7.5)

BAI = Beck Anxiety Inventory; BDI = Beck Depression Inventory; CBT = cognitive behavioural therapy; HAM-A = Hamilton Rating Scale for Anxiety; HAM-D = Hamilton Rating Scale for Depression; PQoL = perceived quality of life

Adapted from Ursuliak et al., 2008.

11. Summary of Evidence for Psychotherapy in Older Adults

- The largest volume and strongest evidence for psychotherapy is regarding the treatment of depression.
- In terms of specific psychotherapies, the strongest evidence is for CBT.
- Less evidence for IPT, but promising
- Some evidence for problem-solving therapy
- Group therapy efficacy is comparable to individual therapy.
- Small evidence base for short-term psychodynamic psychotherapy: efficacy compared to medication has not been established.
- Reminiscence psychotherapy: research quality remains poor overall; some suggestion it might improve depression, life satisfaction, and self-esteem in older adults; possible modest psychosocial benefits in older adults with dementia.

"Man can change and go on changing as long as he lives."

(K. Horney, 1942)

QUESTIONS

1. List the four categories or major problem areas for therapeutic focus considered in IPT, and provide a senior-specific example for each.
2. Define "distortions" and list some commonly used among older adults. Name the "best-fit" distortion for the following examples:
   a. "If I'm not a success, I am a total failure."
   b. "If I'm late for the appointment with the doctor, it will be a disaster."
   c. "I'm just an old has-been."
   d. "If I fall and need help, no one will help me."
   e. "My children don't call me because they think I'm not worthwhile."
   f. "I should write Christmas cards to all my family and friends."
   g. "I made Christmas dinner for the whole family, but that doesn't mean I'm competent in the kitchen. I kept the meal simple and just got lucky pulling it off this time."
   h. "The landlord was curt to me because I did something wrong."

   i. "I feel guilty about needing my daughter to drive me places. This proves I'm a burden to her."

3. Describe the cognitive triangle and provide an explanation for the CBT model that you might use when socializing a senior patient to the therapy.

4. What are core beliefs? How are core beliefs different from automatic thoughts? Describe the two basic types of core beliefs that a senior with depression might have and give an example of each.

5. Name three different therapeutic factors associated with group therapy and describe how they may offer advantages to senior patients when compared to individual therapy.

6. What are the key components of reminiscence psychotherapy, and what are some key outcomes of this therapy in the elderly population?

7. What are some of the limitations in the literature regarding dynamic psychotherapy treatment in the depressed elderly?

8. When would you choose psychotherapy together with, or instead of, medications in treating depression in the elderly?

9. What are some of the changes made to "enhanced" CBT, modified to meet the needs of older adults, as compared to standard CBT?

10. The goals of CBT are to address "here and now" problems, alleviate symptoms of depression and anxiety, and ultimately alter core beliefs. Describe some of the basic processes and techniques the therapist uses to help the patient alter core beliefs.

11. What might be some of the barriers to prescribing or approaching a course of dynamic psychotherapy in the elderly? Consider patient factors, clinician factors, and psychosocial factors that may limit success.

ANSWERS

1. The four categories or major problem areas for therapeutic focus in IPT are:

   - *Role transition*: retirement (the role transition related to loss of work life and changes in home life); illness or infirmity (changing to a more dependent role); caregiving role to partner/loved one (providing more support to partner, and less reliance on partner, particularly in context of dementia or dementia progression); taking on a range of roles previously filled by partner (having to make decisions previously made together, having to cook/clean or handle finances); decision making/power of attorney role (having to make all major decisions for the partner); a reduced caregiver role (such as after partner is placed, or dies); role changes following a separation, divorce, or death of spouse (taking on roles previously fulfilled by partner); role changes following a move from family home after an illness or death of family or closest friends (with resulting role adjustments)

   - *Interpersonal deficits*: those uncovered by one of the above role transitions are common in older adults (e.g., depression following a retirement, or a move due to the loss of established social network, and difficulty mounting the interpersonal skills to reconnect differently or to establish new relationships); interpersonal crisis experienced following the illness, infirmity, or death of spouse who previously met key social or autonomy functions for the partner (good communication skills, self-assertion, or social skills that maintained key relationships); depression resulting from difficulty reaching out for or accepting help or relying on others following a change in a person's own health/functional status

   - *Loss/grief*: loss and grief in the form of bereavement is commonly experienced by older adults, especially women, who outlive their other family members or friends; there are many other types of losses in late life, including anticipatory grief related to a terminal disease in self or a loved one (such as cancer, dementia), or loss of function or good health (stroke, MI), and loss or grief from other changes in life, such as a move from a long-time home or community (can be the loss of a beloved or symbolic object and/or community itself)

- *Role disputes*: common examples include disagreements over the caregiving role to a dependent spouse and disputes between partners after a major transition such as retirement, loss in functional ability, or health status in a partner, or a move; role disputes might also occur around differing expectations of family and friend loyalties; older adults commonly have role disputes with adult children as well, with changing dependency needs, or due to the family members' interpersonal circumstances due to marriage, divorce, having their children, unemployment, or relocation; role disputes can be simple and practical, such as who takes care of household responsibilities, or might be more complicated and represent exacerbations of a longstanding interpersonal pattern of a couple, worsened or made urgent by an age-related stressor
- These problems areas are applied to depression, and there are no specific modifications to the themes for older adults, but these themes have relevance to the life transitions, losses, and challenges often faced by older adults.

2. Distortions are patterns or types of thoughts that maintain negative thinking. The following are examples of distortions that are common in older adults with depression or anxiety:
    a. *All or nothing* (anxiety and depression)

    Example: "If I'm not a success, I am a total failure."
    b. *Catastrophizing* (GAD/anxiety-based)

    Examples: "My heart racing means I am having a heart attack." "If I'm late for the appointment, it will be a disaster."
    c. *Labelling* (negative view of self, ageist views about loss of personal value with age or infirmity)

    Example: "I am just an old has-been."
    d. *Jumping to conclusions* (GAD/anxiety-based)

    Example: "If I fall and need help, no one will help me."
    e. *Mind reading* (negative view of self, assuming ageist judgments by others)

    Example: "My children don't call me because they think I'm not worthwhile."
    f. *Should statements* (moral reasoning, applying guilt to motivate)

    Example: "I should write Christmas cards to all my friends and family."
    g. *Discounting the positives* (glass half empty, in context of depression)

    Example: "I made Christmas dinner for the whole family, but that doesn't mean I'm competent in the kitchen. I kept the meal simple and just got lucky pulling it off this time."
    h. *Personalizing* (self-blame, in context of social anxiety, and low self-esteem)

    Example: "The landlord was curt to me because I did something wrong."
    i. *Emotional reasoning*

    Example: "I feel guilty about needing my daughter to drive me places. This proves I'm a burden to her."

3. The cognitive triangle illustrates the model of this therapy, and shows the linkages among older adults' thoughts, feelings, and behaviours. These three areas interplay and impact one another; the therapy focuses primarily on older adults' thoughts and examines the impact that negative thoughts have on emotions and behaviours. The senior learns tools to evaluate the accuracy or helpfulness of their thoughts, and patterns of thinking that perpetuate negative thoughts and moods; he or she may then work to change the thoughts to be more constructive and accurate. The senior is challenged with the goal of becoming a more realistic or accurate thinker in order to improve his or her moods and behaviours.

4. Core beliefs are fleeting, primitive, telegraphic thoughts at the deepest level of consciousness thought that we "feel" to be true, and are general, crossing all types of situations (compared to automatic thoughts and conditional assumptions, which are more situation-specific thoughts). The two basic types of core beliefs are sociotropic (interpersonal; e.g., "I am unlovable.") and autonomous (work or performance; e.g., "I am incompetent.").

5. Therapeutic factors of group therapy that may offer advantages to older patients, when compared to individual therapy include:
   - *Instillation of hope* (seeing progress in others in the group and being inspired by them)
   - *Universality* (an experience of "welcome to the human race," by sharing problems in common with other older adults in the group)
   - *Imparting information* (opportunity in groups for older adults to share information with others in the group or provide helpful suggestions, such as "Did you know … ?" and "Why don't you … ?")
   - *Altruism* (group members experience the benefits of receiving by giving to others, which may be helpful in appreciating that when their loved ones help them, they might also find it gratifying and not necessarily a burden)
   - *Developing socializing techniques* (expressing accurate empathy to other older adults in the group)
   - *Role modelling* (imitation as a form of praise of themselves or of others)
   - *Interpersonal learning and corrective emotional experience* (growth in terms of using an appropriate level of self-assertion, joining in, or other adaptive behaviours, thus undoing previous maladaptive behaviours)
   - *Recapitulation of primary family* (re-experiencing the older adults' families of origin, but with improvements, and where interpersonal growth is permitted)
   - *Group cohesiveness* (the group members' collective sense of "we"-ness)
   - *Catharsis* (an opportunity for older adults to vent to each other)
   - *Existential factors* (a notion that we are ultimately alone, that life is not always fair, and that we need to take personal responsibility, regardless of our age or stage in life)

6. a. Key components of reminiscence therapy used working with patients with depressive symptoms include:
   - Expressing feelings about the past
   - Recalling family history and life stories
   - Discussing transitions

- Gaining awareness of personal accomplishments and identifying personal goals
- Reviewing life lessons and integrating a cohesive sense of self
- Appreciating capacity for adaptation

   b. Key components in working with patients with dementia using reminiscence
- Using specific items/triggers (such as photos or letters or albums) to prompt reminiscence
- Recalling family history and life stories

   c. Key outcomes with reminiscence therapy with elderly with depressive symptoms include:
- Reduces depressive symptoms and negative feelings
- Enhances self-integration
- Improves psychological well-being
- Eases feelings of loneliness
- Maintains self-esteem and self-value
- Improves coping skills
- Increases satisfaction with life

   d. Key outcomes with reminiscence therapy with elderly with dementia include:
- Improves mood and behavioural symptoms
- Improves functional status
- Reduces caregiver strain
- Improves attention to personhood in patients with dementia

7. Limitations in the literature regarding dynamic psychotherapy treatment in the depressed elderly include the following:
- Most evidence supporting dynamic interventions is brief psychodynamic therapy.
- Hard to control for comorbidities and reproduce studies
- Literature has never compared dynamic psychotherapy to medication.
- Minor depression/dysthymia has not been examined.

- Psychotherapy trials are difficult to conduct, particularly with less manualized therapies.

8. The following is a list of potential factors that could be considered in choosing psychotherapy as a treatment for a senior, with or without a medication:
- Patient preference
- The total number and types of medications, and presence of other psychotropic medications
- Experience of medication side effects
- Partial response to medication treatment
- Poor prognosis and need to augment treatment
- The severity of depression and need to use several modalities
- Availability of psychotherapy services
- Patient appropriateness for psychotherapy

In choosing psychotherapy alone, factors to consider include frailty, medication contraindications, lack of response to medications, suitability for psychotherapy, and patient preference.

9. The modifications involved in the "enhanced" model of CBT include:
   - Use of larger print for those with visual impairment
   - Fewer writing requirements for those with difficulty writing
   - Simplified concepts to make knowledge transfer easier for patients
   - Use of mnemonics to assist with recall of the concepts
   - Use of repetition to help with memory for concepts
   - Building on concepts gradually to ensure clarity of the teaching and for reinforcement through repetition
   - Teaching in several modalities (verbal, written, flipchart) at once to reinforce learning
   - Mid-week phone calls for homework coaching to ensure homework is completed

10. Basic processes and techniques of CBT for depression and anxiety include the following considerations:
    - In general, the cognitive therapist working with a senior would approach the process of altering core beliefs as he or she would with any other patient: for example, help the senior to identify his or her automatic thoughts (thoughts that are the most accessible to the senior and the most situation-specific); help the senior find and label the patterns of negative thinking he or she tends to use (i.e., the distortions); have the patient repeatedly practice across situations and allow time to alter his or her conditional assumptions, and ultimately to modify core beliefs.
    - The process the CBT therapist uses includes Socratic questioning, collaborative empiricism, and the downward arrow technique to uncover conditional assumptions and core beliefs, and synthesizing statements.
    - The techniques used with the senior patient to help him or her alter maladaptive patterns of thinking (and develop alternative thoughts that are more helpful and accurate) include the use of thought records, identifying distortions, being a scientist to test hypotheses, thinking in shades of grey, use of the double-standard technique, and behavioural experiments.
    - The main adjustments to these techniques and processes for a senior patient are similar to those in question #9 and are recommended approaches that can improve outcomes in older adults undergoing CBT: attending to the older adults' ability to see, write, physically attend sessions, recall or learn new material, and complete homework assignments; use of mnemonics, repetition, simplified concepts, modified and enlarged print materials with reduced writing requirements; and homework coaching through mid-week phone calls.

11. Barriers for dynamic therapy in the elderly include:
Patient factors:
   - Limited psychological mindedness regarding likelihood of treatment working
   - Sensory deficits
   - Medical frailty

- Cognitive impairment
- Transference-based issues
  - Elderly patients may become dependent on the therapist and not reach their full potential.
  - Age difference may lead patient to relate to the therapist as a son or daughter.
  - Frail elderly patients may see the therapist as a rescuer or competitor with whom they cannot compete.

Clinician factors:

- Countertransference-based issues
  - Therapist's fear of aging and regarding the patient as a grandparent
  - Unresolved negative feelings for his or her own parents may lead therapist to view patient negatively.
  - Rescue fantasies of therapist may lead to treatment failure.

Psychosocial factors:

- Transportation (driving and money) and ability to maintain a psychotherapeutic frame
- Dependence on caregivers
- Family involvement

CASE DISCUSSION

1. Since her depression onset was clearly timed with retirement (3 months afterward), and her symptoms are explained as depression, the patient and therapist agree on role transition as focus of therapy.

2. Useful questions to ask include:
   - How did your life change after retirement?
   - How did you feel about the change?
   - What people did you leave behind?
   - What people took their place?
   - What was life like before you retired?
   - What were the good things about your work life?
   - What were the bad things?
   - What are the good and bad aspects of your new situation?

3. Mrs C.'s tasks related to role transitioning include:
   - Giving up old role – routines, colleagues missed
   - Expressing guilt, anger, and fears about loss/change – disappointment with husband's lack of interest in travel
   - Acquiring new skills/interests – needs routine, structure, revival of old interests outside of work and apart from husband
   - Developing new attachments/supports – scheduled contact with friends
   - Recognizing positive aspects of her new role

RECOMMENDED RESOURCES FOR REVIEW

Although these resources may not be specifically cited in the text, their approach informed the contents of the chapter, and they are recommended as useful further reading.

Gallagher-Thompson D, Steffen A, Thompson LW, editors. Handbook of cognitive and behavioural therapies with older adults. New York: Springer Science & Business Media; 2008.

Hinrichsen GA, Clougherty KF. Interpersonal psychotherapy for depressed older adults. Washington, DC: American Psychological Association; 2006.

Laidlaw K, Thompson LW, Dick-Siskin L, et al. Cognitive behavioural therapy with older people. Chichester, UK: John Wiley & Sons; 2003.

Mackin RS, Areán PA. Evidence-based psychotherapeutic interventions for geriatric depression. Psychiatr Clin North Am. 2005;28(4):805–20. http://dx.doi.org/10.1016/j.psc.2005.09.009. Medline:16325730

Morgan AC. Practical geriatrics: psychodynamic psychotherapy with older adults. Psychiatr Serv. 2003;54(12):1592–4. http://dx.doi.org/10.1176/appi.ps.54.12.1592. Medline:14645796

Payman V. Psychotherapeutic treatments in late life. Curr Opin Psychiatry. 2011;24(6):484–8. Medline:21799413

Sadavoy J, Leszcz M, editors. Treating the elderly with psychotherapy: the scope for change in later life. Madison, CT: International Universities Press; 1987.

Yalom ID, Leszcz M. The theory and practice of group psychotherapy. 5th ed. New York: Basic Books; 2005.

REFERENCES

Alexopoulos GS. Depression in the elderly. Lancet. 2005;365(9475):1961–70. http://dx.doi.org/10.1016/S0140-6736(05)66665-2. Medline:15936426

Alzheimer Society. Rising tide: the impact of dementia on Canadian society . Toronto: Alzheimer Society of Canada; 2010 [cited 2014 Oct 21]. No PMID. http://www.alzheimer.ca/~/media/Files/national/Advocacy/ASC_Rising_Tide_Full_Report_e.pdf

Areán PA, Cook BL. Psychotherapy and combined psychotherapy/pharmacotherapy for late life depression. Biol Psychiatry. 2002;52(3):293–303. http://dx.doi.org/10.1016/S0006-3223(02)01371-9. Medline:12182934

Barlow DH, Gorman JM, Shear MK, et al. Cognitive-behavioral therapy, imipramine, or their combination for panic disorder: a randomized controlled trial. JAMA. 2000;283(19):2529–36. http://dx.doi.org/10.1001/jama.283.19.2529. Medline:10815116

Barrowclough C, King P, Colville J, et al. A randomized trial of the effectiveness of cognitive-behavioural therapy and supportive counseling for anxiety symptoms in older adults. J Consult Clin Psychol. 2001;69(5):756–62. http://dx.doi.org/10.1037/0022-006X.69.5.756. Medline:11680552

Beekman AT, Deeg DJ, Smit JH, et al. Predicting the course of depression in the older population: results from a community-based study in The Netherlands. J Affect Disord. 1995;34(1):41–9. http://dx.doi.org/10.1016/0165-0327(94)00103-G. Medline:7622738

Blazer D. Depression in the elderly. N Engl J Med. 1989;320(3):164–6. http://dx.doi.org/10.1056/NEJM198901193200306. Medline:2643044

Darkwa OK. Reforming the Ghanaian social security system: prospects and challenges. J Cross Cult Gerontol. 1997;12:(2):186.

de Beurs E, Beekman AT, van Balkom AJ, et al. Consequences of anxiety in older persons: its effect on disability, well-being and use of health services. Psychol Med. 1999;29(3):583–93. http://dx.doi.org/10.1017/S0033291799008351. Medline:10405079

Engels GI, Verney M. Efficacy of nonmedical treatments of depression in elders: a quantitative analysis. J Clin Geropsychol. 1997;3:17–25.

Garner J. Psychodynamic work and older adults. Adv Psychiatr Treat. 2002;8(2):128–35. http://dx.doi.org/10.1192/apt.8.2.128

Gerson S, Belin TR, Kaufman A, et al. Pharmacological and psychological treatments for depressed older patients: a meta-analysis and overview of recent findings. Harv Rev Psychiatry. 1999;7(1):1–28. http://dx.doi.org/10.3109/hrp.7.1.1. Medline:10439302

Hildebrand HP. Psychotherapy with older patients. Br J Med Psychol. 1982;55(1):19–28. http://dx.doi.org/10.1111/j.2044-8341.1982.tb01477.x. Medline:7059528

Horney K. Self-analysis. International Library of Psychology. London: Routledge; 1942 [reprinted 1999].

Jeste DV, Savla GN, Thompson WK, et al. Association between older age and more successful aging: critical role of resilience and depression. Am J Psychiatry. 2013;170(2):188–96. http://dx.doi.org/10.1176/appi.ajp.2012.12030386. Medline:23223917

Jung CG. The aims of psychotherapy. In: Jung CG. The practice of psychotherapy. Vol. 16, The collected works of C.G. Jung. Edited by Michael Fordham. London: Routledge & Kegan Paul; 1953. p. 38.

Kiosses DN, Leon AC, Areán PA. Psychosocial interventions for late-life major depression: evidence-based treatments, predictors of treatment outcomes, and moderators of treatment effects. Psychiatr Clin North Am. 2011;34(2):377–401. http://dx.doi.org/10.1016/j.psc.2011.03.001. Medline:21536164

Koder D, Brodaty H, Anstey. Cognitive therapy for depression in the elderly. Int J Geriatr Psychiatry. 1996;11(2):97–107. http://dx.doi.org/10.1002/(SICI)1099-1166(199602)11:2<97::AID-GPS310>3.0.CO;2-W

Leszcz M. Group therapy. In: Sadock BJ, Sadock VA, & Ruiz P, editors. Kaplan and Sadock's comprehensive textbook of psychiatry. 9th ed. Philadelphia, PA: Lippencott Williams & Wilkins; 2009. p. 4175–80.

Levy BR, Slade MD, Kunkel SR, et al. Longevity increased by positive self-perceptions of aging. J Pers Soc Psychol. 2002;83(2):261–70. http://dx.doi.org/10.1037/0022-3514.83.2.261. Medline:12150226

MacCourt P, Wilson K, Tourigny-Rivard MF; Mental Health Commission of Canada. Guidelines for comprehensive mental health services for older adults in Canada. Calgary, AB: Mental Health Commission of Canada; 2011 [cited 2014 Oct 03]. No PMID. http://www.mentalhealthcommission.ca/English/document/279/mental-health-commission-canada-seniors-guidelines-print

Miller MD. Using interpersonal therapy (IPT) with older adults today and tomorrow: a review of the literature and new developments. Curr Psychiatry Rep. 2008;10(1):16–22. http://dx.doi.org/10.1007/s11920-008-0005-6. Medline:18269890

Mohlman J, Gorenstein EE, Kleber M, et al. Standard and enhanced cognitive-behavior therapy for late-life generalized anxiety disorder: two pilot investigations. Am J Geriatr Psychiatry. 2003;11(1):24–32. Medline:12527537

Payne KT, Marcus DK. The efficacy of group psychotherapy for older adult clients: a meta-analysis. Group Dynamic Theory Res Pract. 2008;12(4):268–78. http://dx.doi.org/10.1037/a0013519

Pinquart M, Duberstein PR, Lyness JM. Treatments for later-life depressive conditions: a meta-analytic comparison of pharmacotherapy and psychotherapy. Am J Psychiatry. 2006;163(9):1493–501. http://dx.doi.org/10.1176/ajp.2006.163.9.1493. Medline:16946172

Pinquart M, Sörensen S. How effective are psychotherapeutic and other psychosocial interventions with older adults? A meta-analysis. J Ment Health Aging. 2001;7(2):207–43.

Poon LW, Martin P, Bishop A, et al. Understanding centenarians' psychosocial dynamics and their contributions to health and quality of life. Curr Gerontol Geriatr Res. 2010;2010:680657. http://dx.doi.org/10.1155/2010/680657

Sadavoy J. An integrated model for defining the scope of psychogeriatrics: the five Cs. Int Psychogeriatr. 2009;21(5):805–12. http://dx.doi.org/10.1017/S104161020999010X. Medline:19505355

Scogin F, McElreath L. Efficacy of psychosocial treatments for geriatric depression: a quantitative review. J Consult Clin Psychol. 1994;62(1):69–74. http://dx.doi.org/10.1037/0022-006X.62.1.69. Medline:8034832

Sirey JA, Bruce ML, Alexopoulos, GS. The Treatment Initiation Program: an intervention to improve depression outcomes in older adults. Am J Psychiatry. 2005;162(1):184–6. http://dx.doi.org/10.1176/appi.ajp.162.1.184. Medline:15625220

Stanley MA, Beck JG, Novy DM, et al. Cognitive-behavioral treatment of late-life generalized anxiety disorder. J Consult Clin Psychol. 2003;71(2):309–19. http://dx.doi.org/10.1037/0022-006X.71.2.309. Medline:12699025

Thompson LW, Coon DW, Gallagher-Thompson D, et al. Comparison of desipramine and cognitive/behavioral therapy in the treatment of elderly outpatients with mild-to-moderate depression. Am J Geriatr Psychiatry. 2001;9(3):225–40. http://dx.doi.org/10.1097/00019442-200108000-00006. Medline:11481130

Ursuliak Z, Cassidy K, Burke D, et al. An observational study of the effectiveness of group cognitive behavior therapy for late-life depressive and anxiety disorders. Canadian Journal of Geriatrics. 2008;11(2):88–93.

Walker DA, Clarke M. Cognitive behavioural psychotherapy: a comparison between younger and older adults in two inner city mental health teams. Aging Ment Health. 2001;5(2):197–9. http://dx.doi.org/10.1080/1360860120038311. Medline:11511068

Webster JD, Bohlmeijer ET, Westerhof GJ. Mapping the future of reminiscence: a conceptual guide for research and practice. Res Aging. 2010;32(4):527–64. http://dx.doi.org/10.1177/0164027510364122

Weissman MM. The psychological treatment of depression. Evidence for the efficacy of psychotherapy alone, in comparison with, and in combination with pharmacotherapy. Arch Gen Psychiatry. 1979;36(11):1261–9. http://dx.doi.org/10.1001/archpsyc.1979.01780110115014. Medline:485783

Weissman MM, Prusoff BA, Dimascio A, et al. The efficacy of drugs and psychotherapy in the treatment of acute depressive episodes. Am J Psychiatry. 1979;136(4B):555–8. Medline:371421

Wetherell JL, Gatz M, Craske MG. Treatment of generalized anxiety disorder in older adults. J Consult Clin Psychol. 2003;71(1):31–40. http://dx.doi.org/10.1037/0022-006X.71.1.31. Medline:12602423

Wilson KC, Mottram PG, Vassilas CA. Psychotherapeutic treatments for older depressed people. Cochrane Database Syst Rev. 2008;(1):CD004853. Medline:18254062

2.8 Suicide among Older Adults

Marnin J. Heisel, PhD, CPsych

INTRODUCTION

Suicide in older adults is a critically important topic for mental health providers and one that generates a considerable amount of concern, challenge, and controversy. Older adults, and men in particular, have among the highest rates of suicide worldwide, and yet the relative rarity of suicide at a population level renders its prediction exceptionally challenging, if not impossible. Researchers investigating risk factors for death by suicide have thus typically employed population-level mortality data, whereas clinical-level researchers have tended to focus on assessment and intervention targeting suicide ideation and behaviour, as their study samples lack sufficient statistical power to focus on prediction or prevention of death by suicide. For clinicians and family members of suicidal older adults, the uncertainties of suicide prediction and prevention can lead to significant discomfort and fear. This chapter provides an up-to-date review of the evidence, along with a practical approach to suicide risk assessment and intervention, a review of treatment guidelines, as well as a useful discussion of intervention and prevention strategies.

CASE SCENARIO

While consulting in the psychiatric emergency department, you meet Bea, a 72-year-old woman of Eastern European birth, brought in by ambulance after her husband, Abe, found her lying unresponsive on the bathroom floor next to empty bottles of heart medication and antidepressants, and with alcohol on her breath. Her husband reported that Bea had been dreading the upcoming graduation party for their daughter's oldest son, as their ex-son-in-law and his new wife (for whom he left their daughter) would be in attendance. He further noted that Bea had been very upset earlier in the day, and had started an argument with him "for no apparent reason" as he was heading out grocery shopping.

1. How would you describe Bea's risk for suicide over the short and long terms?
2. What are some of the key risk factors apparent in this scenario?
3. What potential resiliency factors can be engaged in order to potentially reduce her risk for suicide?
4. What interventions, with at least some empirical support, might be offered to Bea (and/or Abe) to reduce her risk for suicide and to enhance her mental health and well-being?

OVERVIEW

1. The Epidemiology of Suicide

- The World Health Organization (WHO) estimates that approximately 800 000 lives are lost to suicide worldwide every year (1.5–2% of all deaths; Krug et al., 2002; WHO, 2014).
- This exceeds the number of lives lost to war and homicide combined.
- In the United States, 40 600 people died by suicide in 2012 (Centers for Disease Control and Prevention, 2014).
- In Canada, more people died by suicide in 2012 (3926) than due to transport accidents (2599), homicide (493), and HIV (276) combined (3368 total), making suicide the ninth leading cause of death among Canadians (Statistics Canada, 2012, 2014).

1.1 The Epidemiology of Late-Life Suicide

- Older adults have high rates of suicide and employ lethal means of self-harm (Heisel, 2006).
- This is especially true among older men who have among the highest rates of suicide of all demographics in North America and worldwide.
- Older adults may end their lives by refusing food and/or needed medications; these deaths are typically not classified as suicide.
- The ratio of suicidal behaviour to death by suicide in older adults may be as low as 1–4:1 (McIntosh et al., 1994).

2. Some Barriers to Late-Life Suicide Prevention
(Canadian Coalition for Seniors' Mental Health, 2006; Heisel, 2006)

- Suicide is a low base-rate occurrence; Canada's overall suicide rate of 11.3/100 000 amounts to roughly 1 death by suicide for every 8850 Canadians (Statistics Canada, 2014).
- Compared with the study of suicide among adults and/or adolescents, there is a relative paucity of the following:
  - Relevant research
  - Assessment tools and approaches for risk detection, assessment, and monitoring
  - Intervention trials and associated clinical literature
- There is a paucity of highly trained care providers.

2.1 Some Systemic Limitations

- Older adults often do not directly access mental healthcare services, and downplay psychological symptoms (Duberstein et al., 1999; Kjølseth, Ekeberg, & Steihaug, 2010; Lyness et al., 1995).
- There are long waits to see provincially funded providers; most older adults cannot afford private care psychologists or other mental healthcare.
- The demand on family doctor time is great, and there is a scarcity of available providers, especially in northern, rural, and/or remote communities.

- Approximately 45% of people who die by suicide visited a primary care provider in the month prior to death; this figure exceeds 70% for older adults (Luoma, Martin, & Pearson, 2002).
- The primary care system was not designed for assessment and treatment of mental health issues.
- Enhanced detection and referral to clinical mental health care is critical, as are outreach and community-based care.

2.2 *Clinical Implications/Opportunities*

- Innovative models of outreach and health service delivery and training are needed, including:
  - Collaborative care (e.g., the Prevention of Suicide in Primary Care Elderly: Collaborative Trial [PROSPECT; Bruce et al., 2004] and the Improving Mood-Promoting Access to Collaborative Treatment Study [IMPACT; Unützer et al., 2006])
  - Use of non-provincially funded providers
  - Use of social service providers and peer supports
  - Telemedicine/telehealth services, including distress/crisis services
  - Local providers and distant consultants
  - Innovative educational programs and scholarships
  - Distance learning, webinars, conferences, and use of social media
  - Knowledge Translation (KT) to reduce the lag time between dissemination of new clinical findings and implementation in frontline care

3. Guidelines

- Developed by members of the Canadian Coalition for Seniors' Mental Health (CCSMH, 2008; available online at www.ccsmh.ca)
- Resources in the CCSMH project include:
  - Quick reference clinician pocket-card
  - Interactive case-based DVD
  - Facilitator's manual
  - Guide for family members
- The CCSMH guideline format was loosely based on guidelines from the University of Iowa Gerontological Nursing Interventions Research Center (Holkup, 2002); the Iowa guidelines focused on assessment and not intervention, and are currently being updated.
- Additional guidelines include:
  - The American Psychiatric Association's *Practice guideline for the assessment and treatment of patients with suicidal behaviors* (Jacobs et al., 2003); these guidelines are not specific to older adults
  - The US Substance Abuse and Mental Health Services Administration or SAMHSA's *Promoting emotional health and preventing suicide: A toolkit for senior living communities (SPARK kit)* (Substance Abuse and Mental Health Services Administration, 2010)
  - The US Veterans Administration has also recently developed a set of KT tools (http://www.mentalhealth.va.gov/suicide_prevention/)

4. Suicide Risk Assessment

Can suicide be predicted?
- Suicide is a low base-rate phenomenon, and is thus extremely difficult to predict.
- This creates a challenge when screening for those at risk for suicide.
- Prediction of suicide requires immense sample sizes and long follow-up periods.
- Most studies of those who died by suicide did not differentiate imminent from lifetime risk (Fawcett et al., 1990 is an exception) and encountered the problem of establishing an appropriate control condition.
- Available information on this question is thus very limited.
- Pokorny (1996) tried to build a predictive model of suicide in psychiatric inpatients ("first admissions") at the Houston Veterans Affairs Medical Center.
  - He followed 4800 consecutively admitted patients for 4–6 years, at which point 67 had died by suicide.
  - Despite this large sample size, and use of elegant analyses, he could not predict a single death by suicide.
  - He concluded that individual cases of suicide cannot be predicted.
- We thus instead must focus on sensitive assessment of risk rather than on prediction of suicide.

4.1 Why Not Just Ask Patients if They Are Suicidal?

- This is a necessity; however, older adults often downplay psychological symptoms (Duberstein et al., 1999).
- With older adults, we initially need to gently approach the issue of suicide; however, we *must* ask the question, even if risk is not apparent (Grek, 2007).
- We should consider use of collateral source information (Heisel et al., 2011).
- Suicide risk assessment must be carried out in a sensitive fashion, in the context of a trusting therapeutic relationship.
- Clumsy assessment of suicide ideation may be worse than not asking the question at all, as an at-risk older adult's denial of suicide ideation might create a false sense of security in a provider.
- Recent research indicates that 78% of current or recently discharged mental health patients who died by suicide denied suicide ideation as a last communication before death; some did so as little as 5–10 minutes before dying by suicide (Busch, Fawcett, & Jacobs, 2003).
- This suggests a need to improve processes of risk detection, enhance the establishment of clinical rapport, and consider the use of validated population-specific tools.

4.2 Suicide Risk and Resiliency Factors

- Suicide is a complex phenomenon with multiple determinants and contributing factors.
- Identification of suicide risk factors may aid in the detection of those at risk and inform intervention.
- Common risk factors (age, sex, and ethnicity) are non-modifiable; therapeutics need to focus on modifiable factors, such as reducing suicide ideation, treating psychological and physical symptoms, providing support, and enhancing well-being.

- We also need to focus on *resiliency* and *protective* factors (Heisel, 2006; CCSMH, 2008; Heisel & Flett, 2016a; Heisel & The Meaning-Centered Men's Group Project Team, 2016).

4.2.1 Suicide Risk Factors

Suicide ideation and/or behaviour
- Prior suicide behaviour (including suicide attempt), prior self-harm behaviour, previous expression of suicide ideation
- Feels tired of living and/or wishes to die
- Thinks about suicide, has suicide-related wishes and/or desires
- Has a suicide plan/note

Family history
- Family history of suicide, suicide ideation, mental disorder

Mental health problems (can include)
- Any mental disorder, comorbidity
- Major depressive disorder
- Any mood disorder
- Psychotic disorder
- Substance misuse disorder/addictions

Personality factors
- Personality disorders
- Emotional instability
- Rigid personality
- Poor coping skills, introversion

Medical illness
- Pain, chronic illness
- Sensory impairment
- Perceived or anticipated/feared illness

Negative life events and transitions
- Family discord, separation, death, or other losses
- Financial or legal difficulties
- Employment/retirement difficulties
- Relocation stresses

Functional impairment
- Loss of independence
- Problems with activities of daily living

Suicide and terminal illness
- Kleespies, Hughes, and Gallacher (2000) reported that 30–40% of US older adults who died by suicide were medically ill at the time, yet only 2–3% were terminally ill.
- Receiving a terminal prognosis can be psychologically overwhelming and temporarily induce suicide ideation (Silverman, 2000).
- Be vigilant to expressions of an extreme need for perceived autonomy and be aware of high-risk periods, including following communication of a severe/

frightening diagnosis or a terminal prognosis; proceed with sensitivity whenever communicating diagnoses, and especially regarding potentially deteriorating conditions.

4.2.2 Suicide Resiliency Factors

- Religious (or spiritual) practice
- Perceptions of meaning and purpose in life
- Sense of hope or optimism
- Active social networks and support from family and friends
- Good healthcare practices
- Positive help-seeking behaviours
- Engagement in activities of personal interest

4.3 Limitations to Risk-Factor Approach

- Reliance upon
    - Retrospective reports
    - Self-report methodology
    - Proxy informants
- There is a paucity of research on resiliency/protective factors.
- No research study has shown that risk assessment procedures prevent deaths by suicide.
- We cannot (nor should we) indicate the percentage likelihood of someone dying by suicide.
- Assessment of suicide risk should ideally include consideration of imminent-, moderate-, and longer-term risk (Hatton, Valente, & Rink, 1977).

4.4 Should We Screen for Suicide Risk?

- The Gotland study (Rutz, von Knorring, & Wålinder, 1989) indicated that teaching providers to better identify and treat depression in primary care led to a reduction in the community rate of suicide.
- This study has yet to be effectively replicated.
- More research is needed on the subject of screening for suicide risk in primary care.
- We found that use of screening items derived from a depression screening tool (Geriatric Depression Scale [GDS]) effectively identified older primary care patients with suicide ideation (Heisel et al., 2010).
- The US Preventive Services Task Force (USPSTF) recently indicated that "Minimal evidence (2 studies) suggested that screening tools can identify adults and older adults in primary care who are at increased risk for suicide, although these tools produce many false-positive results" and concluded that "primary care-feasible screening tools might help to identify some adults at increased risk for suicide" (O'Connor et al., 2013).

4.5 Assessment Process
(CCSMH, 2008)

- Establish rapport and assess for suicide risk in a sensitive and respectful fashion.
- Respect the dignity of older adults; acknowledge their experiences and validate their feelings.

- Assess for suicide risk factors.
- Assess for psychological resiliency.
- Assess for suicide warning signs: IS PATH WARM*.
- Where appropriate, access collateral information (medical chart, family members, other providers).
- Be mindful of ambivalent wishes to live and to die.
- Develop a risk-management/action plan.
- Seek consultation and/or assistance if you do not have specialized training in mental health or in suicide prevention.

* Remember the mnemonic "IS PATH WARM?"
  - **I** – Ideation
  - **S** – Substance abuse
  - **P** – Purposelessness
  - **A** – Anxiety
  - **T** – Trapped
  - **H** – Hopelessness
  - **W** – Withdrawal
  - **A** – Anger
  - **R** – Recklessness
  - **M** – Mood change

Source: American Association of Suicidology [website], www.suicidology.org.

4.6 Suicide Warning Signs

- In addition to the warning signs outlined above (IS PATH WARM), clinicians may consider the following set of warning signs in the context of an older adult's history and life circumstances (i.e., some may be normative).
- Communication
  - Talks about "the end" and makes other vague reference to not being around much longer
  - Talks a great deal about death (longingly, glorifies death)
  - Refers to self as a burden/better off dead
  - Discusses suicide intent or plan, or
  - Is unwilling to discuss suicide symptoms
- Behaviour
  - Gives away prized possessions
  - Has death-related plans/puts affairs in order (insurance policy, will, pets, etc.)
  - Engages in risky or self-harm behaviour
  - Stockpiles pills, knives, ropes, or other lethal implements
  - Self-imposes isolation/withdraws socially
  - Ceases taking medication or food
  - Stops seeing a medical provider or therapist
  - Suddenly (and perhaps inexplicably) seems much better
  - Suddenly stops talking about death, wanting to die, and/or suicide, especially in the absence of mental healthcare

- Affective/cognitive
  - Depressed, or, if having been depressed, suddenly appears brighter, more energetic, calm
  - Hopelessness/helplessness
  - Anxious or mixed emotional states (e.g., agitated depression)
  - Impulsive/aggressive/angry/homicidal
  - Wistful (especially re: loss/grief)
  - Delusional
  - In pain

4.7 Key Questions
(CCSMH, 2008)

- Ask about their feelings.
  - Do you feel tired of living?
  - Have you been thinking about suicide?
  - Have you been thinking about hurting or killing someone else?
- Ask about a suicide plan.
  - Have you made any specific plans or preparations (giving away possessions, tying up "loose ends")?
  - Do you have access to lethal means such as a gun or other implements?
- Ask about their reasons to live.
  - Who or what makes life so worth living that you would not harm yourself?

4.8 Risk Assessment Scales

- **Geriatric Suicide Ideation Scale** (GSIS; Heisel & Flett, 2006)

    The GSIS is a 31-item, 5-point, Likert-scored, multidimensional measure of suicide ideation and associated factors among older adults. The GSIS contains 4 subscales, assessing Suicide Ideation (e.g., *"I want to end my life"*), Death Ideation (*"I welcome the thought of drifting off to sleep and never waking up"*), Loss of Personal and Social Worth (*"I frequently feel useless"*), and Perceived Meaning in Life (*"I am certain that I have something to live for"*). Research findings have shown strong reliability and validity for the GSIS and its subscales (Heisel & Flett, 2016b). Additional research is needed evaluating risk identification using these tools in standard practice in clinical and community settings.

- **Harmful Behaviours Scale** (HBS; Draper et al., 2002)

    The HBS is a 20-item, 5-point, Likert-scored, observer rating scale of recent direct and indirect self-destructive behaviour for nursing home residents. It has demonstrated good internal consistency and inter-rater reliability (Draper et al., 2002, 2003); however, it requires administration by trained observers in residential care settings.

- **Reasons for Living Scale–Older Adults** (RFL-OA; Edelstein et al., 2009)

    The RFL-OA is a 69-item Likert-scored measure of reasons for not killing oneself when feeling suicidal. It has demonstrated good internal consistency and construct validity. As of the present, there are few published studies using this scale. It is fairly lengthy, and brief subscales have not yet been identified in the literature (Heisel, Neufeld, & Flett, 2016).

- **Suicidal Older Adult Protocol** (SOAP; Fremouw et al., 2009)

    The SOAP is an 18-item clinical interview measure assessing static (demographic and historical variables) and dynamic factors (clinical, contextual, and protective variables). Items are scored as being at "low, medium, or high" levels of risk; four "extreme risk" items are included. The interviewer makes an overall determination of risk and can select from a list of potential actions to take in order to mitigate suicide risk. It was derived from tools developed for adolescents and adults. No validation study appears to have been completed as yet.

5. Intervention

- In referring to stages of intervention with suicidal individuals, suicidologists differentiate among the following terms:
    - "Prevention" (referring to efforts to reduce the likelihood that an individual begins thinking of suicide or engages in self-injurious or suicidal behaviour)
    - "Intervention" (referring to care provision for those with current suicide ideation and/or who have engaged in or are at heightened risk of engaging in suicidal behaviour)
    - "Postvention" (this term has historically been employed to refer to care provided for individuals bereaved by suicide; this term has more recently been used to refer to care provided to those who have engaged in suicidal behaviour)
- Prevention scientists differentiate among "universal" (i.e., population-level), "selected" (i.e., for groups at elevated likelihood of having/developing a problem), and "indicated" (i.e., for those with the problem) interventions (e.g., Knox, Conwell, & Caine, 2004).
- Although few suicide prevention interventions have been tested empirically, the literature supports a set of interventions in reducing suicide risk and/or preventing deaths by suicide (see Mann et al., 2005); few, however, focused exclusively on at-risk older adults (Lapierre et al., 2011; Links, Heisel, & Quastel, 2005).

5.1 What Works?

- A set of public health initiatives (universal-level interventions) have empirical support for decreasing risk for suicide. These include:
    - Restricting access to the means or methods of suicide, such as detoxifying home-based gas and limiting pack sizes for analgesics and other medications in the United Kingdom (Gunnell, Middleton, & Frankel, 2000; Hawton et al., 2001)
    - Convening a program of depression screening and aggressive intervention by general medical practitioners on the island of Gotland, Sweden (Rutz, von Knorring, & Wålinder, 1989)
    - Suicide prevention strategies and professional practice guidelines are being developed and disseminated with the aim of reducing risk for suicide in populations; although more research is needed in order to demonstrate "cause and effect" relationships, implementation of suicide prevention guidelines has been associated with a decline in suicide rates (e.g., Knox, Conwell, & Caine, 2004).
- A set of community initiatives (selected-level interventions) have also demonstrated empirical support for decreasing suicide risk. These include:
    - *Gatekeeper programs* (e.g., Florio et al., 1996). Efforts are underway to train individuals who come into daily contact with older adults (so-called "gatekeepers")

to identify mental health problems and potential suicide risk and to connect at-risk individuals with healthcare services; although these initiatives have not yet demonstrated effectiveness in preventing deaths by suicide, they are likely useful adjuncts when implemented alongside outreach screening and clinical interventions.

- *Outreach initiatives* (Japan; Oyama et al., 2005). Oyama and colleagues reported a reduction in the rate of suicide among older adults in Japan in the context of a program of public presentations and outreach screenings and counselling for those with depression.
- *Telehealth/Telecheck* (Italy; De Leo, Dello Buono, & Dwyer, 2002). A quasi-experimental research study has offered support for a program involving telephone-based support for older adults struggling with psychological distress; clients of this service could both call in for support from distress-line staff and would receive periodic phone calls from staff at pre-arranged times.

• Clinical initiatives (indicated-level interventions). Few trials exist testing clinical interventions with suicidal older adults (Heisel, 2006; Links, Heisel, & Quastel, 2005), necessitating additional research; examples of existing clinical initiatives appear below.

5.2 Clinical Initiatives

• Effective treatment of associated forms of psychopathology may decrease suicide risk.
• However, Waern and colleagues (1996, 1999, 2002) found high rates of mental healthcare utilization among older adults who died by suicide.
• Interventions are needed targeting suicidal older adults, and not simply treatment for depression.
• Few randomized controlled trials (RCTs) exist (suicidal individuals are typically excluded from clinical intervention trials for depression and other disorders; Pearson et al., 2001).
• Existing data support combination medication and psychotherapy in reducing late-life suicide ideation (see Alexopoulos et al., 2009; Bruce et al., 2004; Heisel et al., 2009, 2015; Unützer et al., 2006).

5.3 Medical Interventions to Reduce Risk for Suicide

• Medical interventions have been shown effective in potentially helping reduce risk for suicide, including:
  - Lithium for individuals with bipolar disorder (Angst, Angst, & Stassen, 1999; Baldessarini, Tondo, & Hennen, 1999; Goodwin, 1999)
  - Clozapine for individuals with schizophrenia or schizoaffective disorder (Meltzer et al., 2003)
  - Other antipsychotics for individuals with psychotic disorders (Hawton et al., 1998; Palmer, Henter, & Wyatt, 1999)
  - Antidepressants for mood-disordered individuals (Angst, Angst, & Stassen, 1999)
  - Electroconvulsive therapy (ECT) in reducing suicide ideation (Prudic & Sackeim, 1999)
• However, these studies were not specific to older adults, necessitating controlled intervention trials focusing on at-risk older individuals.

5.4 Psychotherapeutic Interventions to Reduce Risk for Suicide

- Brief psychotherapy has been shown effective in reducing suicide ideation and/or behaviour, including:
  - Cognitive approaches:
    - Cognitive therapy (Brown et al., 2005)
    - Dialectical behaviour therapy (Linehan et al., 1991, 2006)
    - Problem-solving therapy (Salkovskis, Atha, & Storer, 1990)
  - Interpersonal approaches:
    - Brief psychodynamic interpersonal therapy (Guthrie et al., 2001)
    - Interpersonal problem-solving (McLeavey et al., 1994)
- However, these studies were not specific to older adults, necessitating controlled intervention trials focusing on at-risk older individuals.

5.5 Psychotherapeutic Interventions with At-Risk Older Adults

- A review of the randomized controlled treatment literature identified a paucity of clinical trials focusing explicitly on suicidal older adults (Links, Heisel, & Quastel, 2005). Studies have demonstrated some empirical support for the following interventions in reducing suicide ideation:
  - Problem-solving treatment (PST) and antidepressants (Unützer et al., 2006)
  - Interpersonal psychotherapy (IPT) and antidepressants (Bruce et al., 2004; Heisel et al., 2009, 2015; Szanto et al., 2003, 2007)
- Multisite collaborative care trials involved mental health clinicians collaborating with primary care clinicians to treat depressed older adults; treatment typically involved an antidepressant and evidence-based psychotherapy (interpersonal psychotherapy in PROSPECT and behavioural activation and problem-solving treatment in IMPACT). These were effective in significantly enhancing mental health treatment uptake and both the detection and reduction/resolution of depressive symptom severity and suicide ideation (Alexopoulos et al., 2009; Bruce et al., 2004; Hunkeler et al., 2006; Unützer et al., 2006).
- Cognitive therapy research is underway, including an adaptation of dialectical behaviour therapy for older adults at risk for suicide (see Lynch et al., 2003).

5.6 Recommendation: Treatment and Management – The Therapeutic Relationship
(CCSMH, 2006)

- Develop a trusting and genuine therapeutic relationship with at-risk older adults. Actively and attentively listen to the client, and take your time. When present, these elements help contribute to a person feeling heard and respected, and can help contribute to the older client feeling connected.

5.7 Some Common Factors in Psychotherapy with Suicidal People

- Leenaars (2006) identified a set of important common factors in psychotherapy with suicidal individuals from a person-centered perspective, including:
  - Establishing a strong therapeutic relationship
  - Striving for a genuine "human exchange"

- Collaborating with the client and setting goals consensually
- Using multi-modal therapeutic approaches given underlying complexities involved in working with at-risk individuals

5.8 Psychotherapy: Adaptive and Maladaptive Hope – Guideline Recommendations
(CCSMH, 2006)

- Foster hope in clients who are suicidal. Healthcare providers may promote hope by initiating hope-focused conversations.
- Healthcare providers should explore strategies to assist older persons to find and maintain meaning and purpose in their lives.

5.9 Problems in Psychotherapy with Suicidal Patients
(Hendin et al., 2006)

- Based on a retrospective study with 36 therapists who lost a patient to suicide while in therapy
- Identified six common problems:
    - Poor communication with other therapists involved
    - Permitting clients to control the therapy
    - Avoidance of issues related to sexuality
    - Ineffective or coercive actions resulting from the therapist's anxieties about a patient's potential suicide
    - Not recognizing the meaning of patient communications
    - Untreated/undertreated symptoms

6. Risk Management

6.1 Risk-Management Strategies
(CCSMH, 2008)

6.1.1 Immediate Risk Management

- Do not leave the person alone until you have arranged for the involvement of another appropriate care provider or source of protection.
- Establish an immediate safety plan that includes:
    - Family support; 24-hour (or in-home) care providers
    - Police intervention (if needed)
- Consider care needs:
    - Emergency services
    - Telephone and/or in-person distress/support services
    - Mental health services
    - Medical services
    - Social service providers, community supports
- Ensure that follow-up care is arranged.
- Where possible, restrict access to lethal means.

6.1.2 Ongoing Risk Management

- Address underlying issues:
  - Medical, psychological, social, and environmental
- Continually assess suicide risk, resiliency, and warning signs.
- Continue to build and sustain the therapeutic relationship.
- Foster hope and enhance a sense of meaning in life.
- Develop a safety plan that includes after-hours support.
- Read and review CCSMH and other treatment guidelines.
- Work within a culturally competent model of care.
- Work in an interdisciplinary care model where possible.
- Develop relationships with mental health teams for support and ongoing follow-up.
- Be aware of community resources and referral sites/processes.

6.2 Guideline Recommendations on Risk-Management Strategies
(CCSMH, 2006)

- Don't feel you have to work alone. Suicide prevention requires a team approach. Providers are ideally encouraged to connect with a registered mental health professional. If mental healthcare professionals are unavailable, providers should connect with another member of a healthcare team within the community.
- Providers working with suicidal individuals require networks of support to ensure their own emotional well-being and to avoid burnout.
- For those designing and administrating systems of care, it is recommended that interdisciplinary and collaborative care models be established and supported.

6.3 Elements of the Treatment Plan with Suicidal Patients

Slaby (1998) articulated a number of elements that are ideally present in a treatment plan with suicidal individuals. These include:
- Assessing the presence of suicide thoughts and plans on an ongoing basis
- Considering factors that increase or decrease that person's risk for suicide
- Considering the need for different levels of care, potentially including a hospital admission
- Helping the patient access care when at risk (including after hours)
- Making efforts to enhance interpersonal support in the individual's life
- Considering the roles of psychotherapy, pharmacotherapy, and/or ECT as required
- Providing psychoeducation for the patient and members of his/her support network
- Maintaining good clinical records

6.4 Outpatient Suicide: Common Failure Scenarios

Bongar and colleagues (1998) identified a number of common problems in providing care for individuals at risk for suicide, including failing to:
- Evaluate the need for medications and review/revise prescribed medication
- Consider hospitalization and to identify appropriate criteria and goals for hospital admissions
- Assess for suicide risk, conduct a mental status exam, and diagnose psychopathology
- Maintain appropriate relationships with the patient and/or trainees involved in patient care

- Establish a treatment plan
- Appropriately take a history and document clinical interventions and judgment

6.5 *What Should Providers Do?*

- Engage the patient; develop rapport by sitting and listening non-judgmentally, showing interest, and being supportive and approachable.
- Find out about the person's situational/interpersonal issues, listen intently, and follow-up on hints.
- Don't assume all is well … Question!
- Assess psychopathology and suicide risk, and plan appropriate care (and follow-up).
- Involve others!!! Communicate!
- Keep detailed notes; documentation is critical, but avoid "no-harm contracts" (Lewis, 2007). Contracts do not decrease risk for suicide and may inadvertently increase risk (Edwards & Sachmann, 2010). Kroll (2000) reported that 41% of psychiatrists who used no-harm contracts lost a patient to suicide while on a contract. Moreover, calling it a contract raises the legal bar, and the consequent risk of a lawsuit. Develop a "safety plan" instead (Brown et al., 2005).
- Provide follow-up and supportive aftercare.

6.6 *Treatment Implications*

- We cannot predict who will die by suicide; however, we can and must assess suicide risk (and resiliency).
- Outreach is critical for detecting at-risk individuals; don't forget to follow through.
- Make suicide risk assessment part of usual practice, even when you don't think it's present.
- Routinely assess access to firearms and other lethal means.
- Assess history of suicidal behaviour, one of the strongest risk factors for death by suicide.
- Be open to discussions of suicide; it takes time and should.
- Consider use of rating scales.
- Work in teams wherever possible, ideally including a psychologist and other healthcare specialists.
- Communication among providers is absolutely critical.

7. Summary

- Suicide is a significant mental health and public health problem.
- Older adults have high rates of suicide, and the older adult population is growing.
- Treatment guidelines and other KT resources now exist for assessment and intervention with at-risk older adults.
- Suicide risk and resiliency factors must be assessed; this is to be done with sensitivity and attending to contextual factors in the life of an older adult.
- Use of validated measures and approaches can help.
- Promising clinical and community interventions exist.
- Improved access to appropriate and highly trained healthcare services is sorely needed.

- Collaborative care is strongly encouraged, as are focused outreach approaches and aftercare.
- More work is needed in terms of developing, implementing, and evaluating approaches to suicide risk detection and intervention, and enhancing systems of care to respond to the needs of at-risk older adults.
- Additional research and KT efforts are clearly needed.

QUESTIONS

1. List five of the leading demographic and/or clinical risk factors for suicide among older adults.
2. Briefly discuss two community-level interventions that have been shown empirically to help reduce risk for suicide behaviour and/or death by suicide among older adults.
3. What clinical interventions have been shown empirically to help reduce or resolve suicide ideation, behaviour, and/or death among older adults?
4. The presence of one or more mental disorders is nearly ubiquitous among older adults with suicide ideation and/or behaviour, and mental health trainees frequently encounter suicidal patients in the course of their training rotations. How can we revise mental health training programs to enhance provider knowledge and skill in working with individuals at risk for suicide?
5. How might provider attitudes positively or negatively impact the detection and/or delivery of sensitive clinical services to older adults at risk for suicide?

ANSWERS

1. Risk factors for suicide in older adults include:

Demographic risk factors:

- Age (older; this is primarily the case for men)
- Sex (male)
- Ethnicity (white/Euro-American)
- Marital status (widowed, divorced, or separated)
- Socioeconomic status (SES) (lower SES, generally)

Clinical risk factors:

- History of suicidal behaviour (suicide attempt)
- Presence of suicide ideation and/or a wish to die
- Presence of one or more mental disorders, especially:
  - Mood disorders
  - Psychotic disorders
  - Substance misuse disorders
  - Risk is higher with multiple comorbidities
- Rigid personality traits and personality disorders
- Medical illness and pain (experienced or anticipated)
- Losses, transitions, and other psychosocial stressors, including:
  - Financial stressors
  - Interpersonal stressors
  - Residential stressors

- Occupational stressors
- Environmental stressors
- Functional impairment

2. Helpful community-level interventions that reduce risk include:
   - Referring depressed, socially isolated, or otherwise at-risk older adults to a telephone distress outreach and support service (e.g., Telehealth/Telecheck in Padua, Italy; see De Leo, Dello Buono, & Dwyer, 2002)
   - Community outreach depression lectures, screenings, and counselling for those with depression (e.g., Oyama et al., 2005, in Japan)

   The reader might also note other effective strategies:
   - Collaborative/shared care programs (e.g., PROSPECT [Bruce et al., 2004] and IMPACT [Unützer et al., 2006] studies)
   - Means restriction (e.g., bridge barriers, restricting access to alcohol and firearms, detoxifying gas ovens, and restriction of medication-pack sizes; see Mann et al., 2005)

3. Regarding helpful clinical interventions that reduce risk:
   - Few intervention trials exist with older adults explicitly at risk for suicide, and fewer still RCTs.
   - Existing trials support combination antidepressant pharmacotherapy and empirically supported psychotherapy, including:
     - Interpersonal psychotherapy (e.g., Bruce et al., 2004; Heisel et al., 2009; Heisel et al., 2015)
     - Problem-solving treatment (e.g., Unützer et al., 2006)
   - Although not specific to older adults, some support exists for use of:
     - Lithium (Angst, Angst, & Stassen, 1999; Baldessarini, Tondo, & Hennen, 1999; Goodwin, 1999)
     - Clozapine (Meltzer et al., 2003)
     - Other antipsychotics (Hawton et al., 1998; Palmer, Henter, & Wyatt, 1999)
     - Antidepressants (Angst, Angst, & Stassen, 1999)
     - ECT (Prudic & Sackeim, 1999)
     - Cognitive therapy (Brown et al., 2005; Linehan et al., 1991, 2006; Salkovskis, Atha, & Storer, 1990)
     - Interpersonal/psychodynamic psychotherapy (Guthrie et al., 2001; McLeavey et al., 1994)

4. Options for revising mental health training programs include the following:
   - Dedicated half- or full-year courses in suicidology could be provided at the undergraduate level for students interested in entering the healthcare workforce, or at colleges in diploma programs in health services fields.
   - Students could be encouraged (e.g., through the offer of extra credit and/or improved likelihood of acceptance into advanced training programs) to engage in volunteer positions with potentially suicidal individuals (e.g., on a distress line or in a mental health clinic).
   - More advanced-level courses focusing on theories of suicide and clinical skills training courses focusing on suicide risk detection and intervention could be

offered in graduate school and in healthcare profession training programs, including in medical school.

- Clinical examples of suicidal individuals (and/or those who lost a loved one to suicide) could be woven into clinical skills training throughout residencies and/or internships and practica in psychiatry, psychology, and other medical specialties and health professions.
- Professional examinations could include an example of a suicidal individual in order to evaluate trainee thinking and practice with individuals potentially at risk for suicide.

5. Provider attitudes are critical for the detection and management of suicide risk.
- Provider attitudes can have an appreciable impact on varied aspects of healthcare services, from the wish to see (or not see) certain types of patients, interest in learning about factors contributing to suicide risk and up-to-date approaches for assessment and treatment, the amount of time allocated for clinical appointments (and duration of time between appointments), subtle nonverbal cues, and even direct statements regarding the anticipated success of treatment.
- Providers holding negativistic views towards suicidal older adults, including believing that such individuals cannot be successfully treated or aren't adherent to treatment, that they drain or waste clinician time, are a medico-legal or financial threat, or are selfish or manipulative, may inadvertently communicate these impressions to the patient, negatively impacting the patient's self-perception of worth and hope for therapeutic change.
- Providers holding overly engaged or enmeshed approaches towards suicidal individuals may inadvertently send their patients a negative message regarding the patient's own ability to care for him- or herself or the provider's tolerance of the patient's suicidal thoughts or feelings, and may threaten therapeutic rapport and the effectiveness of treatment.
- Given the impact that our attitudes can have on the way in which we think about and offer care to our patients, it behooves us to identify and evaluate our attitudes towards our suicidal patients in order to ensure that we are offering effective and appropriately sensitive care.

CASE DISCUSSION

1. Given that Bea has just engaged in an apparent overdose, her imminent risk for suicide appears to be fairly high. It is unclear whether the acute interpersonal stressors that might have triggered her self-injurious behaviour have now subsided, or remain an ongoing concern. If her interpersonal stressors have now subsided, she may have overcome the highest risk period; if not, risk may remain high for the foreseeable future. Her apparent alcohol use could complicate this picture. Her clinician would be wise to assess the context in which she drinks and whether her drinking pattern meets criteria for an alcohol misuse diagnosis. If, for instance, Bea drank in order to overcome a reticence to take the medication overdose, provided the interpersonal and situational stressors can be managed and overcome, her long-term suicide risk may be reasonably low. If, however, she frequently drinks excessively or in dangerous situations, then long-term risk for suicide would be higher (and intervention for substance misuse clearly warranted).

2. Although not clear from the case description, Bea appears to have been prescribed antidepressants, suggesting that she may have been diagnosed with a mood disorder (presence of a mental disorder increases risk for suicide).

Additional considerations:

- Although not clear from the case description, Bea appears to have been prescribed heart medication (presence of medical illness, and attendant fear of pain, decline, and functional impairment may increase risk for suicide).
- Although not clear from the case description, Bea may struggle with alcohol misuse (alcohol misuse can increase risk for suicide).
- Bea may be experiencing interpersonal conflict (with her ex-son-in-law, and possibly with Abe, her husband).
- Bea may struggle with emotional expression (she appears to have had difficulty expressing herself to her husband in such a manner as to enhance the likelihood of having her emotional needs met; granted, it may be the case that the problem lay in his reception rather than in her transmission of her emotional upset, but either way this had a negative outcome).
- Bea is of Eastern European birth (suicide rates are high in this part of the world; research suggests that individuals who immigrate to a new country bring the suicide rate of their country of origin with them).

3. Resiliency factors that may be able to be engaged to reduce her risk of suicide include the following:

- Bea is married (marriage can protect against suicide risk; her husband Abe seems concerned about her).
- Bea appears to have at least one child (her daughter) and more than one grandchild. The case description did not comment on the nature of her relationship with her offspring; however, it suggests that she has family who might be engaged to provide her with support (however, this can quickly be conceptualized as a risk factor if, in fact, she has poor or strained relations with her offspring).
- Although her possible mental health and cardiac problems were mentioned as potential risk factors, the fact that she (apparently) has been prescribed medication suggests that she is amenable to healthcare and may have one or more physicians (utilization of healthcare services can be protective against suicide).

4. Helpful interventions with empirical support include the following:

- Conduct a complete psychosocial assessment and provide her with appropriate treatment.
- Consider (and offer if deemed appropriate) combination psychotherapy and antidepressant medication, as supported by the clinical literature.
- Her mental healthcare provider(s) would ideally work in conjunction with Bea's primary care medical provider.
- Her husband Abe might be encouraged to attend one or more of her therapy sessions in order to teach him how to more fully participate in Bea's care and to help him learn the warning signs that indicate Bea might be struggling emotionally and could benefit from additional support.
- Her husband might also be engaged to serve a gatekeeper function, contacting Bea's clinicians or taking her for emergency care when she is at imminent risk.

RECOMMENDED RESOURCES FOR REVIEW

Although these resources may not be specifically cited in the text, their approach informed the contents of the chapter, and they are recommended as useful further reading.

Grek A. Clinical management of suicidality in the elderly: an opportunity for involvement in the lives of older patients. Can J Psychiatry. 2007;52(6 Suppl 1):47S–57S. Medline:17824352

Heisel MJ. Suicide and its prevention among older adults. Can J Psychiatry. 2006;51(3):143–54. Medline:16618005

Heisel MJ, Duberstein PR. Working sensitively and effectively to reduce suicide risk among older adults. In: Kleespies PM, editor. The Oxford handbook of behavioral emergencies and crises. Oxford, UK; New York, NY: Oxford University Press; 2016. http://dx.doi .org/10.1093/oxfordhb/9780199352722.001.0001

Lapierre S, Erlangsen A, Waern M, et al; International Research Group for Suicide among the Elderly. A systematic review of elderly suicide prevention programs. Crisis. 2011;32(2):88–98. http://dx.doi.org/10.1027/0227-5910/a000076. Medline:21602163

REFERENCES

Alexopoulos GS, Reynolds CF III, Bruce ML, et al.; PROSPECT Group. Reducing suicidal ideation and depression in older primary care patients: 24-month outcomes of the PROSPECT study. Am J Psychiatry. 2009;166(8):882–90. http://dx.doi.org/10.1176/appi.ajp.2009.08121779. Medline:19528195

Angst J, Angst F, Stassen HH. Suicide risk in patients with major depressive disorder. J Clin Psychiatry. 1999;60(Suppl 2):57–62, discussion 75–6, 113–6. Medline:10073389

Baldessarini RJ, Tondo L, Hennen J. Effects of lithium treatment and its discontinuation on suicidal behavior in bipolar manic-depressive disorders. J Clin Psychiatry. 1999;60(Suppl 2):77–84, discussion 111–6. Medline:10073392

Bongar B, Maris RW, Berman AL, et al. Outpatient standards of care and the suicidal patient. In: Bongar B, Berman AL, Maris RW, et al., editors. Risk management with suicidal patients. New York: Guilford; 1998. p. 4–33.

Brown GK, Ten Have T, Henriques GR, et al. Cognitive therapy for the prevention of suicide attempts: a randomized controlled trial. JAMA. 2005;294(5):563–70. http://dx.doi.org/10.1001/jama.294.5.563. Medline:16077050

Bruce ML, Ten Have TR, Reynolds CF III, et al. Reducing suicidal ideation and depressive symptoms in depressed older primary care patients: a randomized controlled trial. JAMA. 2004;291(9):1081–91. http:// dx.doi.org/10.1001/jama.291.9.1081. Medline:14996777

Busch KA, Fawcett J, Jacobs DG. Clinical correlates of inpatient suicide. J Clin Psychiatry. 2003;64(1):14–9. http://dx.doi.org/10.4088/JCP.v64n0105. Medline:12590618

Canadian Coalition for Seniors' Mental Health (CCSMH). National guidelines for seniors' mental health: the assessment of suicide risk and prevention of suicide. Toronto: Canadian Coalition for Seniors' Mental Health; 2006. http://www.ccsmh.ca/en/natlGuidelines/initiative.cfm

– Suicide: assessment & prevention for older adults. Based on: Canadian Coalition for Seniors' Mental Health (CCSMH) national guidelines: the assessment of suicide risk and prevention of suicide. Toronto: Canadian Coalition for Seniors' Mental Health; 2008. http://www.ccsmh.ca/en/resources/resources.cfm

Centers for Disease Control and Prevention; National Center for Injury Prevention and Control. WISQARS (Web-based Injury Statistics Query and Reporting System) fatal injury reports, national and regional, 1999–2014. Data file. http://webappa.cdc.gov/sasweb/ncipc/mortrate10_us.html

De Leo D, Dello Buono M, Dwyer J. Suicide among the elderly: the long-term impact of a telephone support and assessment intervention in northern Italy. Br J Psychiatry. 2002;181(3):226–9. http://dx.doi.org/10.1192/ bjp.181.3.226. Medline:12204927

Draper B, Brodaty H, Low LF, Richards V. Prediction of mortality in nursing home residents: impact of passive self-harm behaviors. Int Psychogeriatr. 2003;15(2):187–96. http://dx.doi.org/10.1017/S1041610203008871. Medline:14620077

Draper B, Brodaty H, Low LF, Richards V, et al. Self-destructive behaviors in nursing home residents. J Am Geriatr Soc. 2002;50(2):354–8. http://dx.doi.org/10.1046/j.1532-5415.2002.50070.x. Medline:12028220

Duberstein PR, Conwell Y, Seidlitz L, et al. Age and suicidal ideation in older depressed inpatients. Am J Geriatr Psychiatry. 1999;7(4):289–96. http://dx.doi.org/10.1097/00019442-199911000-00003. Medline:10521160

Edelstein BA, Heisel MJ, McKee DR, et al. Development and psychometric evaluation of the reasons for living–older adults scale: a suicide risk assessment inventory. Gerontologist. 2009;49(6):736–45. http://dx.doi.org/10.1093/geront/gnp052. Medline:19546114

Edwards SJ, Sachmann MD. No-suicide contracts, no-suicide agreements, and no-suicide assurances: a study of their nature, utilization, perceived effectiveness, and potential to cause harm. Crisis. 2010;31(6):290–302. http://dx.doi.org/10.1027/0227-5910/a000048. Medline:21190927

Fawcett J, Scheftner WA, Fogg L, et al. Time-related predictors of suicide in major affective disorder. Am J Psychiatry. 1990;147(9):1189–94. http://dx.doi.org/10.1176/ajp.147.9.1189. Medline:2104515

Florio ER, Rockwood TH, Hendryx MS, et al. A model gatekeeper program to find the at-risk elderly. J Case Manag. 1996;5(3):106–14. Medline:9257625

Fremouw W, McCoy K, Tyner E, et al. Suicidal older adult protocol–SOAP. [unpublished manuscript, West Virginia University; 2009]. http://gerocentral.org/reference/fremouw-w-mccoy-k-tyner-e-musick-r-2009-suicide-older-adult-protocol-soap-unpublished-manuscript-west-virginia-university-access-manual-here/

Goodwin FK. Anticonvulsant therapy and suicide risk in affective disorders. J Clin Psychiatry. 1999;60(Suppl 2):89–93, discussion 111–6. Medline:10073394

Gunnell D, Middleton N, Frankel S. Method availability and the prevention of suicide–a re-analysis of secular trends in England and Wales 1950-1975. Soc Psychiatry Psychiatr Epidemiol. 2000;35(10):437–43. http://dx.doi.org/10.1007/s001270050261. Medline:11127717

Guthrie E, Kapur N, Mackway-Jones K, et al. Randomised controlled trial of brief psychological intervention after deliberate self poisoning. BMJ. 2001;323(7305):135–8. http://dx.doi.org/10.1136/bmj.323.7305.135. Medline:11463679

Hatton CL, Valente SM, Rink A. Suicide assessment and intervention. New York: Appleton Century Croft; 1977.

Hawton K, Arensman E, Townsend E, et al. Deliberate self harm: systematic review of efficacy of psychosocial and pharmacological treatments in preventing repetition. BMJ. 1998;317(7156):441–7. http://dx.doi.org/10.1136/bmj.317.7156.441. Medline:9703526

Hawton K, Townsend E, Deeks J, et al. Effects of legislation restricting pack sizes of paracetamol and salicylate on self poisoning in the United Kingdom: before and after study. BMJ. 2001;322(7296):1203–7. http://dx.doi.org/10.1136/bmj.322.7296.1203. Medline:11358770

Heisel MJ, Conwell Y, Pisani AR, et al. Concordance of self- and proxy-reported suicide ideation in depressed adults 50 years of age or older. Can J Psychiatry. 2011;56(4):219–26. Medline:21507278

Heisel MJ, Duberstein PR, Lyness JM, et al. Screening for suicide ideation among older primary care patients. J Am Board Fam Med. 2010;23(2):260–9. http://dx.doi.org/10.3122/jabfm.2010.02.080163. Medline:20207936

Heisel MJ, Duberstein PR, Talbot NL, et al. Adapting interpersonal psychotherapy for older adults at risk for suicide: preliminary findings. Prof Psychol Res Pr. 2009;40(2):156–64. http://dx.doi.org/10.1037/a0014731. PMID:20574546

Heisel MJ, Flett GL. The development and initial validation of the geriatric suicide ideation scale. Am J Geriatr Psychiatry. 2006;14(9):742–51. http://dx.doi.org/10.1097/01.JGP.0000218699.27899.f9. Medline:16943171

– Does recognition of meaning in life confer resiliency to suicide ideation among community-residing older adults? A longitudinal investigation. Am J Geriatr Psychiatry. 2016a;24(6):455–66. http://dx.doi.org/10.1016/j.jagp.2015.08.007. PMID:26880611

– Investigating the psychometric properties of the Geriatric Suicide Ideation Scale (GSIS) among community-residing older adults. Aging Ment Health. 2016b;20(2): 208–21. http://dx.doi.org/10.1080/13607863.2015.1072798

Heisel MJ, The Meaning-Centered Men's Group Project Team. Enhancing psychological resiliency in older men facing retirement with Meaning-Centered Men's Groups. In: Batthyány A, editor. Logotherapy and existential analysis: proceedings of the Viktor Frankl Institute, Vienna. vol. 1. Switzerland: Springer International; 2016. p. 165–73.

Heisel MJ, Neufeld E, Flett GL. Reasons for living, meaning in life, and suicide ideation: investigating the roles of key positive psychological factors in reducing suicide risk in community-residing older adults. Aging Ment Health. 2016;20(2):195–207. http://dx.doi.org/10.1080/13607863.2015.1078279

Heisel MJ, Talbot NL, King DA, et al. Adapting interpersonal psychotherapy for older adults at risk for suicide. Am J Geriatr Psychiatry. 2015;23(1):87–98. http://dx.doi.org/10.1016/j.jagp.2014.03.010. PMID:24840611

Hendin H, Haas AP, Maltsberger JT, et al. Problems in psychotherapy with suicidal patients. Am J Psychiatry. 2006;163(1):67–72. http://dx.doi.org/10.1176/appi.ajp.163.1.67. Medline:16390891

Holkup P. Evidence-based protocol. Elderly suicide: secondary prevention. Iowa City, IA: University of Iowa Gerontological Nursing Interventions Research Center, Research Dissemination Core; 2002.

Hunkeler EM, Katon W, Tang L, et al. Long term outcomes from the IMPACT randomised trial for depressed elderly patients in primary care. BMJ. 2006;332(7536):259–63. http://dx.doi.org/10.1136/bmj.38683.710255.BE. Medline:16428253

Jacobs DG, Baldessarini RJ, Conwell Y, et al. American Psychiatric Association practice guidelines: Practice guidelines for the assessment and treatment of patients with suicidal behaviors. Arlington, VA: American Psychiatric Association; 2003.

Kjølseth I, Ekeberg Ø, & Steihaug S. Elderly people who committed suicide— their contact with the health service. What did they expect, and what did they get? Aging Ment Health. 2010;14(8):938– 46. http://dx.doi.org/10.1080/13607863.2010.501056. Medline:21069599

Kleespies, PM, Hughes, DH, Gallacher, FP. Suicide in the medically and terminally ill: psychological and ethical considerations. J Clin Psychol. 2000;56(9):1153–71. Medline:10987689

Knox KL, Conwell Y, Caine ED. If suicide is a public health problem, what are we doing to prevent it? Am J Public Health. 2004;94(1):37–45. http://dx.doi.org/10.2105/AJPH.94.1.37. Medline:14713694

Kroll J. Use of no-suicide contracts by psychiatrists in Minnesota. Am J Psychiatry. 2000;157(10):1684–6. http://dx.doi.org/10.1176/appi.ajp.157.10.1684. Medline:11007726

Krug EG, Dahlberg LL, Mercy JA, et al, editors. World report on violence and health. Geneva, CH: World Health Organization; 2002. http://www.who.int/violence_injury_prevention/violence/world_report/en/

Leenaars AA. Psychotherapy with suicidal people: the commonalities. Arch Suicide Res. 2006;10(4):305–22. http://dx.doi.org/10.1080/13811110600790710. Medline:16920682

Lewis LM. No-harm contracts: a review of what we know. Suicide Life Threat Behav. 2007;37(1):50–7. http://dx.doi.org/10.1521/suli.2007.37.1.50. Medline:17397279

Linehan MM, Armstrong HE, Suarez A, et al. Cognitive-behavioral treatment of chronically parasuicidal borderline patients. Arch Gen Psychiatry. 1991;48(12):1060–4. http://dx.doi.org/10.1001/archpsyc.1991.01810360024003. Medline:1845222

Linehan MM, Comtois KA, Murray AM, et al. Two-year randomized controlled trial and follow-up of dialectical behavior therapy vs therapy by experts for suicidal behaviors and borderline personality disorder. Arch Gen Psychiatry. 2006;63(7):757–66. http://dx.doi.org/10.1001/archpsyc.63.7.757. Medline:16818865

Links PS, Heisel MJ, Quastel A. Is suicide ideation a surrogate endpoint for geriatric suicide? Suicide Life Threat Behav. 2005;35(2):193–205. http://dx.doi.org/10.1521/suli.35.2.193.62870. Medline:15843336

Luoma JB, Martin CE, Pearson JL. Contact with mental health and primary care providers before suicide: a review of the evidence. Am J Psychiatry. 2002;159(6):909–16. http://dx.doi.org/10.1176/appi.ajp.159.6.909. Medline:12042175

Lynch TR, Morse JQ, Mendelson T, et al. Dialectical behavior therapy for depressed older adults: a randomized pilot study. Am J Geriatr Psychiatry. 2003;11(1):33–45. http://dx.doi.org/10.1097/00019442-200301000-00006. Medline:12527538

Lyness JM, Cox C, Curry J, et al. Older age and the underreporting of depressive symptoms. J Am Geriatr Soc. 1995;43(3):216–21. http://dx.doi.org/10.1111/j.1532-5415.1995.tb07325.x. Medline:7884106

Mann JJ, Apter A, Bertolote J, et al. Suicide prevention strategies: a systematic review. JAMA. 2005;294(16):2064–74. http://dx.doi.org/10.1001/jama.294.16.2064. Medline:16249421

McIntosh JL, Santos JF, Hubbard RW, et al. Elder suicide: research, theory, and treatment. Washington, DC: American Psychological Association; 1994.

McLeavey BC, Daly RJ, Ludgate JW, et al. Interpersonal problem-solving skills training in the treatment of self-poisoning patients. Suicide Life Threat Behav. 1994;24(4):382–94. Medline:7740595

Meltzer HY, Alphs L, Green AI, et al.; International Suicide Prevention Trial Study Group. Clozapine treatment for suicidality in schizophrenia: International Suicide Prevention Trial (InterSePT). Arch Gen Psychiatry. 2003;60(1):82–91. http://dx.doi.org/10.1001/archpsyc.60.1.82. Medline:12511175

O'Connor E, Gaynes BN, Burda BU, et al. Screening for and treatment of suicide risk relevant to primary care: a systematic review for the U.S. Preventive Services Task Force. Ann Intern Med. 2013;158(10):741–54. http://dx.doi.org/10.7326/0003-4819-158-10-201305210-00642. Medline:23609101

Oyama H, Watanabe N, Ono Y, et al. Community-based suicide prevention through group activity for the elderly successfully reduced the high suicide rate for females. Psychiatry Clin Neurosci. 2005;59(3):337–44. http://dx.doi.org/10.1111/j.1440-1819.2005.01379.x. Medline:15896228

Palmer DD, Henter ID, Wyatt RJ. Do antipsychotic medications decrease the risk of suicide in patients with schizophrenia? J Clin Psychiatry. 1999;60(Suppl 2):100–3, discussion 111–6. Medline:10073396

Pearson JL, Stanley B, King C, et al. Intervention research with persons at high risk for suicidality: safety and ethical considerations. J Clin Psychiatry. 2001;62(Suppl 25):17–26. MEDLINE:11765091

Pokorny AD. Prediction of suicide in psychiatric patients: report of a prospective study. In: Maltsberger JT, Goldblatt MJ, editors. Essential papers on suicide. New York: New York University Press; 1996. p. 480–507.

Prudic J, Sackeim HA. Electroconvulsive therapy and suicide risk. J Clin Psychiatry. 1999;60(Suppl 2):104–10, discussion 111–6. Medline:10073397

Rutz W, von Knorring L, Wålinder J. Frequency of suicide on Gotland after systematic postgraduate education of general practitioners. Acta Psychiatr Scand. 1989;80(2):151–4. http://dx.doi.org/10.1111/j.1600-0447.1989.tb01318.x. Medline:2801163

Salkovskis PM, Atha C, Storer D. Cognitive-behavioural problem solving in the treatment of patients who repeatedly attempt suicide. A controlled trial. Br J Psychiatry. 1990;157(6):871–6. http://dx.doi.org/10.1192/bjp.157.6.871. Medline:2289097

Silverman MM. Rational suicide, hastened death, and self-destructive behaviors. Couns Psychol. 2000;28(4):540–50. http://dx.doi.org/10.1177/0011000000284004

Slaby AE. Outpatient management of suicidal patients. In: Bongar B, Berman AL, Maris RW, et al, editors. Risk management with suicidal patients. New York: Guilford; 1998. p. 34–64.

Statistics Canada. Mortality summary, list of causes. Catalogue number 84F0209X. Ottawa: Statistics Canada; 2012.

– Table 102–0551: Deaths and mortality rate, by selected grouped causes, age group and sex, Canada, annual, CANSIM (database); 2014. http://www5.statcan.gc.ca/cansim/a26?lang=eng&id=1020551

Substance Abuse and Mental Health Services Administration (SAMHSA). Promoting emotional health and preventing suicide: a toolkit for senior living communities. Rockville, MD: Center for Mental Health Services, Substance Abuse and Mental Health Services Administration; 2010.

Szanto K, Mulsant BH, Houck PR, Dew MA, Dombrovski A, et al. Emergence, persistence, and resolution of suicidal ideation during treatment of depression in old age. J Affect Disord. 2007;98(1–2):153–61. http://dx.doi.org/10.1016/j.jad.2006.07.015. Medline:16934334

Szanto K, Mulsant BH, Houck P, Dew MA, Reynolds CF. Occurrence and course of suicidality during short-term treatment of late-life depression. Arch Gen Psychiatry. 2003;60(6):610–7. http://dx.doi.org/10.1001/archpsyc.60.6.610. Medline:12796224

Unützer J, Tang L, Oishi S, et al.; IMPACT Investigators. Reducing suicidal ideation in depressed older primary care patients. J Am Geriatr Soc. 2006;54(10):1550–6. http://dx.doi.org/10.1111/j.1532-5415.2006.00882.x. Medline:17038073

Waern M, Beskow J, Runeson B, et al. High rate of antidepressant treatment in elderly people who commit suicide. BMJ. 1996;313(7065):1118. http://dx.doi.org/10.1136/bmj.313.7065.1118. Medline:8916699

– Suicidal feelings in the last year of life in elderly people who commit suicide. Lancet. 1999;354(9182):917–8. http://dx.doi.org/10.1016/S0140-6736(99)93099-4. Medline:10489955

Waern M, Runeson BS, Allebeck P, et al. Mental disorder in elderly suicides: a case-control study. Am J Psychiatry. 2002;159(3):450–5. http://dx.doi.org/10.1176/appi.ajp.159.3.450. Medline:11870010

World Health Organization (WHO). Preventing suicide: a global imperative. Geneva: WHO; 2014. http://www.who.int/mental_health/suicide-prevention/world_report_2014/en/

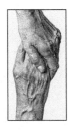

SECTION 3:
OTHER DISORDERS

3.1 Primary Psychotic Disorders in Older Adults

Tarek K. Rajji, MD, FRCPC

INTRODUCTION

Psychosis is a common presentation of many mental illnesses in older adults and includes primary psychotic disorders such as schizophrenia along with psychotic presentations of other illnesses such as mood disorders, delirium, and dementia. Geriatric psychiatrists will encounter individuals with long-standing schizophrenia that developed during early adulthood as well as individuals who develop schizophrenia or psychotic disorders later in life. In this chapter, Dr Rajji reviews the epidemiology and some of the unique features of schizophrenia with onset in older adulthood and contrasts it to schizophrenia with onset earlier in life. A review of pharmacological treatment strategies and psychosocial interventions for schizophrenia are then presented.

CASE SCENARIO

Ms V. is a 72-year-old female with a 40-year history of schizophrenia. She is supported by Old Age Security, lives in supportive housing, and follows up once a month in an outpatient clinic. She has a community agency worker who supports her with some of her instrumental activities of daily living (IADLs). She has no next of kin available. She has been maintained for about 20 years on clozapine 250 mg qhs. Psychiatrically she is relatively stable with persistent auditory hallucinations, hearing family members from childhood talking to her at times. She is on no other medications except vitamin D and a multivitamin. Over the past 1–2 years she has been developing a chronic cough and shortness of breath. She is a chronic smoker and has been trying to cut down with the support of staff in her clinic and her housing. Her housing staff has been noticing over the past 6 months that she has been more forgetful and at times confused. They also noted that she has been awake at night several times, talking to herself and having distressful arguments at times. She continues to be independent with her activities of daily living but needs more prompting than before. There are no acute safety concerns.

1. What is the differential of the changes in her cognitive and functional state?
2. What are the necessary assessments?
3. What are some potential interventions?
4. What measures need to be implemented in her future care after treating her current illness?

OVERVIEW

1. Natural History of Schizophrenia

(Leiberman, 2003)

- Three phases: prodrome; onset/deterioration; residual/stable
- Prodrome: typically in the teens; focus on primary prevention
- Onset/deterioration: typically in the 20s; focus on secondary prevention and remediation
- Residual/stable: typically in the 40s and later; focus on rehabilitation

1.1 Long-Term Studies of Schizophrenia

(Cohen, 2003)

- Ten long-term studies
- A total of 2429 patients
- Follow-up: 20 to 37 years
- Significant clinical improvement: 46–84% (median = 53%)
- Social recovery: 21–77% (median = 49%)
- About 20% remain institutionalized or quasi-institutionalized

2. Epidemiology

- 12% of persons with schizophrenia were age 50 or older in 2004 (Goeree et al., 2005).
- The number of older persons with schizophrenia will double in the next 20 years (Cohen et al., 2008).
- 0.6–1% prevalence (Gurland & Cross, 1982)
- 12% live in long-term homes
- 3% in hospitals
- 85% in the community
- The costs of schizophrenia are highest early in life around the time of onset and later in life, after age 65 (Cuffel et al., 1996).

3. Types of Schizophrenia in Late Life

3.1 Early-Onset Schizophrenia

- Onset before the age of 40
- Vast majority of older patients with schizophrenia

3.2 Late-Onset Schizophrenia

- Onset between age 40 and 60
- 23.5% of all patients with schizophrenia
- Incidence: 12.6 per 100 000 population per year are diagnosed with schizophrenia with first onset after 44 years (van Os et al., 1995)

3.3 Very-Late-Onset Schizophrenia-Like Psychosis

- Onset after the age of 60
- 3% of all patients with schizophrenia

3.4 Early vs Late-Onset Schizophrenia
(Jeste, Lanouette, & Vahia, 2009; Rajji, Ismail, & Mulsant, 2009)

- More women are among those with late-onset schizophrenia.
- Late-onset schizophrenia is associated with positive rather than negative symptoms.
- There is more variability in the profile of the cognitive deficits of patients with late-onset schizophrenia, with some domains less impacted than others; in contrast, those with early-onset schizophrenia tend to have a more generalized deficit.
- Patients with late-onset schizophrenia tend to respond to lower doses of antipsychotics than those with early-onset.

3.5 Risk Factors for Late- and Very-Late-Onset Schizophrenia

- Psychosocial isolation
- Female gender
- Bereavement
- Sensory deficits
- Immigration

(See also question 2 at the end of this chapter.)

4. Delusional Disorder

- 0.03% prevalence
- About 25% are older than 65 years
- Types:
    - Erotomanic
    - Grandiose
    - Jealous
    - Persecutory
    - Somatic
    - Mixed

5. Differentiating Chronic Schizophrenia vs Alzheimer's Disease with Psychosis

Table 3.1.1 describes key clinical features that differentiate an older person with Alzheimer's disease vs an older person with schizophrenia.

6. Medical Comorbidities in Older Patients with Schizophrenia

Little information is available on the medical comorbidities observed in older patients with schizophrenia. This is thought to be due to:

- Discrimination
- Poor reporting due to increase in pain tolerance
- Poor insight into medical problems
- Pain sensitivity reduced by antipsychotics
- Not more physical problems than same-age peers
- Severity of problems may be worse
- Survival bias
- Lifespan reduced by 10–15 years

Table 3.1.1: Alzheimer's Disease vs Schizophrenia in Late Life

Symptoms	Alzheimer's Disease	Schizophrenia
Delusions: Someone stealing; thought control	 +++ +/–	 ++ ++/+++
Hallucinations: Auditory Visual	 +/++ ++/+++	 ++/+++ +
Family history	Alzheimer's disease	Major mental illness
Course	Progressive decline	Variable
Social situation	Married, widowed, divorced, not socially isolated	Single, socially isolated

+ = present; ++ = common; +++ = highly common; +/– = more or less present

Adapted from Desai & Grossberg, 2003.

7. Cognition in Late-Life Schizophrenia

Given the focus on rehabilitation in an older person with schizophrenia, cognitive function is a major factor affecting the success of any rehabilitation intervention.

7.1 Institutionalized Older Patients with Schizophrenia

(e.g., Waddington & Youssef, 1996; Harvey et al., 1999; Friedman et al., 2001)

- Cognition declines after at least 2 years of follow-up.
- After age 65, Mini Mental State Examination (MMSE) score declines by 1 point/year vs 3 points/year in Alzheimer disease.

7.2 Community-Dwelling Older Patients with Schizophrenia

- Overall cognition is stable (Heaton et al., 2001; Palmer et al., 2003).
- One study suggests decline in visuospatial ability (Nayak Savla et al., 2006).
- Cognitive decline in older patients with schizophrenia parallels that of normal aging; there is no evidence for an acceleration (Rajji et al., 2013).

7.3 Factors that Affect Cognition in Late-Life Schizophrenia

7.3.1 Medical Comorbidities

- Hypertension → decline in global cognition (Yaffe et al., 2007)
- Diabetes → information processing speed, memory (Stewart & Liolitsa, 1999; Awad, Gagnon, & Messier, 2004)
- Hypothyroidism → attention, executive function, and verbal and visual memory (Burmeister et al., 2001; Davis, Stern, & Flashman, 2003)
- Vascular disease

7.3.2 Anticholinergic Burden

- High serum anticholinergic burden is associated with impaired cognition among older community-dwelling adults (Mulsant et al., 2003).
- Serum anticholinergic burden negatively correlates with verbal working memory and verbal learning and memory among patients with schizophrenia (Vinogradov et al., 2009).
- High serum anticholinergic activity negatively impacts the ability to benefit from cognitive training (Vinogradov et al., 2009).

7.3.3 Age at Onset
(Rajji, Ismail, & Mulsant, 2009)

- Patients with youth or adult onset tend to have more generalized and severe cognitive impairments.
- Patients with a late onset tend to have more specific deficits.

8. Treatments

8.1 Service Needs for Older Patients with Schizophrenia

- Chronic care model
- Medications management
- Mood and cognition monitoring
- Coordination of care with primary care providers
- Accessible services
- Social integration
- Social rehabilitation services

8.2 Antipsychotic Medications

- Best evidence is for olanzapine or risperidone.
- Consider risperidone as first line, given the high anticholinergic burden of olanzapine.
- Consider other atypical antipsychotics with low anticholinergic burden, e.g., aripiprazole and ziprasidone.
- Most clozapine studies avoided older patients.
    - Still, worth considering clozapine in treatment-resistant patients instead of trying, for example, olanzapine, with equally high anticholinergic burden.
- See Table 3.1.2 for the dosing of common antipsychotics.

Table 3.1.2: Dosing of Common Antipsychotics for Older Persons with Schizophrenia

Medication	Initial dose (mg)	Titration step (mg)	Maintenance target dose (mg)	Half-life (hours)
Aripiprazole	2–5	2–5	10–15	75
Clozapine	6.25–12.5	12.5–25	100–200	4–66
Olanzapine	2.5–5	2.5–5	5–20	21–54
Quetiapine	12.5–50	25–50	100–450	6
Risperidone	0.25–0.5	0.25–0.5	1–4	3–20

8.3 Assertive Community Treatment

• Six studies included a substantial group of older patients with schizophrenia.
• No age-based analysis
• No evidence that older patients benefit less than younger patients

8.4 Case Management

• Eight studies included patients aged 50 or above.
• Less evidence supporting case management for older patients with schizophrenia
• More variability in outcomes: four studies were positive and the others were negative or showed mixed results

QUESTIONS

1. List five characteristics that differentiate late-onset schizophrenia from early-onset schizophrenia in older adults.
2. List five risk factors for late- and very-late-onset schizophrenia.
3. Describe the pharmacokinetic and pharmacodynamic changes that could impact treatment of late-life schizophrenia.
4. Describe a cognitive test that could assist in differentiating between memory deficits associated with schizophrenia and memory deficits associated with dementia in an older patient with schizophrenia.
5. Describe a psychosocial intervention that has been shown to improve function in patients with late-life schizophrenia.
6. How do we improve our current medical care system to engage older patients with schizophrenia on one hand, and the medical community on the other, for a better quality of care?
7. How can we promote healthy aging in older patients with schizophrenia and promote aging in the community while delaying transition to institutions such as long-term care homes?

ANSWERS

1. Characteristics that differentiate between late-onset schizophrenia and early-onset schizophrenia in older adults include the following:
   • The proportion of women among those with late-onset schizophrenia is higher than those with early-onset schizophrenia.
   • Those with late-onset schizophrenia tend to have primarily positive rather than negative symptoms.
   • There is more variability in the profile of the cognitive deficits experienced by those with late-onset schizophrenia, with some domains less impacted than others, whereas those with early-onset schizophrenia tend to have a more generalized deficit.
   • Patients with late-onset schizophrenia tend to respond to lower doses of antipsychotics than those with early-onset schizophrenia.
   • Patients with late-onset schizophrenia seem to have larger thalamic volumes than those with early-onset schizophrenia.
   • Higher prevalence of paranoid subtype in late-onset schizophrenia

- More organized delusions in late-onset schizophrenia
- Higher premorbid functioning in late-onset schizophrenia
- Sensory deficits more common in late-onset schizophrenia
- Higher prevalence of persecutory and partition delusions in late-onset schizophrenia

2. Risk factors for late- and very-late-onset schizophrenia include:
   - Psychosocial isolation and lower social supports
   - Female gender
   - Bereavement
   - Sensory deficits (especially hearing loss)
   - Immigration
   - Family history (late-onset only)
   - Childhood maladjustment
   - Abnormal social functioning
   - Abnormal premorbid personality (e.g., paranoid, schizoid, type A)
   - Presence of delusions in the absence of medical conditions that may cause delirium
   - Cerebrovascular abnormalities (very-late-onset)

3. Pharmacokinetic changes with potential impact include:
   - Lower volume of distribution
   - More blood-brain barrier permeability
   - Less D2 receptors to block
   - Lower hepatic and renal function, leading to slower metabolism and clearance
   - Muscle mass decreases and fat stores increase, leading to longer elimination half-lives of lipid-soluble drugs.
   - Together, these changes suggest that for any given dose, an older person may have a higher brain concentration of the drug and therefore may need a lower dose given at less frequent intervals than younger patients.

   Pharmacodynamic changes include:
   - The receptors in the brain may be less sensitive to blockade, suggesting higher doses are needed.
   - Age-related decline in receptor reserve, increasing susceptibility to clinical and adverse effects

4. While no single test can differentiate cognitive deficits associated with dementia from those associated with schizophrenia, there have been interesting studies looking at the "saving score" in verbal learning tests.
   - These tests typically consist of reading to an individual a list of X number of words (e.g., 10), and asking them to recall as many as possible. This is repeated several (e.g., 3) times, and more words are recalled with each trial. Then, after a delay of typically 20 minutes, the person is asked to recall as many words as he or she can. What has been observed in adult and older patients with schizophrenia compared to those with Alzheimer's disease (AD) is the following:
     - An individual with AD may learn 8/10 words by the third trial; then, after 20 min, he or she may recall 4 – in this case, the saving score is 50% (if the 4 words recalled were out of the 8 encoded after the third trial).

- An individual with schizophrenia (possibly because of severe executive deficits) may encode only 5 out of 10 by the third trial; however, out of these 5 words, 4 are recalled, giving a saving score of 80%.
- Thus, just by looking at the number of words recalled, these two individuals would appear to have similar deficits. However, based on the saving scores, an individual with schizophrenia is more likely to recall what he or she learned even though he or she would have been impaired in the initial learning phase.

5. Psychosocial interventions that improve function in patients with late-life schizophrenia include:
   - Cognitive behavioural social skills training
     - Aims to increase social functioning and cognitive insight
     - The major advantage is that it is manualized and delivered in group settings, making it efficient clinically.
     - Its limitation is that it has not yet been tested among truly older persons with schizophrenia (the original study included only patients in their 50s, and thus its ability to help improve function among those in their 60s or above is unclear [Granholm et al., 2005]).
   - Cognitive behavioural therapy to help reduce and deal with psychotic symptoms
   - Functional adaptation skills training
   - Cognitive training/remediation
   - Supportive employment or volunteerism
   - Community-based case management

6. In optimizing the medical system and quality of care, the following are points to consider:
   - Use of a chronic care model in delivering care to older persons with schizophrenia
   - Use of care coordinators
   - Providing primary care within a psychiatric setting given the preference of patients to be assessed in a psychiatric setting rather than a general medical practice setting
   - Collaboration with primary care clinics, possibly through the use of a nurse practitioner who would consult with them
   - Providing a flexible outreach team
   - Mandatory geriatric psychiatry training for family medicine residents
   - Advocating that more services be available for older patients with mental illness

7. To promote healthy aging at home in older adults with schizophrenia, consider the following interventions:
   - Transitional housing programs to increase success in transitioning between inpatient and outpatient settings
   - Psychosocial rehabilitation programs that target issues related to aging among patients with schizophrenia
   - Increased supports for functional disabilities within the environments where older patients with schizophrenia live
   - Careful review of vascular risk factors and antipsychotic medications, with the aim of reducing antipsychotic dose due to metabolic side effects

- Increased communication with primary care providers
- Promoting a healthy lifestyle that includes exercise, intellectual activity, and social engagement

CASE DISCUSSION

1. The differential diagnosis of her cognitive and functional changes could include:
   - Relapse of schizophrenia
   - Delirium due to infection
   - Increase in clozapine levels (secondary to a reduction in smoking, which is an inducer of clozapine metabolism), which could result in anticholinergic toxicity and confusion
   - Infection, which could lead to lower levels of clozapine by inducing clozapine metabolism, and cause worsening of psychotic symptoms
   - Dementia
   - Chronic cough and shortness of breath may be due to smoking history
   - Chest infection secondary to agranulocytosis
   - Depression
   - Delirium due to other causes (e.g., neurological, cardiac, syndrome of inappropriate antidiuretic hormone section [SIADH])
   - Metastases or paraneoplastic syndrome related to lung carcinoma
   - Non-adherence to medication
   - Drug-drug interaction with new medication(s)
   - Cognitive effects of potential chronic obstructive pulmonary disease and congestive heart failure

2. The following should be assessed:
   - Vital signs
   - Bloodwork including liver function tests, white blood count, and neutrophil counts
   - Urinalysis and culture
   - Chest X-ray
   - Clozapine levels
   - Safety and IADL assessments
   - Cognitive assessment (e.g., MMSE and clock drawing, or MoCA)
   - ECG to rule out arrhythmia
   - Confusion Assessment Method (CAM) to assess for delirium
   - CT head
   - Collateral history from caregiver(s)
   - Polysomnography to assess for sleep apnea

3. Potential interventions include:
   - Treating underlying cause of delirium if delirium is diagnosed
   - Adjusting clozapine dose (may need to be abruptly discontinued if there is evidence of agranulocytosis, myocarditis, or congestive heart failure)
   - Smoking cessation interventions
   - Consider cholinesterase inhibitor if dementia is diagnosed

- Increase environmental supports to accommodate for her functional decline
- Nonpharmacologic interventions for delirium if delirium is diagnosed

4. Aspects of future care that should be implemented include:
   - Consider alternative housing options
   - Consider increasing supports over the long term to promote aging at home
   - Regular checking of clozapine levels
   - Regular reassessment of cognitive function
   - Discussion about substitute decision maker and advanced care planning
   - Implement measures to improve medication adherence

RECOMMENDED RESOURCES FOR REVIEW

Although these resources may not be specifically cited in the text, their approach informed the contents of the chapter, and they are recommended as useful further reading.

Breitner JC, Husain MM, Figiel GS, et al. Cerebral white matter disease in late-onset paranoid psychosis. Biol Psychiatry. 1990;28(3):266–74. http://dx.doi.org/10.1016/0006-3223(90)90582-M. PMID:2378929

Brodaty H, Sachdev P, Koschera A, et al. Long-term outcome of late-onset schizophrenia: 5-year follow-up study. Br J Psychiatry. 2003;183(3):213–9. http://dx.doi.org/10.1192/bjp.183.3.213. Medline:12948993

Folsom DP, Lebowitz BD, Lindamer LA, et al. Schizophrenia in late life: emerging issues. Dialogues Clin Neurosci. 2006;8(1):45–52. Medline:16640113

Howard R, Rabins PV, Seeman MV, et al.; International Late-Onset Schizophrenia Group. Late-onset schizophrenia and very-late-onset schizophrenia-like psychosis: an international consensus. Am J Psychiatry. 2000;157(2):172–8. http://dx.doi.org/10.1176/appi.ajp.157.2.172. Medline:10671383

Jeste DV, Harris MJ, Krull A, et al. Clinical and neuropsychological characteristics of patients with late-onset schizophrenia. Am J Psychiatry. 1995;152(5):722–30. http://dx.doi.org/10.1176/ajp.152.5.722. Medline:7726312

Loewenstein DA, Czaja SJ, Bowie CR, et al. Age-associated differences in cognitive performance in older patients with schizophrenia: a comparison with healthy older adults. Am J Geriatr Psychiatry. 2012;20(1):29–40. http://dx.doi.org/10.1097/JGP.0b013e31823bc08c. Medline:22130385

Ting C, Rajji TK, Ismail Z, et al. Differentiating the cognitive profile of schizophrenia from that of Alzheimer disease and depression in late life. PLoS One. 2010;5(4):e10151. http://dx.doi.org/10.1371/journal.pone.0010151. Medline:20405043

Tsuboi T, Suzuki T, Uchida H. A tipping point in drug dosing in late-life schizophrenia. Curr Psychiatry Rep. 2011;13(3):225–33. http://dx.doi.org/10.1007/s11920-011-0189-z. Medline:21327902

REFERENCES

Awad N, Gagnon M, Messier C. The relationship between impaired glucose tolerance, type 2 diabetes, and cognitive function. J Clin Exp Neuropsychol. 2004;26(8):1044–80. Medline:15590460

Burmeister LA, Ganguli M, Dodge HH, et al. Hypothyroidism and cognition: preliminary evidence for a specific defect in memory. Thyroid. 2001;11(12):1177–85. Medline:12186506

Cohen CI, editor. Schizophrenia into later life: treatment, research, and policy. Arlington, VA: American Psychiatric Publishing; 2003.

Cohen CI, Vahia I, Reyes P, et al. Focus on geriatric psychiatry: schizophrenia in later life: clinical symptoms and social well-being. Psychiatr Serv. 2008;59(3):232–4. http://dx.doi.org/10.1176/appi.ps.59.3.232. Medline:18308900

Cuffel BJ, Jeste DV, Halpain M, et al. Treatment costs and use of community mental health services for schizophrenia by age cohorts. Am J Psychiatry. 1996;153(7):870–6. Medline:8659608

Davis JD, Stern RA, Flashman LA. Cognitive and neuropsychiatric aspects of subclinical hypothyroidism: significance in the elderly. Curr Psychiatry Rep. 2003;5(5):384–90. Medline:13678560

Desai AK, Grossberg GT. Differential diagnosis of psychotic disorders in the elderly. In: Cohen CI, editor. Schizophrenia into later life: treatment, research, and policy. 1st ed. Arlington, VA: American Psychiatric Publishing; 2003. p. 55–75.

Friedman JI, Harvey PD, Coleman T, et al. Six-year follow-up study of cognitive and functional status across the lifespan in schizophrenia: a comparison with Alzheimer's disease and normal aging. Am J Psychiatry. 2001;158(9):1441–8. Medline:11532729

Goeree R, Farahati F, Burke N, et al. The economic burden of schizophrenia in Canada in 2004. Curr Med Res Opin. 2005;21(12):2017–28. Medline:16368053

Granholm E, McQuaid JR, McClure FS, et al. A randomized, controlled trial of cognitive behavioral social skills training for middle-aged and older outpatients with chronic schizophrenia. Am J Psychiatry. 2005;162(3):520–9. http://dx.doi.org/10.1176/appi.ajp.162.3.520. Medline:15741469

Gurland BJ, Cross PS. Epidemiology of psychopathology in old age. Some implications for clinical services. Psychiatr Clin North Am. 1982;5(1):11–26.

Harvey PD, Silverman JM, Mohs RC, et al. Cognitive decline in late-life schizophrenia: a longitudinal study of geriatric chronically hospitalized patients. Biol Psychiatry. 1999;45(1):32–40. Medline:9894573

Heaton RK, Gladsjo JA, Palmer BW, et al. Stability and course of neuropsychological deficits in schizophrenia. Arch Gen Psychiatry. 2001;58(1):24–32. Medline:11146755

Jeste, DV, Lanouette, MN, Vahia IV. Schizophrenia and paranoid disorders. In: Blazer DG, Steffens DC, editors. The American Psychiatric Publishing textbook of geriatric psychiatry. 4th ed. Arlington, VA: American Psychiatric Publishing; 2009. p. 317–32.

Mulsant BH, Pollock BG, Kirshner M, et al. Serum anticholinergic activity in a community-based sample of older adults: relationship with cognitive performance. Arch Gen Psychiatry. 2003;60(2):198–203. Medline:12578438

Nayak Savla G, Moore DJ, Roesch SC, et al. An evaluation of longitudinal neurocognitive performance among middle-aged and older schizophrenia patients: use of mixed-model analyses. Schizophr Res. 2006;83(2–3):215–23. PMID:16507344

Palmer BW, Bondi MW, Twamley EW, et al. Are late-onset schizophrenia spectrum disorders neurodegenerative conditions? Annual rates of change on two dementia measures. J Neuropsychiatry Clin Neurosci. 2003;15(1):45–52. Medline:12556570

Rajji TK, Ismail Z, Mulsant BH. Age at onset and cognition in schizophrenia: meta-analysis. Br J Psychiatry. 2009;195(4):286–93. http://dx.doi.org/10.1192/bjp.bp.108.060723. Medline:19794194

Rajji TK, Voineskos AN, Butters MA, et al. Cognitive performance of individuals with schizophrenia across seven decades: a study using the MATRICS consensus cognitive battery. Am J Geriatr Psychiatry. 2013;21(2):108–18. http://dx.doi.org/10.1016/j.jagp.2012.10.011. Medline:23343484

Stewart R, Liolitsa D. Type 2 diabetes mellitus, cognitive impairment and dementia. Diabetic Med. 1999;16(2):93–112. Medline:10229302

van Os J, Howard R, Takei N, et al. Increasing age is a risk factor for psychosis in the elderly. Soc Psychiatry Psychiatr Epidemiol. 1995;30(4):161–4.

Vinogradov S, Fisher M, Warm H, et al. The cognitive cost of anticholinergic burden: decreased response to cognitive training in schizophrenia. Am J Psychiatry. 2009;166(9):1055–62. http://dx.doi.org/10.1176/appi.ajp.2009.09010017. Medline:19570929

Waddington JL, Youssef HA. Cognitive dysfunction in chronic schizophrenia followed prospectively over 10 years and its longitudinal relationship to the emergence of tardive dyskinesia. Psychol Med. 1996;26(4):681–8. Medline:8817702

Yaffe K. Metabolic syndrome and cognitive disorders: is the sum greater than its parts? Alzheimer Dis Assoc Disord. 2007;21(2):167–71. Medline:17545744

3.2 Delirium in Older Adults

Peter Chan, MD, FRCPC

INTRODUCTION

Delirium, an acute confusional state, is a common outcome of medical illness or other stressors in older adults, and other mental health conditions such as dementia can increase the risk of developing delirium. Also, many of the pharmacological treatments that are used for management of psychiatric disorders can trigger delirium. Delirium can also mimic a number of other psychiatric disorders such as dementia, depression, or primary psychotic disorders. In this chapter, Dr Chan provides an overview of the epidemiology and features of delirium followed by an approach to its evaluation and treatment.

CASE SCENARIO

Mr F. is a 71-year-old widower, retired police officer, and former military veteran who has been admitted to hospital for the past two days with increasing "confusion" manifesting over several days after a fall at home, according to family. He was diagnosed with a non-displaced pubic ramus fracture and urosepsis. Ciprofloxacin and morphine were started. He has been having gastroesophageal reflux, and his family doctor has prescribed lansoprazole and metoclopramide, which were continued in hospital. He is also known to have benign prostatic hyperplasia, with history of transurethral resection of prostate (TURP). He was initially settled, but today you are asked to see him due to agitation, as he is "picking at the air," disoriented, and very restless. Limb myoclonus is occasionally manifested.

1. What are the differential diagnoses?
2. What more information is needed from collateral sources?
3. What are the comorbid medical and psychiatric conditions that are unrecognized, and may be contributing to his presentation?
4. Outline a management strategy.
5. Over what time frame should there be a reassessment of whether he is at "baseline"?
6. What strategies can enhance outcome and improve long-term prognosis?

OVERVIEW

1. Overall Framework

• Think predisposing, precipitating, perpetuating, and preventive factors.

- Use an interdisciplinary, biopsychosocial model for assessment and treatment.
- Prognosis differs in geriatric delirium compared to younger adults, and therefore a high index of suspicion combined with early detection and management may improve outcome for some seniors.

2. Epidemiology
(Tropea et al., 2008; Voyer et al., 2008)

- Surgery
    - 40.5–55.9% incidence in hip fracture surgery patients 60 years and over
    - 14.7% incidence in elective hip surgery patients 60 years and over without severe dementia
    - 32–46% incidence in patients 65 years or older who have undergone coronary artery bypass graft (CABG) surgery
- General medical
    - 15–20% prevalence at time of admission to ward
    - 18% prevalence of patients 65 years and older within 72 hours of admission, and a further 2% incident delirium up to 1 week following admission
- Intensive care unit (ICU)
    - 70% prevalence of delirium of all patients 65 years or older, during their ICU stay and up to 7 days post-discharge
- Long-term care
    - 40.5% 14-day period prevalence from US state minimum data set
    - 71.5% in Quebec City cohort of 4 long-term care (LTC) facilities with 6 month prospective follow-up
    - 52.6% of older hospitalized patients from LTC facilities developed delirium

3. Subtypes of Delirium
(Meagher, 2009)

- Hyperactive ("agitated"):
    - Must be differentiated from anxiety, dementia
    - May have underlying geriatric depression leading to delirium from general medical condition (GMC)
    - Alcohol withdrawal may cause this (delirium tremens = adrenergic outflow)
- Hypoactive ("apathetic"):
    - Must be differentiated from depression
    - Less sleep-wake reversal
    - Particularly in hepatic encephalopathy, dehydration
- Mixed hypoactive/hyperactive
- Normal psychomotor activity

4. Pathophysiology
(Maldonado, 2008)

- Classic theory
    - Acetylcholine (Ach)

- Anticholinergics (e.g., atropine) can induce delirium and can slow electro-encephalogram (EEG)
    - Reversed by physostigmine (experimental)
  - Dopamine (DA)
    - Dopamine agonists can induce (e.g., L-Dopa)
    - Antipsychotics can treat
- Other neurochemicals implicated
  - GABA (γ-aminobutyric acid): decreased
  - Glutamate: increased
  - Noradrenaline: increased; monotherapy with IV dexmedetomidine, an α2 agonist, in critical care settings can be effective
  - Melatonin
- Postoperative oxidative stress, perfusion problems, hypoxemia (Fricchione et al., 2008)
- Inflammation (Cunningham, 2011): systemic inflammatory factors affecting central nervous system (CNS)
- Possible factors
  - Serotonin: delirium in serotonin syndrome; low L-tryptophan levels can be found (in some), esp. in critically ill? Replace L-tryptophan??
  - Histamine: antihistamines can precipitate delirium

5. Diagnosis

- DSM remains the standard (DSM-IV and DSM-5 [American Psychiatric Association, 2000, 2013]).
- DSM-5: "A disturbance in attention (ie: reduced ability to direct, focus, sustain, or shift attention) and awareness (reduced orientation to the environment)."
- DSM-5: "Attenuated delirium syndrome" (under "other specified delirium"). This is analogous to the term "subsyndromal delirium." These are symptoms characteristic of delirium that cause clinically significant distress or impairment in social, occupational, or other important areas of functioning predominate but do not meet full criteria for delirium (Levkoff et al., 1996; Cole et al., 2013).
- EEG may aid in diagnosis in select cases (Lipowski, 1992):
  - Diffuse slowing of the EEG correlating with reduced cerebral metabolic rate for glucose or oxygen, or cerebral blood flow
  - Look for diffuse EEG slowing (delta and/or theta waves)
    - Exception: alcohol-withdrawal delirium, which presents with fast activity
  - May aid in the diagnosis when presentation is puzzling (e.g., catatonia, recurrent seizures, or non-convulsive status epilepticus, apathetic depression) but generally not indicated
  - Can be difficult to interpret in presence of advanced dementia due to some EEG slowing, which can occur at these stages of dementia; delirium more likely to produce marked slowing on EEG
  - EEG slowing should normalize or return back to baseline once delirium resolves, even in those with dementia
- Practical tips and subtle manifestations occurring:
  - 24-hour observation, including sleep-wake cycle

- – Anxiety
- – New incontinence
- – Unsteady gait, falls
- – Dysarthria or incoherence
- – Mood or affective lability
- – Subtle paranoia and hypervigilance
- – Ask specifically about vivid dreams or nightmares!

6. Screening

- Various evidence-based delirium screening tools (Wong et al., 2010):
    - – Confusion Assessment Method (CAM)
    - – Global Attentiveness Rating (GAR): 2 minute interview, visual analogue scale
    - – Memorial Delirium Assessment Scale (MDAS)
    - – Delirium Rating Scale Revised-98 (DRS-R-98)
    - – Clinical Assessment of Confusion (CAC)
    - – Delirium Observation Screening Scale (DOSS)
- *Mini Mental State Examination (MMSE) is a poor screening tool for delirium.*
- Delirium vs dementia
    - – No reliable screening tool to differentiate delirium and dementia
    - – Adding psychomotor change to CAM-short form may improve specificity to dementia with comorbid delirium (Thomas et al., 2012)
    - – "Spatial span forwards" < 4 may distinguish delirium from dementia? (Meagher et al., 2010). Digit span tests??
- Under-recognition, especially in those:
    - – Over 80 years with hypoactive delirium with visual impairment and/or pre-existing dementia (Inouye et al., 2001)
    - – Long-term care residents, esp. over age 85 (Voyer et al., 2008)
- CAM (Inouye et al., 1990)
    - – CAM has high sensitivity and specificity (> 90%) in trained front-line healthcare professionals
    - – Has been validated for use in detecting delirium in those with dementia
    - – Has been adapted to the ICU setting (CAM-ICU)

7. Differentiating Delirium from Dementia and Dementia with Lewy Bodies (DLB)

This can be difficult due to fluctuation in attention on/consciousness in DLB and due to attention deficits in some with more advanced stages of other types of dementia, but some features can help distinguish (Cole, 2004):

- Attentional processes generally preserved in those with dementia
- Acute onset in delirium, while insidious onset in dementia
- Visual hallucinations in DLB often prolonged, complex, and not necessarily distressing; less diurnal variation compared to delirium
- Parkinsonism usually absent in delirium; can be present in DLB as a core feature

- Infrequent neuroleptic sensitivity with judicious use of antipsychotics in delirium, whereas frequent Parkinsonism with typical antipsychotics and certain atypical antipsychotics when prescribed in DLB
- Insight into symptoms may be present in lucid intervals in delirium, but insight often lacking in dementia

8. Predisposing Factors

(Canadian Coalition for Seniors' Mental Health [CCSMH], 2006, 2010, 2014)

- Inouye's "big 6" (Inouye et al., 1993)
  - Cognitive impairment/dementia
  - Sleep deprivation
  - Immobility
  - Visual impairment: ask whether the patient wears glasses!
  - Hearing impairment: ask about hearing; carry a portable voice amplifier
  - Dehydration: BUN:Creat > 18 (US units)
- Others (supported by some studies; Inouye, Westendorp, & Saczynski, 2014)
  - Age 75 or greater
  - Male
  - History of delirium
  - Depression
  - Pre-existing functional impairments/ disability
  - Severity medical illness
  - Alcohol use disorders
  - History of transient ischemic attack (TIA) or stroke
  - Medications with significant anticholinergic activity
  - Fracture on admission
  - Critical care settings
  - Terminal cancer

9. Precipitating Factors

Conditions are numerous; consider "DIMS-R (drugs, infection, metabolic, structural, retention)" approach for common conditions (Chan, 2011)

- Check for urinary retention with a bladder scanner!

9.1 DIMS-R: Common Precipitating Factors for Delirium

- Drugs
  - Prescribed (narcotics, steroids, anticholinergic, NSAIDs)
  - Over-the-counter (dimenhydrinate, diphenhydramine)
  - Drug intoxication or withdrawal (alcohol, sedative-hypnotics, narcotics)
- Infection (urinary tract, lungs, skin, blood)
- Metabolic disturbances
  - Fluid (dehydration, hypovolemia)
  - Electrolyte (sodium, potassium, magnesium)
  - Nutrition (malnutrition, thiamine deficiency, anemia)
- Structural insults
  - Cardiovascular (angina, infarction, congestive heart failure)
  - Central nervous system (stroke or ischemia, concussion)

  – Pulmonary (hypoxia; e.g., chronic obstructive pulmonary disease exacerbation)
  – Gastrointestinal (bleeding with anemia, *C. difficile*, colitis)
- Retention problems (urinary retention, constipation)

10. Strategies around Medications That May Be Contributing to Delirium

- Discontinuing/substituting anticholinergic medications
  – Diphenhydramine (Benadryl), dimenhydrinate (Gravol), hydroxyzine (Atarax)
  – Benztropine (Cogentin), etc.
  – Oxybutynin (Ditropan), or other urinary anticholinergics
- Avoid amitriptyline (Elavil); nortriptyline is better tolerated.
- Avoid the use of cimetidine (Tagamet) in the elderly!
- Monitoring the effects of steroids (prednisone equivalent ≥ 40mg/d; Fardet, Petersen, & Nazareth, 2012), which can lead to delirium, psychosis, or mania
- Monitoring the effects of quinolones, especially ciprofloxacin
- Switching narcotics to (avoid meperidine = Demerol):
  – Hydromorphone (Dilaudid)
  – Oxycodone
  – Fentanyl (chronic pain)
- Evidence-based factors precipitating delirium once in hospital = incident delirium (Inouye & Charpentier, 1996)
  – Physical restraints (RR = 4.4)
  – Malnutrition (RR = 4.0)
  – More than three medications added (RR = 2.9)
  – Use of bladder catheter (RR = 2.4)
  – Any iatrogenic event (RR = 1.9)
- Physical restraints
  – Increase risk of:
    ▪ *Developing* delirium
    ▪ *Developing* additional morbidities (e.g., pneumonia, deep vein thrombosis, stasis ulcers), and death
  – Avoid limb or Posey restraints in the elderly; use least restrictive restraint if restraint is needed.
  – In 2001, the Ontario government passed Bill 85, the *Patient Restraints Minimization Act*, defining when to use restraints.
  – Clinical practice guidelines (CPGs) for geriatric delirium discuss restraint use (CCSMH, 2006, 2010, 2014):
    "Physical restraints for older persons suffering from delirium should be applied only in exceptional circumstances. Specifically this is when:
    a) There is a serious risk for bodily harm to self or others; OR
    b) Other means for controlling behaviours leading to harm have been explored first, including pharmacologic treatments, but were ineffective; AND
    c) The potential benefits outweigh the potential risks of restraints."

11. Nonpharmacological Management
(Popeo, 2011; CCSMH, 2006, 2010, 2014; Flaherty, 2011)

- Minimize use of physical restraints.
- Minimize use of bladder catheters.
- Minimize room transfers.
- Maintain adequate nutrition and hydration.
- Optimize sensory input.
- Maintain orientation.
- Decrease environmental stimuli.
- Increase mobility earlier.
- Consider family member or 1:1 sitter.
- Detect and manage pain.
- Implement an educational program to inform hospital staff and an algorithmic treatment protocol.
- Nonpharmacological multicomponent, often interdisciplinary-based, prevention or management randomized controlled trials (RCTs) have shown mixed results, usually only a modest benefit.

12. Pharmacological Management

12.1 General Overview

- Recommendations based on evidence from RCTs with limited numbers
- No evidence that a particular antipsychotic is more effective than another
- Although haloperidol is considered the "standard," there are no published placebo-controlled RCTs involving haloperidol, only haloperidol RCTs in comparison to other meds. Comparator to atypicals (3 RCTs in Cochrane). Prolonged QTc risk, especially IV, so baseline electrocardiogram (ECG) ideal. Risk of extrapyramidal symptoms, esp. elderly > 4.5 mg/day in Cochrane Review (Lonergan et al., 2007)
- Various CPGs have recommended haloperidol or atypicals as alternatives (Table 3.2.1).

Table 3.2.1: National Practice Guidelines and Antipsychotic Recommendations for Delirium Management

Country	Year	Antipsychotic Recommendations
Canada (geriatric delirium)	2006, 2010, 2014	Haldol; alternative risperidone, olanzapine, quetiapine
Australia	2006, 2011	Haldol, olanzapine, risperidone
NICE (United Kingdom)	2010	Haldol, olanzapine
United States (APA)	1999	Haldol

Sources: Canadian Coalition for Seniors' Mental Health (CCSMH) 2006, 2010, 2014; Australian Health Ministers Advisory Council (AHMAC), 2006, 2011; National Institute for Health and Care Excellence (NICE), 2010; American Psychiatric Association, 1999.

- Antipsychotic for delirium (Flaherty, 2011; Peritogiannis et al., 2009; Seitz, Gill, & van Zyl, 2007; Chan, 2011)
    - Haloperidol
    - Other conventional antipsychotics
        - Loxapine (Loxapac)
        - Chlorpromazine
        - Methotrimeprazine (Nozinan)
        - Perphenazine
    - Atypical antipsychotics
        - Risperidone, olanzapine, quetiapine, aripiprazole, ziprasidone
- See Table 3.2.2 for antipsychotic dosages and routes of administration for delirium management.

Table 3.2.2: Antipsychotic Dosages and Routes of Administration for Delirium Management

Medication	Trade Name	Category	Starting Dose (mg)	Usual Dose Range (mg)	Routes of Administration
Loxapine	Loxapac	Conventional	5–15	5–100	IM, SC, PO
Methotrimeprazine	Nozinan	Conventional	2.5–10	2.5–100	IV, IM, SC, PO
Chlorpromazine	Largactil	Conventional	6.25–12.5	2.5–100	IM, SC, PO
Perphenazine	Trilafon	Conventional	1–2	2–16	IV, IM, PO
Haloperidol	Haldol	Conventional	0.5–1.0	0.5–5	IV, IM, SC, PO
Risperidone	Risperdal	Atypical	0.5–1.0	0.25–3	PO liq/tabs, SL
Olanzapine	Zyprexa	Atypical	1.25–5	2.5–15	PO, SL, IM
Quetiapine	Seroquel	Atypical	12.5–50	12.5–200	PO (IR, XR)

IM = intramuscular; IR = instant release; IV = intravenous; PO = by mouth; SC = subcutaneous; SL = sublingually; XR = extended release

12.2 General Principles and Recommendations
(CCSMH, 2006, 2010, 2014; levels of evidence in brackets)

- Psychotropic medications should be reserved for patients who are in distress due to agitation or psychotic symptoms in order to carry out essential investigations or treatment and to prevent patients from endangering themselves or others. (D)
- The use of psychotropic medications for the specific purpose of controlling wandering in delirium is not recommended. (D)
- Antipsychotics are the treatment of choice to manage the symptoms of delirium (with the exception of alcohol or benzodiazepine withdrawal delirium). (B)
- Haloperidol is suggested as the antipsychotic of choice based on the best available evidence to date. (B) Initial dosages are in the range of 0.25–0.5 mg. Od-bid. (D)
- Atypical antipsychotics may be considered as alternative agents as they have lower rates of extrapyramidal signs. (B)
- Benzatropine should not be used prophylactically with haloperidol in the treatment of delirium. (D)

- In older persons with delirium who also have Parkinson's disease or dementia with Lewy bodies, atypical antipsychotics are preferred over typical antipsychotics. (D)
- Sedative-hypnotic agents are recommended as the primary agents for managing alcohol-withdrawal delirium (B). Their use in other forms of delirium should be avoided. (D)
- Aim for monotherapy, the lowest effective dose, and tapering as soon as possible. (D)

12.3 Prescribing Antipsychotics

- Frequency: regular vs prn; evening dosing of more sedating types of antipsychotics (e.g., loxapine, methotrimeprazine, quetiapine, olanzapine) may help with sleep-wake disturbance; consider dosing at 4 p.m., then 8 p.m., rather than morning dose
- Route: PO (tabs, sl, liquid) vs SC vs IM vs IV. Clinical experience is that SC route can be just as quickly absorbed as IM antipsychotic, with less pain in elderly with SC route of administration
- Common initial dosages (CCSMH, 2006, 2010, 2014) in the frail elderly:
  - Haloperidol at 0.25–0.5 mg bid
  - Risperidone at 0.25 mg od-bid
  - Olanzapine at 1.25–2.5 mg per day
  - Quetiapine at 12.5–50 mg per day
- Considerations and caveats
  - Risks of atypical antipsychotics: "black box" warning (mortality risk), and risk of cerebrovascular accident (CVA) or CVA-like events (Health Canada, 2005)
  - Metabolic syndrome (less likely if short duration) possible but uncommon
  - Be alert for anticholinergic effects of antipsychotics
  - Prolonged QTc and torsade de pointe; much riskier 500 msec and above
  - Use of cholinesterase inhibitors? – may be hazardous in critically ill (van Eijk et al., 2010) so not usually considered; some case reports show that they can be effective in select cases when refractory to other agents (Mukadam, Ritchie, & Sampson, 2008)
  - Treatment of hypoactive delirium: stimulants? – black box warning tempers use; may help in terminal illness (Gagnon, Low, & Schreier, 2005); evidence for olanzapine use in hypoactive delirium in cancer populations (Breitbart, Tremblay, & Gibson, 2002), but current CPGs do not suggest treating this pharmacologically unless associated distress or behavioural disturbance
  - Melatonin? No clear evidence for use, but can have a hypnotic effect at standard doses; some clinical experience that it can be helpful for those with residual sleep-wake disturbance when other symptoms of delirium remitted

13. Evidence-Based Preventive Measures for Geriatric Delirium
(Tabet & Howard, 2009; Holroyd-Leduc, Khandwala, & Sink, 2010)

13.1 Hospital Elder Life Program (HELP) for Prevention of Delirium
(Inouye et al., 1999)

- Targeted intervention: mobilization, correcting sensory impairments, reorientation, activation through a comprehensive volunteer program, addressing hydration and nutrition, avoidance of restraints and psychotropics

- RCT with n = 850 elderly medical inpatients, intervention vs usual care group
- Incidence of delirium developed in 9.9% of the intervention group compared to 15% of the usual care group (OR 0.6, CI95 0.39–0.92)
- Reduction in the days of delirium and number of episodes in the intervention group; no reduction in the severity and recurrence rates
- Subsequent studies have shown cost savings, though some costs to initially starting the program and training staff including volunteers
- Resources to develop the program is free (www.hospitalelderlifeprogram.org)
- Quite a few HELPs worldwide; a number (around 20) of HELPs within Canadian hospitals, mostly in Ontario

13.2 Melatonin
(Al-Aama et al., 2011, de Jonghe et al., 2014)

- Al-Aama's Canadian RCT with n = 145 geriatric patients from emergency, admitted to internal medicine units, and followed prospectively for 14 days
  - Mean age = 84 years, 35–38% with pre-existing cognitive impairment
  - Randomized to placebo or melatonin 0.5 mg qhs
  - Reduction in incidence of delirium from 31% (placebo) to 12% (melatonin). P = 0.014
  - Odds ratio = 0.19 (adjusted for dementia)
  - Needs further study before recommending routine use
- de Jonghe's Dutch RCT in 378 hip fracture surgery patients showed no difference in placebo vs melatonin on the incident rates of delirium and no differences at 3 months
- Melatonin generally well tolerated but some can get nightmares, and there can be certain drug interactions

13.3 Perioperative Antipsychotics
(Fok et al., 2015)

- Five published and one unpublished RCTs to date with most studies showing a lower incidence of delirium in a variety of settings with different antipsychotics in surgical settings (Table 3.2.3)
- Pooled relative risk of the five studies resulted in weighted odds ratio of 0.44 in the reduction of the relative risk of delirium among those receiving antipsychotic medication compared with placebo (P-Value 0.0005; $I^2 = 69\%$).
- Interesting findings but not routinely indicated as yet; needs further study
- High risk elderly group may benefit more? (e.g., multiple predisposing factors); Fok's paper estimates beneficial effect occurring when the baseline surgical delirium risk is 18% or above.
- Concern in the olanzapine prophylaxis RCT, as those who developed delirium had longer duration and more severity

13.4 Other Considerations

- Proactive geriatric medicine consultation post–hip fracture may help (Marcantonio et al., 2001), though study not replicated

Table 3.2.3: Placebo-controlled RCTs of Antipsychotics for the Prophylaxis of Geriatric Delirium

Authors	TX (n)	Placebo (n)	Site	Age	Dose	Outcome
Wang et al., 2012	229	228	ICU	≥ 65	Haldol IV 0.5 mg load then 0.1 mg/hr IV x 12 hrs, on ICU admission	• Lower incidence of delirium (15.3% vs 23.2%)
Kalisvaart et al., 2005	212	218	Hip Surg.	≥ 70	Haldol po 1.5 mg/d preoperative and up to 3 days postoperative	• Similar incidence of delirium (15.1% vs 16.5%) • Fewer # delirium days (5.4 days vs 11.8 days) • Fewer # days in hospital (17.1 days vs 22.6 days) • Less severity of delirium
Kaneko et al., 1999	38	40	GI Surg.	Mean 72	Haldol IV 5 mg/d x 5 days postoperative	• Lower incidence of delirium (10.5 48,805098196493184v% vs 32.5%)
Prakanrattana & Prapaitrakool, 2007	63	63	CABG	Mean 61	Risperidone sublingual 1 mg/d on 1st post-operative day only	• Lower incidence of delirium (11.1% vs 31.7%)
Larsen et al., 2010	196	204	Hip, Knee Surg.	Mean 74	Olanzapine 5 mg/d preoperative and postoperative (2d)	• Lower incidence of delirium (14.3% vs 40.2%); BUT in olanzapine group: • Longer duration of delirium • More severe delirium

CABG = coronary artery bypass graft; GI = gastrointestinal; ICU = intensive care unit; IV = intravenous; po = by mouth; RCT = randomized controlled trial; TX = treatment

- Multidisciplinary geriatric intervention programs (including education of the involved health professionals, assessment of the patients' risk factors, improved postoperative alertness to medical problems, interdisciplinary case evaluation, and specific recommendations): mixed results (reviewed in Flaherty, 2011)
- Relatives? An intervention program delivered by family members and based on caregiver education, avoidance of patients' sensorial deprivation, reorientation using aids like clocks and calendars, and encouraging family members to visit the patients at least 5 hours daily and to apply preventive strategies has been shown to reduce delirium rates in elderly medical patients (Martinez et al., 2012)
- Earplugs may help in critical care settings (Alway et al., 2013)

14. Prognosis

- Unlike younger adults, older adults may not return to baseline
- Increased mortality in hospital and up to 2 year post-delirium (Leslie et al., 2005; McCusker et al., 2003; McAvay et al., 2006)
- Increased morbidity: more length of stay, functional decline, or institutional care (Rockwood et al., 1999; McCusker et al., 2003; McAvay et al., 2006)
- More cognitive deficits: up to 30–60% at 1 month (Rockwood, 1993; McCusker et al., 2003; Marcantonio et al., 2003); lingering impairment at 6 months post-cardiac surgery (Saczynski et al., 2012)

- More likely to be persistently delirious (Cole et al., 2009)
- Those with dementia and delirium less likely to achieve pre-delirium cognitive and functional baseline status (McCusker et al., 2001) and have a longer course of delirium (Dasgupta & Hillier, 2010; Boettger, Passik, & Breitbart, 2011)
- Increased risk of developing dementia? (Rockwood et al., 1999)
    - Witlox et al., 2010; meta-analysis
        - Odds ratio = 12.52 (95% CI 1.86–84.21), mean follow-up = 4 years
        - Based on two studies: Bickel et al., 2008; Lundström et al., 2003
    - Krogseth et al., 2011
        - Odds ratio = 10.5 (95%CI 1.6–76.3), follow-up = 6 months
    - Davis et al., 2012
        - Cohort of 553 seniors, aged 85 or over, Vantaa, Finland
        - Odds ratio = 8.7 (95% CI 2.1–35), followed up to 10 years
        - Delirium was associated with worsening dementia severity

QUESTIONS

1. List four evidence-based predisposing factors for geriatric delirium.
2. Identify four subtle manifestations of delirium or subsyndromal delirium in the elderly.
3. How would you help design an interdisciplinary program in your institution to systematically detect and manage geriatric delirium by employing multicomponent interventions?

ANSWERS

1. Evidence-based predisposing factors for geriatric delirium include:
    - Pre-existing dementia or cognitive impairment
    - Severity and duration of underlying medical illness
    - BUN:Cr greater than 18 (US units) (i.e., dehydration)
    - Sensory impairment (visual or hearing)
    - Sleep deprivation
    - Immobility or physical restraints
    - Advanced age such as age 75 or greater (some studies)
    - Male gender (some studies)
    - Severity of medical illness
    - History of delirium
    - Substance dependence
    - Bladder catheter use
    - Malnutrition
    - Depression
    - Pre-existing functional impairments/disability
    - History of TIA or stroke
    - Medications with significant anticholinergic activity
    - Fracture on admission
    - Critical care settings
    - Terminal cancer

2. Subtle manifestations of delirium or subsyndromal delirium in the elderly include:
    - Restlessness
    - Anxiety/irritability
    - Hypersensitivity to stimuli or hypervigilance
    - Nightmares
    - New-onset urinary incontinence
    - Unsteady gait/falls
    - Dysarthria or word-finding difficulty

- Difficulty with English (or French) if this is their second language
- Mood/affect lability
- Subtle paranoia and hypervigilance
- Fatigue/lethargy/apathy
- Psychomotor disturbance
- Impaired sleep-wake cycle

- Attentional difficulties
- Visuospatial abnormalities
- Illusions (e.g., visual)
- Mild disorientation
- Slight personality changes
- Fluctuating cognitive abilities

3. A multicomponent interdisciplinary program for delirium detection and management would include the following considerations:
   - Establishing a preventive program along the lines of the Hospital Elder Life Program (HELP) initiative (e.g., keeping calendars and clocks updated, visual and hearing enhancements, proper lighting during the day, quiet environment at night)
   - Education of staff in ER, ICU, and surgical/medical units on delirium symptoms, predisposing and precipitating factors, and having a high index of suspicion for patients at risk
   - Identifying where the prevalence of delirium is the highest in the hospital (e.g., ICU, post-surgery)
   - Establishing a protocol for using the CAM to screen patients at risk in all settings
   - Education and protocol on factors that reduce morbidity and facilitate faster resolution of delirium (e.g., early mobilization)
   - Avoiding catheters, iatrogenic causes, restraints
   - Minimizing unnecessary psychotropic or anticholinergic medications
   - Encouraging consultation of geriatric medicine, geriatric psychiatry, and internal medicine if the patient is complex or challenging
   - Measuring outcomes with protocol use (e.g., length of stay, morbidity, mortality)
   - Making the identification and management of delirium part of clinical pathways on the various hospital units
   - Having a champion(s) for recognition and management
   - Helping establish acute care for elders units in hospitals may be beneficial

CASE DISCUSSION

1. The differential diagnoses include the following:
   - Delirium
   - Underlying dementia
   - Head injury or subdural hematoma
   - Breakthrough pain
   - Uremic encephalopathy (urosepsis)
   - Neurodegenerative disorder (e.g., corticobasilar degeneration or Creutzfeldt-Jakob disease as suggested by myoclonus)
   - Hepatic encephalopathy
   - Alcohol-withdrawal delirium
   - Urinary retention or constipation (DIMS-R mnemonic, R = retention)
   - Meningoencephalitis

- Medication-induced akathisia (metoclopramide)
- Neoplasm

2. On collateral history, it will be important to explore the following topics:
   - Pre-existing cognitive impairment and baseline function
   - Pre-existing sensory impairments
   - Substance abuse
   - Medication non-adherence vs misuse
   - Over-the-counter medication abuse
   - Suicidality
   - Risk of harm to others (firearms)
   - Informal and formal supports, if any
   - Caregiver burden
   - Living environment
   - Recent urinary and bowel patter
   - Recurrent falls and/or head trauma recently

3. Comorbid conditions that may be unrecognized may include the following:
   - Post-traumatic stress disorder
   - Depression
   - Anxiety disorders
   - Dementia/major cognitive disorder
   - Minor cognitive impairment (MCI)/Minor cognitive disorder
   - Substance abuse or dependence, especially alcohol or narcotic (e.g., Tylenol #3)
   - Unstable gait or syncope that may have led to his fall; closed head injury or traumatic brain injury (TBI)
   - Encephalopathy from sexually transmitted diseases (e.g., HIV, herpes simplex)
   - Coronary or cerebral arterial insufficiency
   - Urinary tract infection or generalized sepsis
   - Urinary retention (benign prostatic hyperplasia)
   - Constipation
   - GI Bleed
   - Other cardiac causes (e.g., arrhythmias)
   - Nephritis and acute kidney injury
   - Acute or chronic hepatic injury
   - Medication-induced delirium (narcotics, ciprofloxacin)
   - Underlying electrolyte disturbance
   - Hypocalcemia or hypomagnesemia (lansoprazole)
   - Ciprofloxacin-induced confusion and/or myoclonus
   - Thyroid abnormalities
   - B12 deficiency
   - Inadequate calorie and/or fluid intake
   - Inadequate pain management

4. The management strategy would include the following ideas:
   - Rule out underlying medical conditions and treat
   - CT scan of head
   - Consider EEG in complex and/or persistent cases despite treatment
   - Bladder scan
   - Check for constipation
   - Switch morphine to hydromorphone or oxycodone (may combine with acetaminophen)
   - Consider switch of antibiotic and/or judicious use of lorazepam if cipro-induced toxicity
   - Consider discontinuation of metoclopramide or switch to domperidone
   - Clinical Institute Withdrawal Assessment of Alcohol Scale, Revised (CIWA-Ar) protocol for possible alcohol withdrawal, with awareness that it is somewhat non-specific as it can also screen positive for delirium secondary to a general medical condition
   - Give thiamine +/– magnesium if alcohol involved
   - Nonpharmacological management of delirium, including optimizing sensory input, early mobilization, ensuring hydration, reorientation, and sleep hygiene
   - Avoiding physical restraints
   - Consider 1:1 sitter
   - Antipsychotics regularly and as needed
   - Ensure safety and medical stability

5. Regarding the assessment of his baseline, the following concepts should be considered:
   - Correction of physical condition does not necessarily lead to immediate resolution of delirium.
   - Postoperative delirium tends to be shorter in duration than delirium occurring in the frail medically ill older adults (which is often multifactorial in cause), but no clear time frame for any one patient – could be weeks or even months.
   - Resolution of sleep disturbance and other features is suggestive of subsyndromal delirium.
   - Functional and cognitive recovery can be much slower in frail older adults, so early discharge home may be ill-advised, especially if there are inadequate supports at home.
   - Collateral history can be useful to determine when patient has returned to baseline.

6. Strategies to improve his outcome and long-term prognosis include:
   - Nonpharmacological management as above
   - No clear evidence for pharmacological strategies for improving long-term prognosis
   - Falls assessment and rehab
   - Home assessment for environmental hazards and any needed additional supports
   - Blister-packing and supervision of medications if there are lingering cognitive deficits
   - Alcohol or substance abuse treatment/counselling

- Ultimately, geriatric delirium confers a rather poor or guarded prognosis in many, as associated with enhanced morbidity and mortality.
- Consider referral to community specialists (e.g., geriatric psychiatrists, geriatricians) and/or interdisciplinary teams for follow-up for those with lingering deficits.

RECOMMENDED RESOURCES FOR REVIEW

Although these resources may not be specifically cited in the text, their approach informed the contents of the chapter, and they are recommended as useful further reading.

Flaherty JH. The evaluation and management of delirium among older persons. Med Clin North Am. 2011;95(3):555–77, xi. http://dx.doi.org/10.1016/j.mcna.2011.02.005. Medline:21549878

Inouye SK, Westendorp RG, Saczynski JS. Delirium in elderly people. Lancet. 2014;383(9920): 911–22. Medline:23992774

Mattappalil A, Mergenhagen KA. Neurotoxicity with antimicrobials in the elderly: a review. Clin Ther. 2014;36(11):1489–1511.e4. http://dx.doi.org/10.1016/j.clinthera .2014.09.020. Medline:25450476

CLINICAL PRACTICE GUIDELINES AND POSITION PAPERS

American Psychiatric Association. Practice guideline for the treatment of patients with delirium. Am J Psychiatry. 1999;156(5 Suppl):1–20. Medline:10327941

Australian Health Ministers Advisory Council (AHMAC); Health Care of Older Australians Standing Committee (HCOASC). Clinical practice guidelines for the management of delirium in older people. Developed by the Clinical Epidemiology and Health Service Evaluation Unit, Melbourne Health in collaboration with the Delirium Clinical Guidelines Expert Working Group for the AHMAC. Melbourne, AU: Victorian Government Department of Human Services; 2006. https://www2.health.vic.gov.au/about/ publications/policiesandguidelines/?q=delirium&pn=1

– Delirium care pathways 2010. Melbourne, AU: Commonwealth of Australia; 2011. https://www2.health.vic .gov.au/about/publications/policiesandguidelines/?q=delirium&pn=1

Canadian Coalition for Seniors' Mental Health (CCSMH). National guidelines for senior's mental health: the assessment and treatment of delirium. Toronto: CCSMH; 2006. http://www.ccsmh.ca/en/projects/ delirium.cfm

– Guideline on the assessment and treatment of delirium in older adults at the end of life. Adapted from the CCSMH national guidelines for seniors' mental health: the assessment and treatment of delirium. Toronto: CCSMH; 2010. http://www.ccsmh.ca/pdf/guidelines/NatlGuideline_DeliriumEOLC.pdf

– 2014 guideline update: the assessment and treatment of delirium. Toronto: CCSMH; 2014. http://www.ccsmh .ca/en/projects/delirium.cfm

UK National Institute for Health and Care Excellence (NICE). Delirium: prevention, diagnosis and management. UK National Institute for Health and Care Excellence (NICE) Clinical Guidelines, No. 103. London: NICE: 2010. https://www.nice.org.uk/guidance/cg103

REFERENCES

Al-Aama T, Brymer C, Gutmanis I, et al. Melatonin decreases delirium in elderly patients: a randomized, placebo-controlled trial. Int J Geriatr Psychiatry. 2011;26(7):687–94. http://dx.doi.org/10.1002/gps.2582. Medline:20845391

Alway A, Halm MA, Shilhanek M, et al. Do earplugs and eye masks affect sleep and delirium outcomes in the critically ill? Am J Crit Care. 2013;22(4):357–60. http://dx.doi.org/10.4037/ajcc2013545. Medline:23817826

American Psychiatric Association (APA). Diagnostic and statistical manual of mental disorders. 4th ed. text revision. (DSM IV-TR). Washington, DC: APA; 2000.

– Diagnostic and statistical manual of mental disorders. 5th ed. (DSM-5). Washington, DC: APA: 2013.

Bickel H, Gradinger R, Kochs E, et al. High risk of cognitive and functional decline after postoperative delirium: a three-year prospective study. Dement Geriatr Cogn Disord. 2008;26(1):26–31. http://dx.doi .org/10.1159/000140804. Medline:18577850

Boettger S, Passik S, Breitbart W. Treatment characteristics of delirium superimposed on dementia. Int Psychogeriatr. 2011;23(10):1671–6. http://dx.doi.org/10.1017/S1041610211000998. Medline:21729412

Breitbart W, Tremblay A, Gibson C. An open trial of olanzapine for the treatment of delirium in hospitalized cancer patients. Psychosomatics. 2002;43(3):175–82. Medline:12075032

Chan PK. Clarifying the confusion about confusion: current practices in managing geriatric delirium. B C Med J. 2011;53(8):409–13.

Cole MG. Delirium in elderly patients. Am J Geriatr Psychiatry. 2004;12(1):7–21. http://dx.doi.org/10.1097/ 00019442-200401000-00002. Medline:14729554

Cole MG, Ciampi A, Belzile E, Dubuc-Sarrasin M. Subsyndromal delirium in older people: a systematic review of frequency, risk factors, course and outcomes. Int J Geriatr Psychiatry. 2013;28(8):771–80. http://dx.doi .org/10.1002/gps.3891. Medline:23124811

Cole MG, Ciampi A, Belzile E, Zhong L. Persistent delirium in older hospital patients: a systematic review of frequency and prognosis. Age Ageing. 2009;38(1):19–26. http://dx.doi.org/10.1093/ageing/afn253. Medline:19017678

Cunningham C. Systemic inflammation and delirium: important co-factors in the progression of dementia. Biochem Soc Trans. 2011;39(4):945–53. http://dx.doi.org/10.1042/BST0390945. Medline:21787328

Dasgupta M, Hillier LM. Factors associated with prolonged delirium: a systematic review. Int Psychogeriatr. 2010;22(3):373–94. http://dx.doi.org/10.1017/S1041610209991517. Medline:20092663

Davis DH, Muniz Terrera G, Keage H, et al. Delirium is a strong risk factor for dementia in the oldest-old: a population-based cohort study. Brain. 2012;135(Pt 9):2809–16. http://dx.doi.org/10.1093/brain/aws190. Medline:22879644

de Jonghe A, van Munster BC, Goslings JC, et al.; Amsterdam Delirium Study Group. Effect of melatonin on incidence of delirium among patients with hip fracture: a multicentre, double-blind randomized controlled trial. CMAJ. 2014;186(14):E547–56. http://dx.doi.org/10.1503/cmaj.140495. Medline:25183726

Fardet L, Petersen I, Nazareth I. Suicidal behavior and severe neuropsychiatric disorders following glucocorti-coid therapy in primary care. Am J Psychiatry. 2012;169(5):491–7. http://dx.doi.org/10.1176/appi.ajp.2011 .11071009. Medline:22764363

Fok MC, Sepehry AA, Frisch L, et al. Do antipsychotics prevent postoperative delirium? A systematic review and meta-analysis. Int J. Geriatric Psychiatry. 2015;30(4):333–44. http://dx.doi.org/10.1002/gps.4240. Medline:25639958

Fricchione GL, Nejad SH, Esses JA, et al. Postoperative delirium. Am J Psychiatry. 2008;165(7):803–12. http:// dx.doi.org/10.1176/appi.ajp.2008.08020181. Medline:18593786

Gagnon B, Low G, Schreier G. Methylphenidate hydrochloride improves cognitive function in patients with advanced cancer and hypoactive delirium: a prospective clinical study. J Psychiatry Neurosci. 2005;30(2):100–7. Medline:15798785

Health Canada. Atypical antipsychotic drugs and dementia – advisories, warnings, and recalls for health professionals. Ottawa: Health Canada; 2005. http://www.healthycanadians.gc.ca/recall-alert-rappel-avis/ hc-sc/2005/14307a-eng.php

Hewko RA. Recognition, assessment, and management of delirium in the geriatric patient. BC Med J. 1996;39(9):480–3.

Holroyd-Leduc JM, Khandwala F, Sink KM. How can delirium best be prevented and managed in older patients in hospital? CMAJ. 2010;182(5):465–70. http://dx.doi.org/10.1503/cmaj.080519. Medline:19687107

Inouye SK, Bogardus ST Jr, Charpentier PA, et al. A multicomponent intervention to prevent delirium in hospitalized older patients. N Engl J Med. 1999;340(9):669–76. http://dx.doi.org/10.1056/ NEJM199903043400901. Medline:10053175

Inouye SK, Charpentier PA. Precipitating factors for delirium in hospitalized elderly persons. Predictive model and interrelationship with baseline vulnerability. JAMA. 1996;275(11):852–7. http://dx.doi.org/10.1001/ jama.1996.03530350034031. Medline:8596223

Inouye SK, Foreman MD, Mion LC, et al. Nurses' recognition of delirium and its symptoms: comparison of nurse and researcher ratings. Arch Intern Med. 2001;161(20):2467–73. http://dx.doi.org/10.1001/ archinte.161.20.2467. Medline:11700159

Inouye SK, van Dyck CH, Alessi CA, et al. Clarifying confusion: the confusion assessment method. A new method for detection of delirium. Ann Intern Med. 1990;113(12):941–8. http://dx.doi.org/10.7326/0003-4819-113-12-941. Medline:2240918

Inouye SK, Viscoli CM, Horwitz RI, et al. A predictive model for delirium in hospitalized elderly medical patients based on admission characteristics. Ann Intern Med. 1993;119(6):474–81. http://dx.doi.org/10.7326/ 0003-4819-119-6-199309150-00005. Medline:8357112

Kalisvaart KJ, de Jonghe JF, Bogaards MJ, et al. Haloperidol prophylaxis for elderly hip-surgery patients at risk for delirium: a randomized placebo-controlled study. J Am Geriatr Soc. 2005;53(10):1658–66. Medline:16181163

Kaneko T, Cai J, Ishikura T, et al. Prophylactic consecutive administration of haloperidol can reduce the occurrence of postoperative delirium in gastrointestinal surgery. Yonago Acta Med. 1999;42(3):179–84.

Krogseth M, Wyller TB, Engedal K, et al. Delirium is an important predictor of incident dementia among elderly hip fracture patients. Dement Geriatr Cogn Disord. 2011;31(1):63–70. http://dx.doi.org/10.1159/000322591. Medline:21212674

Larsen KA, Kelly SE, Stern TA, et al. Administration of olanzapine to prevent postoperative delirium in elderly joint-replacement patients: a randomized, controlled trial. Psychosomatics. 2010;51(5):409–18. http://dx.doi.org/10.1176/appi.psy.51.5.409. Medline:20833940

Leslie DL, Zhang Y, Holford TR, et al. Premature death associated with delirium at 1-year follow-up. Arch Intern Med. 2005;165(14):1657–62. http://dx.doi.org/10.1001/archinte.165.14.1657. Medline:16043686

Levkoff SE, Liptzin B, Cleary PD, et al. Subsyndromal delirium. Am J Geriatr Psychiatry. 1996;4(4):320–9. http://dx.doi.org/10.1097/00019442-199622440-00006.

Lipowski ZJ. Update on delirium. Psychiatr Clin North Am. 1992;15(2):335–46. Medline:1603727

Lonergan E, Britton AM, Luxenberg J, et al. Antipsychotics for delirium. Cochrane Database Syst Rev. 2007;(2):CD005594. Medline:17443602

Lundström M, Edlund A, Bucht G, et al. Dementia after delirium in patients with femoral neck fractures. J Am Geriatr Soc. 2003;51(7):1002–6. http://dx.doi.org/10.1046/j.1365-2389.2003.51315.x. Medline:12834522

Maldonado JR. Pathoetiological model of delirium: a comprehensive understanding of the neurobiology of delirium and an evidence-based approach to prevention and treatment. Crit Care Clin. 2008;24(4):789–856, ix. http://dx.doi.org/10.1016/j.ccc.2008.06.004. Medline:18929943

Marcantonio ER, Flacker JM, Wright RJ, et al. Reducing delirium after hip fracture: a randomized trial. J Am Geriatr Soc. 2001;49(5):516–22. http://dx.doi.org/10.1046/j.1532-5415.2001.49108.x. Medline:11380742

Marcantonio ER, Simon SE, Bergmann MA, et al. Delirium symptoms in post-acute care: prevalent, persistent, and associated with poor functional recovery. J Am Geriatr Soc. 2003;51(1):4–9. http://dx.doi.org/10.1034/j.1601-5215.2002.51002.x. Medline:12534838

Martinez FT, Tobar C, Beddings CI, et al. Preventing delirium in an acute hospital using a non-pharmacological intervention. Age Ageing. 2012;41(5):629–34. http://dx.doi.org/10.1093/ageing/afs060. Medline:22589080

McAvay GJ, Van Ness PH, Bogardus ST Jr, et al. Older adults discharged from the hospital with delirium: 1-year outcomes. J Am Geriatr Soc. 2006;54(8):1245–50. http://dx.doi.org/10.1111/j.1532-5415.2006.00815.x. Medline:16913993

McCusker J, Cole M, Dendukuri N, Belzile E, et al. Delirium in older medical inpatients and subsequent cognitive and functional status: a prospective study. CMAJ. 2001;165(5):575–83. Medline:11563209

McCusker J, Cole M, Dendukuri N, Han L, et al. The course of delirium in older medical inpatients: a prospective study. J Gen Intern Med. 2003;18(9):696–704. http://dx.doi.org/10.1046/j.1525-1497.2003.20602.x. Medline:12950477

Meagher D. Motor subtypes of delirium: past, present and future. Int Rev Psychiatry. 2009;21(1):59–73. http://dx.doi.org/10.1080/09540260802675460. Medline:19219713

Meagher DJ, Leonard M, Donnelly S, et al. A comparison of neuropsychiatric and cognitive profiles in delirium, dementia, comorbid delirium-dementia and cognitively intact controls. J Neurol Neurosurg Psychiatry. 2010;81(8):876–81. http://dx.doi.org/10.1136/jnnp.2009.200956. Medline:20587481

Mukadam N, Ritchie CW, Sampson EL. Cholinesterase inhibitors for delirium: what is the evidence? Int Psychogeriatr. 2008;20(2):209–18. http://dx.doi.org/10.1017/S1041610207006205. Medline:18411423

Peritogiannis V, Stefanou E, Lixouriotis C, et al. Atypical antipsychotics in the treatment of delirium. Psychiatry Clin Neurosci. 2009;63(5):623–31. http://dx.doi.org/10.1111/j.1440-1819.2009.02002.x. Medline:19674385

Popeo DM. Delirium in older adults. Mt Sinai J Med. 2011;78(4):571–82. http://dx.doi.org/10.1002/msj.20267. PMID:21748745

Prakanrattana U, Prapaitrakool S. Efficacy of risperidone for prevention of postoperative delirium in cardiac surgery. Anaesth Intensive Care. 2007;35(5):714–19. Medline:17933157

Rockwood K. The occurrence and duration of symptoms in elderly patients with delirium. J Gerontol. 1993;48(4):M162–6. http://dx.doi.org/10.1093/geronj/48.4.M162. Medline:8315229

Rockwood K, Cosway S, Carver D, et al. The risk of dementia and death after delirium. Age Ageing. 1999;28(6):551–6. http://dx.doi.org/10.1093/ageing/28.6.551. Medline:10604507

Saczynski JS, Marcantonio ER, Quach L, et al. Cognitive trajectories after postoperative delirium. N Engl J Med. 2012;367(1):30–9. http://dx.doi.org/10.1056/NEJMoa1112923. Medline:22762316

Seitz DP, Gill SS, van Zyl LT. Antipsychotics in the treatment of delirium: a systematic review. J Clin Psychiatry. 2007;68(1):11–21. http://dx.doi.org/10.4088/JCP.v68n0102. Medline:17284125

Tabet N, Howard R. Pharmacological treatment for the prevention of delirium: review of current evidence. Int J Geriatr Psychiatry. 2009;24(10):1037–44. http://dx.doi.org/10.1002/gps.2220. Medline:19226527

Thomas C, Kreisel SH, Oster P, et al. Diagnosing delirium in older hospitalized adults with dementia: adapting the confusion assessment method to international classification of diseases, tenth revision, diagnostic criteria. J Am Geriatr Soc. 2012;60(8):1471–7. http://dx.doi.org/10.1111/j.1532-5415.2012.04066.x. Medline:22881707

Tropea J, Slee JA, Brand CA, et al. Clinical practice guidelines for the management of delirium in older people in Australia. Australas J Ageing. 2008;27(3):150–6. http://dx.doi.org/10.1111/j.1741-6612.2008.00301.x. Medline:18713175

van Eijk MM, Roes KC, Honing ML, et al. Effect of rivastigmine as an adjunct to usual care with haloperidol on duration of delirium and mortality in critically ill patients: a multicentre, double-blind, placebo-controlled randomised trial. Lancet. 2010;376(9755):1829–37. http://dx.doi.org/10.1016/S0140-6736(10)61855-7. Medline: 21056464

Voyer P, Richard S, Doucet L, et al. Detection of delirium by nurses among long-term care residents with dementia. BMC Nurs. 2008;7:4. http://dx.doi.org/10.1186/1472-6955-7-4. PMID:18302791

Wang W, Li HL, Wang DX, et al. Haloperidol prophylaxis decreases delirium incidence in elderly patients after noncardiac surgery: a randomized controlled trial*. Crit Care Med. 2012;40(3):731–9. http://dx.doi.org/10.1097/CCM.0b013e3182376e4f. Medline:22067628

Witlox J, Eurelings LS, de Jonghe JF, et al. Delirium in elderly patients and the risk of postdischarge mortality, institutionalization, and dementia: a meta-analysis. JAMA. 2010;304(4):443–51. http://dx.doi.org/10.1001/jama.2010.1013. Medline:20664045

Wong CL, Holroyd-Leduc J, Simel DL, et al. Does this patient have delirium? Value of bedside instruments. JAMA. 2010;304(7):779–86. http://dx.doi.org/10.1001/jama.2010.1182. Medline:20716741

ADDITIONAL E-RESOURCES

Canadian Coalition for Seniors' Mental Health (CCSMH): www.ccsmh.ca

Care for Elders. [Internet]. Vancouver, BC: University of British Columbia, Division of Geriatric Psychiatry; n.d. www.careforelders.ca

Vancouver Island Health Authority (VIHA). [Internet]. Victoria, BC: VIHA;2014. Delirium in the older person. www.viha.ca/mhas/resources/delirium

3.3 Sleep Difficulties and Disorders in Older Adults, and Their Management

Jonathan Fleming, MB, FRCPC

INTRODUCTION

Sleep-related problems are part of normal aging and represent some of the most common complaints among older adults in primary care and specialty settings. Changes in older persons' sleep can reflect normal aging, primary sleep disorders, or other underlying psychiatric or medical disorders. Understanding the epidemiology of sleep changes and disorders is important for practicing clinicians, along with an understanding of pharmacological and nonpharmacological management. In this chapter Dr Fleming presents an overview of normal changes in sleep associated with aging followed by a discussion of primary sleep disorders and their treatment.

CASE SCENARIO

Your family physician colleague, Dr S., with whom you are having lunch, asks your advice about one of his patients that he saw this morning. He has known Mr and Mrs R. for over 30 years. They are both retired teachers and in fairly good health; Mrs R. has hypercholesterolemia and is on a statin with benefit, and Mr R. has various aches and pains from having been a semi-professional rugby player in his youth. They always come together for their appointments. Mr R. seems impatient generally and is sometimes abrupt with his wife, but behaves similarly with the female office staff. Last year Mrs R. complained that her husband said "bad things at night," by which she means he utters expletives that he would never say even at his most irritated. He had never done this before, and it is infrequent. She thought it might be alcohol related, as it seemed to always happen after he came home from choir practice and had a couple of beers with his friends. But when she tracked it, it was quite random. Later she thought it might be related to his prostate, as it seems to happen only after he goes back to sleep "after his pee break" at about 4:00 a.m.

Last night he was making similar noises as he has done before with some clearly spoken words among mumbling, but his body seemed to be twitching. She turned on the light, and he was clearly asleep. Then he started to shout. She couldn't understand what he was saying at first, but among the mumbling she clearly heard the name George. Then suddenly he said, "F – off you bastard!" and hit Mrs R. in the face with his fist. She yelled of course, and he woke up immediately. She was badly hurt and crying; he comforted her appropriately and said that he was very sorry but that he was having a dream about a bullying schoolmate who picked on him at school. He told her, "In my dream I took a swing at him and must have hit you." There is no history of abuse and both are shocked by this event. Dr S. asks, "What's happening? Should I encourage her to press charges?"

OVERVIEW

1. Changes in Sleep Performance in the Elderly

Complaints about sleep are common in the elderly.

- 70% non-dementing seniors reported frequently or regularly having at least one insomnia symptom (Jaussent et al., 2011).

Common subjective complaints include:

- A relative advance of the sleep phase (Monk, 2005)
- Fall asleep earlier; awaken earlier
- Increased snoring
- Disturbing dream content associated with awakenings

The four consistent age-related changes in polysomnographic studies are (Ohayon et al., 2004):

- Decreased total sleep time
- Decreased sleep efficiency
- Decreased slow-wave sleep (stage 3 and 4 or N3)
- Increased wake after sleep onset

2. DSM-5 Defined Sleep Disorders

Excluding the other specified and unspecified sleep disorders, the DSM-5 identifies twelve sleep disorders:

- Insomnia disorder
- Hypersomnolence disorder
- Narcolepsy
- Obstructive sleep apnea/hypopnea
- Central sleep apnea
- Sleep-related hypoventilation
- Circadian rhythm sleep-wake disorders
- Non–rapid eye movement sleep arousal disorders
- Nightmare disorder
- Rapid eye movement sleep behaviour disorder
- Restless legs syndrome
- Substance/medication-induced sleep disorder

2.1 Insomnia Disorder

2.1.1 Characteristics

- A durable, frequent complaint (> 3 months; > 3 nights per week) of sleep dissatisfaction that is associated with:
    - Difficulty initiating or maintaining sleep OR
    - Early-morning awakening with inability to return to sleep
- Distressing and/or impairing

2.1.2 Exclusions

Insomnia disorder is NOT diagnosed if:

- There is inadequate opportunity to sleep.
- It is caused by substance use or medications known to cause sleep disruption.

- It is better explained by and occurs exclusively during the course of another sleep-wake disorder, for example a circadian rhythm sleep-wake disorder.
- It is explained by medical or psychiatric disorders.

2.1.3 Epidemiology

Insomnia *symptoms* are:
- Common (~30% of the population)
- Frequently comorbid with psychiatric disorders

Insomnia *disorder* is:
- Less prevalent than symptoms (~6–10%)
- Can occur at any time in the life-cycle (first episode is usually in young adulthood)
- The disorder becomes chronic in 45–75% cases and extends into old age (Buysse et al., 2008; Morin et al., 2009).

2.1.4 Functional Consequences

- Mood changes (dysphoria and irritability)
- Decreased attention and concentration (higher rates of accidents)
- Interpersonal, social, and occupational problems

Persistent insomnia has long-term consequences particularly affecting quality of life (Roth et al., 2006) and increasing risk of:
- Major depressive disorder (Skapinakis et al., 2013)
- Hypertension (Meng, Zheng, & Hui, 2013)
- Myocardial infarction (Sofi et al., 2014)

The differential diagnosis of insomnia disorder includes:
- Normal sleep variations (short sleepers) and age-related sleep changes
- Situational/acute insomnia
- Circadian rhythm sleep-wake disorder
- Restless legs syndrome
- Breathing-related sleep disorders
- Narcolepsy
- Parasomnias
- Substance/medication-induced sleep disorder, insomnia type

2.2 Hypersomnolence Disorder (HD)

2.2.1 Characteristics

Hypersomnolence is a broad clinical term that includes:
- Protracted or prolonged sleep periods (during the night or – usually irresistibly – during the day)
- Impaired wakefulness with difficulty staying awake when required or expected
- Sleep inertia on any awakening
- Sleep inertia is highly specific to HD yet is not reported by all (Anderson et al., 2007)

HD is characterized by a durable and frequent complaint (> 3 months; > 3 nights per week) of excessive sleepiness despite at least 7 hours sleep that causes distress and/or impairment with one of the following:

- A prolonged main sleep episode of more than 9 hours per day that is non-restorative or unrefreshing, OR
- Recurrent periods of sleep or lapses into sleep within the same day, OR
- Difficulty in coming to full alertness after an abrupt awakening

Characteristically and unlike sleep deprivation states, recovery naps are unrefreshing and non-restorative (Vernet et al., 2010).

2.2.2 Exclusions

Other causes of hypersomnolence must be excluded:

- Substance use or medications known to cause sleepiness
- Another sleep-wake disorder, for example a breathing-related sleep disorder
- The hypersomnia is not explained by medical or psychiatric disorders

2.2.3 Epidemiology

- Community prevalence of HD is unknown.
- About 5–10% of sleepy patients seen at sleep clinics are diagnosed with HD (Ohayon, Dauvilliers, & Reynolds, 2012).
- Where possible a sleep study – overnight study followed by a Multiple Sleep Latency Test (Bodkin & Manchanda, 2011) – should be completed to differentiate HD from other sleep disorders, particularly narcolepsy and obstructive sleep apnea/hypopnea (OSAH).
- HD begins in young adulthood and is a chronic disorder (Anderson et al., 2007) continuing into old age.
- Its expression in old age has not been extensively studied, but comorbid sleep conditions such as respiratory sleep disorders co-occur.

2.2.4 Functional Consequences

- Functional impairments associated with HD have been less well studied than insomnia disorder and narcolepsy, but persistent hypersomnia affects quality of life and social and occupational functioning (Vernet et al., 2010).
- Persistent hypersomnolence can cause automatic behaviours (typically routine, uncomplicated activities and, rarely, driving) with partial or complete amnesia.
- Mood changes not qualifying for a mood disorder diagnosis may precede or follow the onset of HD.
- Depressive symptoms have been noted in 15–25% of patients with HD (Dauvilliers et al., 2013).

2.2.5 Differential Diagnosis of HD

- Normal variation in sleep need – long sleeper getting inadequate sleep
- Poor sleep quantity or quality and fatigue
- Breathing-related sleep disorders
- Circadian rhythm sleep-wake disorders
- Parasomnias
- Other mental disorders

2.3 Narcolepsy

2.3.1 Characteristics

- Characterized by recurrent, irresistible urges to sleep with involuntary lapses into sleep or elective napping occurring at least 3 times per week over the past 3 months

In addition the DSM-5 requires *one of three* markers associated with this condition to be present:

- Cataplexy, characterized by brief (seconds to minutes) episodes of sudden bilateral loss of muscle tone with maintained consciousness, specifically precipitated by laughter or joking
- A sleep study showing a rapid eye movement (REM) sleep latency less than or equal to 15 minutes or a mean sleep latency, on a Multiple Sleep Latency Test, of less than or equal to 8 minutes and two or more sleep-onset REM periods
- Low cerebrospinal fluid (CSF) hypocretin levels in the absence of acute brain injury, inflammation, or infection

Sleepiness in narcolepsy is characterized by:

- Involuntary lapses into sleep, OR
- Frequent, elective daytime naps to maintain alertness
- Refreshing sleep periods (unlike in HD)
- Rare sleep inertia (seen in HD)
- Occurrence of automatic behaviours (similar to HD)
- Cataplexy

Cataplexy can be difficult to diagnose, but when present is one of the core tetrad symptoms (Akintomide & Richards, 2011) of narcolepsy:

- Sleepiness
- Cataplexy
- Sleep paralysis
- Hypnogogic hallucinations

2.3.2 Epidemiology

- The prevalence of narcolepsy-cataplexy is 0.02–0.067%, affecting both genders with a slight male preponderance (Dauvilliers, Arnulf, & Mignot, 2007).

2.3.4 Mechanism

- It is an auto-immune disease affecting the orexin/hypocretin system (Li, Hu, & de Lecea, 2014) with a typical onset in young adulthood but late onsets do occur.

2.3.5 Functional Impairments

- There are significant functional impairments associated with narcolepsy (Broughton & Broughton, 1994) and comorbidity in later life with medical, psychiatric, and other sleep disorders.
- Cognitive difficulties are more frequent in older narcoleptic patients than in controls (Ohayon et al., 2005).

2.3.6 Differential Diagnosis of Narcolepsy

- Sleep deprivation and insufficient nocturnal sleep
- Sleep apnea syndromes
- Major depressive disorder
- Conversion disorder
- Hypersomnolence disorder
- Seizures
- Schizophrenia (because of hypnogogic hallucinations)

2.4 Obstructive Sleep Apnea/Hypopnea (OSAH)

Airway obstruction causes snoring but no one symptom or sign is sufficiently precise to diagnose OSAH clinically (Myers, Mrkobrada, & Simel, 2013), so DSM-5 requires polysomnographic evidence of at least:

- Five obstructive apneas (total absence of airflow measured at the nose and mouth lasting 10 seconds or more), OR
- Five hypopneas (a reduction of airflow) per hour of sleep with O2 desaturations of 3% or greater and/or an arousal on the electroencephalogram (EEG)

In addition the patient may experience:

- Snoring, snorting/gasping
- Frank breathing pauses during nocturnal sleep
- Unrefreshing sleep
- Daytime sleepiness
- Fatigue

OSAH has complicated and variable effects on cognition (Scheltens et al., 1991).

- The associated hypoxemia is a risk factor for mild cognitive impairment (MCI) and dementia (Yaffe et al., 2011; Chang et al., 2013).

2.4.1 Severity Classification

On the basis of the apnea/hypopnea index (number of events/hour), OSAH is classified as:
- Mild (index < 15/hr)
- Moderate (index 15–30/hr)
- Severe (index > 30/hr)

2.4.2 Epidemiology

OSAH is a very common disorder; its prevalence is approximately (Punjabi, 2008):
- 3–7% for men
- 2–5% for women
- Prevalence increases with age
    - 70% for men and 56% for women in those 65–95 years (Ancoli-Israel et al., 1991)

2.4.3 Other Risk Factors

Other risk factors for OSAH include:

- Male sex
- Obesity
- Family history
- Craniofacial abnormalities
- Smoking
- Alcohol

2.5 Central Sleep Apnea (CSA)

- CSA is characterized by diminished or absent respiratory effort, coupled with the presence of symptoms including excessive daytime sleepiness, frequent nocturnal awakenings, or both (Aurora et al., 2012).
- The apneas and hypopneas are caused by variability in central respiratory effort rather than airway obstruction.
- Polysomnography is required to demonstrate these events because nocturnal signs (e.g., snoring, gasping) are absent.

2.5.1 DSM-5 Types

DSM-5 identifies three types of CSA:

- Idiopathic
- Cheyene-Stokes breathing
- Central sleep apnea comorbid with opioid use (associated with effects on respiratory rhythm generators and drive)

2.5.2 Comorbidity and Functional Consequences

- CSA can co-occur with OSAH or emerge as it is treated by continuous positive airway pressure (CPAP) (Malhotra & Owens, 2010).
- CSA can cause:
  - Insomnia
  - Daytime sleepiness
  - Mood disturbances
- Neurocognitive changes have not been reported with CSA.
- Older patients with congestive heart failure (CHF) and sleep apnea (particularly CSA) have a 2.7 times greater risk of reduced survival than patients with CHF or apnea alone (Sasayama et al., 2006).

2.6 Sleep-Related Hypoventilation

- Sleep-related hypoventilation requires a sleep study to demonstrate episodes of decreased respiration associated with elevated CO_2 levels or, if CO_2 monitoring is unavailable, episodes of low pO_2 on oximetry that are not caused by apneas or hypopneas.
- Uncommon in adults (Casey, Cantillo, & Brown, 2007), but can result in:
  - Frequent arousals and awakenings from sleep
  - Morning headache
  - Complaints of insomnia/hypersomnia

2.7 Circadian Rhythm Sleep-Wake Disorders

The sleep-wake cycle is generated by a complex interaction (Reid & Zee, 2011) between:
- Endogenous circadian regulation
- External physical light and dark cycles
- The drive to sleep – increases proportionally with time awake
- Social activities
- Environmental factors

2.7.1 DSM-5 Types

The DSM-5 recognizes six types of disruption to the circadian rhythm of sleep diagnosed by sleep diary or actigraphy (Martin & Hakim, 2011):
- Delayed sleep phase type
- Advanced sleep phase type
- Irregular sleep-wake type
- Non-24 hour sleep-wake type
- Shift work type
- Unspecified type

2.7.2 Age and Mechanisms

- Commonly circadian sleep disorders first present in the young but when chronic can continue into old age.
- With age there is a tendency towards earlier sleep times (Carrier et al., 1997) that is distinguished from an advanced sleep phase because it is not locked in (staying up late is possible).
- Multiple mechanisms associated with dementia are considered important in the circadian dysregulation of sleep in these patients:
  - Damage to the circadian pacemaker in the suprachiasmatic nucleus
  - Alterations in the pineal gland and melatonin secretion
  - Changes in melatonin receptors
- The irregular sleep-wake type is seen in patients with dementia (Sack et al., 2007).
  - No clear major sleep period
  - Three or more bouts of sleep of varying length during a 24-hour period

2.8 Parasomnias

- Parasomnias are events that emerge from sleep, and in the DSM-5 are divided into those that arise from non–rapid eye movement (NREM) sleep and those that arise from REM sleep.

2.8.1 NREM Parasomnias

- There are two DSM-5–defined NREM sleep arousal disorders: sleepwalking and sleep terrors.
- Typically these events:
  - Occur in younger individuals (tend to burn out by the 3rd decade)

- Emerge from the first third of the sleep period (where deep or delta wave sleep is prominent)
- Are not associated with prominent dream activity or imagery
- Are associated with amnesia for the event in the morning

2.8.2 Exclusions for NREM Parasomnias

Their rarity in the elderly requires that new-onset NREM parasomnias necessitate a full work-up to eliminate:

- Nocturnal seizures
- Neurological disorders such as Parkinson's disease (Poryazova et al., 2013)
- Sleep-related breathing disorder
- Effects of medications, alone or in combination

First and second generation antidepressants are associated with the development of NREM parasomnias (Kierlin & Littner, 2011).

- Hypnotic medications, particularly zolpidem in the 10 mg dose (Hoque & Chesson, 2009), have also been implicated.
- Withdrawal from centrally acting medications and substances

2.8.3 Differential Diagnosis of NREM Parasomnias

Nightmare disorder:

- Characterized by complete awakenings usually in the last third of the night (when REM sleep predominates) with good recall of the dream narrative

Breathing-related sleep disorders:

- Arousals and awakenings associated with apnea or hypopnea can cause confused arousals and parasomnias

REM sleep behaviour disorder (see below):

- Distinguished from NREM parasomnias by:
  - Timing (REM sleep behaviour disorder tends to occur in the last half of the night when REM predominates, and NREM parasomnias in the first half)
  - Presence of complex movements and vocalizations mirroring the dream content (e.g., repeated striking out at an attacker) with good recall

Parasomnia overlap syndrome:

- A rare condition diagnosed by polysomnography and characterized by an admixture of REM and NREM parasomnias (Schenck, Boyd, & Mahowald, 1997)

Sleep-related seizures:

- Tend to be stereotypical movements expressed throughout the night but can also emerge from naps (Zucconi, 2013)

Alcohol-induced blackouts:

- History of complicated behaviours with amnesia may mimic NREM parasomnias

Dissociative amnesia with dissociative fugue:

- Dissociative events may be extremely difficult to distinguish from sleepwalking and have been noted to emerge during sleep studies (Fleming, 1987).

Panic disorder:
- Nocturnal panic attacks can cause abrupt awakenings from NREM sleep.
- They are NOT accompanied by complex movements.
- The sleeper rapidly comes to complete alertness.
- The sleeper has full awareness (no amnesia) of the event.

Medication-induced complex behaviours:
- Multiple centrally acting medications have been associated with causing or exacerbating NREM parasomnias.

2.8.4 REM Parasomnias

- REM sleep cycles about every 90 minutes, and each episode increases in duration as the night progresses; therefore REM parasomnias are more likely to occur in the last third of the night, whereas NREM parasomnias are more likely to occur in the first third.
    - Arousals from REM sleep are rapid and complete and, unlike arousals from delta/deep sleep, are not characterized by confusion and amnesia.
- The two REM parasomnias are nightmare disorder and REM sleep behaviour disorder (RBD).

2.8.5 REM Parasomnias: Nightmare Disorder

Nightmare disorder is characterized in the DSM-5 by:
- Very distressing, repeated, extended, dysphoric dreams
- Good recall of the content
- Content usually frightening (threats to survival, security, or physical integrity)
- Symptoms of autonomic arousal
- Not caused by substance use or withdrawal

Nightmares are subdivided by duration and severity:
- Acute (duration of 1 month or less), OR
- Subacute (duration is greater than 1 month but less than 6 months), OR
- Persistent (duration is 6 months or greater)
- Mild (< 1 episode per week)
- Moderate (one or more episodes per week but not nightly)
- Severe (nightly episodes)

The prevalence of nightmares among older adults has been shown to be just above 4% (Salvio et al., 1992).

2.8.6 REM Sleep Behaviour Disorder (RBD)

- RBD is characterized by:
    - A full awakening with no confusion or amnesia
    - Vocalizations (usually discernible, unlike the mutterings that can occur with NREM parasomnias) and/or
    - Complex motor behaviours (typically fight or flight behaviours)
    - Loss of normal REM atonia (on a sleep study) picked up from the submentalis electromyogram leads and in the arms and legs
    - If the parasomnia occurs within the context of an established synucleinopathy

diagnosis such as personality disorder or multiple system atrophy, the diagnosis can be made without a sleep study.

- In the general population, the prevalence of RBD is approximately 0.38–0.5% (Kang et al., 2013).
  - RBD is estimated to occur in 25–50% of patients with personality disorder and can precede the onset of the disorder by over 10 years (Schenck et al., 1987).
- The predictive association with neurodegenerative diseases has raised interest in what was once considered an idiopathic disorder and the importance of its subclinical expression (Schenck & Mahowald, 2008).

2.9 Restless Legs Syndrome (RLS)

- Increasingly called Willis-Ekbom disease after the two physicians who described the disorder in different eras
- The Willis-Ekbom Disease Foundation (now called the Restless Legs Syndrome Foundation) is a reliable source of useful physician and patient information: www.willis-ekbom.org

2.9.1 Clinical Features

RLS is a symptom-based diagnosis, and DSM-5 requires:
- Urge to move the legs, usually accompanied by or in response to uncomfortable and unpleasant sensations
- Occurrence or worsening during rest or inactivity
- Partial or total relief by movement
- Occurrence or worsening during the evening or night
- Frequency of ≥ 3 times per week
- Persistence (present for at least 3 months)

2.9.2 Exclusions

- Medical conditions (e.g., neuropathy, renal disease, etc.)
- Psychiatric disorder (e.g., anxiety or agitation)
- Drug of abuse or medication (e.g., akathisia)

2.9.3 Etiology

- Etiological theories emphasize genetics and disturbances in iron and dopamine metabolism (Dauvilliers & Winkelmann, 2013).
- Familial and non-familial forms exist; the former tends to have an early onset (childhood and adolescence) with a slow progression (Zhang et al., 2014).
- Because different severity criteria are used, various prevalence rates are reported (2–10%), but the condition is more prevalent in women and in the elderly (Gupta et al., 2012).
- An association between symptoms of depression (Hornyak et al., 2005), depressive syndromes (Gupta, Lahan, & Goel, 2013), and RLS has been noted in a number of studies.
- But antidepressants (amitriptyline, escitalopram, mianserine, mirtazapine, duloxetine) are known to cause RLS (Perez-Lloret et al., 2012).

2.9.4 Cognitive Dysfunction and Comorbidities

- Disturbances in executive functions (Fulda et al., 2011) and impaired cognition (Celle et al., 2010) have been reported in patients with severe RLS.
- Untreated RLS patients show cognitive deficits similar to that reported for one night of sleep loss (Pearson et al., 2006).
- Over 90% of patients with RLS also have periodic limb movements (PLMs) during sleep and rarely when at quiet rest.
- PLMs – with or without RLS – increase with age and can affect sleep architecture and sleep performance (Claman et al., 2013).

2.9.5 Sleep Study

- A sleep study is required to define their significance.
    - Can be benign OR
    - Cause micro-arousals (EEG changes lasting 3–10 seconds) or awakenings (> 15 seconds)
- PLMs can increase morbidity and mortality in persons with RLS, specifically when associated with cardiovascular disease (Cuellar, 2013).
- Mirza et al., 2013 showed frequent PLMs (periodic movement index > 35/hr of sleep) were a predictor for atrial fibrillation progression, and treatment with dopaminergic drugs was protective of this progression.

2.9.6 Differential Diagnosis

- Habitual foot tapping
- Positional discomfort
- Arthralgia or arthritis
- Leg cramps (Allen & Kirby, 2012)
- Myalgia
- Positional ischemia (numbness)
- Leg edema
- Peripheral neuropathy
- Radiculopathy

2.10 Substance/Medication-Induced Sleep Disorder

- This DSM-5 diagnosis is made when a non-delirious, prominent, and severe sleep disturbance requiring clinical attention is caused by a substance (i.e., a drug of abuse, a medication, toxin exposure) known to cause disrupted sleep.
- It cannot be "better explained" by a sleep disorder that is not substance/medication-induced and results in four types of disturbance:
    - Insomnia type
    - Daytime sleepiness type
    - Parasomnia type
    - Mixed type
- If the disturbance is caused by a substance, there must be:
    - Evidence of intoxication or withdrawal
    - Onset should be noted to have occurred during intoxication or discontinuation
- A plethora of medications can cause prominent sleep disruption including:
    - Adrenergic agonists and antagonists
    - Dopamine agonists and antagonists

- Cholinergic agonists and antagonists
- Serotonergic agonists and antagonists
- Antihistamines
- Corticosteroids
- Drugs known to cause sleep disruption include:
  - Caffeine
  - Nicotine
  - Alcohol
  - Marijuana
  - Opioids
  - Sedatives
  - Stimulants
- Untreated sleep disruption on withdrawal has been implicated in restarting substance use (Brower et al., 2001; Babson et al., 2013).

3. Treatment

3.1 Sleep Hygiene

- Sleep hygiene (SH) refers to optimal behaviours that promote and maintain sound sleep (Roszkowska & Geraci, 2010).
- SH alone is unlikely to be curative of sleep disturbances in the elderly but MUST be practiced consistently to optimize any therapeutic intervention.

3.1.1 Essential SH Behaviours

- Maintain a regular sleep-wake schedule by getting up with an alarm at the same time each and every day (including weekends).
- Failure to do so may contribute to tolerance to the hypnotic effect of any medication.
- Turn clock faces away.
- Knowing the time causes cognitive and affective arousal that delays sleep onset or a return to sleep after an awakening.
- Exercise every day (e.g., 30 minutes walking, Tai Chi, etc.).
  - If exercise is activating, complete it earlier in the day.
  - Exercise can be split (e.g., 3 × 10 minute periods).
- Get out into bright light in the morning hours; in the summer time avoid evening light.
- Ideally eliminate alcohol, nicotine, and caffeine but avoid use after mid-afternoon.
- Have a wind-down period with no stimulating activities for at least an hour before bedtime.
- Avoid spending long periods of time in horizontal rest.
- If a nap is required, limit it to 25 minutes (use an alarm) and complete it by mid-afternoon.

3.2 Insomnia Disorder

A behavioural intervention is always preferred over pharmacotherapy when disrupted sleep is not associated with significant daytime impairment.

- The safest evidence-based intervention for insomnia disorder is CBT-I (cognitive behavioural treatment of insomnia) that incorporates:
  - SH
  - Restricted time in bed

- Cognitive therapy to address unhelpful cognitions (e.g., "I must have 8 hours of sleep to function") (Lichstein et al., 2013)
- CBT-I trials in older adults show sustained effect for up to 2 years (Morin et al., 1999).
  - Access to trained CBT-I therapists is variously available and may not be covered by health insurance plans.
  - Internet-based programs are available at cost (https://www.sleepio.com/; http://www.cbtforinsomnia.com) but may not be accessible or acceptable to all elderly patients.

The first-line medications of choice are the intermediate acting benzodiazepines and benzodiazepine agonists approved by the US Food and Drug Administration and Health Canada (Schutte-Rodin et al., 2008).

- The clinical utility of benzodiazepines and benzodiazepine agonists – their risks and benefits – are currently being re-evaluated for anxiety and sleep disorders (Baldwin et al., 2013), particularly in the light of minimal or no evidence of the efficacy and risks of other pharmacological interventions (Rickels, 2013).
- The available intermediate acting benzodiazepines and benzodiazepine agonists in Canada are:
  - Temazepam
  - Triazolam
  - Zopiclone
  - Zolpidem
- Choice is directed by:
  - Symptom pattern
  - Past treatment responses
  - Treatment goals
  - Comorbid conditions
  - Contraindications
  - Concurrent medication interactions
  - Side effects
  - Patient preference
  - Cost
- All Health Canada–approved hypnotics can be associated with clinically significant adverse effects, especially in the elderly where age can alter pharmacodynamics and pharmacokinetic effects.
- The benefits of the benzodiazepine receptor agonists (the Z drugs) over traditional benzodiazepines with short half-lives is controversial:
  - They are less disruptive to sleep architecture.
  - They cause less tolerance and less rebound on withdrawal.
  - Like the benzodiazepines, Z drugs in a dose dependent manner (Gunja, 2013) affect:
    - Cognition
    - Behaviour
    - Next-day performance
    - Driving ability
- The effective utilization of hypnotics requires (Perlis, Gehrman, & Riemann, 2008):
  - Documenting the significant and impairing daytime complaints related to sleep loss
  - Assessing risk for drug-drug interactions

- Using the lowest effective dose (e.g., 3.75 mg of zopiclone; 5 mg zolpidem) for the shortest period of time
  - Using intermittent dosing (e.g., three nights per week) where practical and effective
  - Noting adverse drug reactions
  - Regularly assessing and noting the response to the intervention
- Psychotropic medication of all types (Bloch et al., 2011) – particularly long-acting benzodiazepines – are one of several risk factors for falls in the elderly.
- BUT disrupted sleep is another risk factor for falling in this age group (Brassington, King, & Bliwise, 2000).
- Discontinuing hypnotics is known to decrease the risk of falls (Tsunoda et al., 2010), but no study of withdrawing Z drugs has assessed sleep parameters, psychological and behavioural adjustment, and quality of life after the withdrawal has been accomplished.

Melatonin is an important endogenous coordinator of the sleep-wake cycle and a melatonin agonist (ramelteon) with proven efficacy in treating insomnia with minimal side effects (Borja & Daniel, 2006) – particularly cognitive or psychomotor side effects – is available in the United States but not in Canada.

- Melatonin is not a controlled substance.
- Ensure the use of active pharmaceutical grade melatonin (available in most large pharmacies in Canada).
- It may be helpful in some patients (Olde Rikkert & Rigaud, 2001).
- It may facilitate withdrawal from benzodiazepine hypnotics in the elderly (Kunz et al., 2012).
- Its secretion is dysregulated in delirium and dementia (Mishima K et al., 1999).
- Exogenous melatonin may be helpful in managing "sundowning" in demented patients (Lammers & Ahmed, 2013).

3.3 Hypersomnolence Disorder

- Treatment response is variable in this disorder and often less than satisfactory (Anderson et al., 2007).
- The primary focus is on pharmacotherapy.
- The same stimulants as for narcolepsy (see section 3.4) but higher dosages are used (Anderson et al., 2007).
- Behavioural recommendations should be made:
  - Attend to diet – avoid high caloric "energy" foods and drinks; they cause weight gain.
  - Ensure adequate nocturnal sleep.
  - Maintain good SH.
  - Minimize napping – unlike in narcolepsy and sleep deprivation from other causes, scheduled naps are ineffective and sleep inertia may impair functioning on awakening.
- Although there are no systematic treatment studies in this patient group, if a concurrent mood disorder is present it should be treated vigorously with an activating antidepressant such as venlafaxine.

3.4 Narcolepsy

- Treatment of narcolepsy targets the impairing symptoms of daytime sleepiness and cataplexy through the use of medications and strategic napping.
- Psychostimulants are the mainstay of treatment for excessive daytime sleepiness, but side effects can limit their use and tolerance to their alerting effect may occur over time.

Common side effects include:
- Irritability and mood changes
- Headaches
- Decreased appetite
- Increased blood pressure
- Irregular heart beat

Modafinil is considered a first-line drug in managing narcolepsy and is started at a dosage of 200 mg per day, increasing if required to 400 mg per day.

- Its R-enantiomer, armodafinil (not available in Canada) has a longer half-life (14–17 hrs), is more potent, and better tolerated.
- The initial dose is 50 mg and can be increased to 250 mg in the morning (De la Herrán-Arita & García-García, 2013).

Methylphenidate causes fewer side effects than dextroamphetamine and is used in a dose range of 10–60 mg per day.

- Dextroamphetamine, in both a slow and regular release preparation, is the most potent, prescribed stimulant and is used in a dose range of 15 to 60 mg per day.

Most antidepressants have anticataplectic effects (e.g., clomipramine, paroxetine, phenelzine, etc.).

- Commonly venlafaxine is used to treat cataplexy in a dose range of 75 mg to 300 mg (Vignatelli, D'Alessandro, & Candelise, 2006).

Gammahydroxybutyrate (GHB) promotes sleep, increases its depth, eliminates cataplexy, and reduces daytime sleepiness (Kalra & Hart, 1992), but due to its use as a date rape drug it was banned worldwide.

- A highly controlled and effective variant – sodium oxybate (Robinson & Keating, 2007) – is available but its cost often precludes its use.
- Timed daytime naps (< 25 minutes each nap to prevent sleep inertia) provides protection from sleepiness for up to 2 hours and is a commonly used behavioural strategy.

In addition to the disrupted nocturnal sleep associated with narcolepsy (Roth et al., 2013), other factors further disrupt sleep in the older patient (Chakravorty & Rye, 2003):
- Age effects
- Medication effects
- Development of PLMs de novo or associated with stimulant/antidepressant use
- Respiratory sleep disorders associated with weight gain
- RBD as a comorbid condition (DelRosso, Chesson, & Hoque, 2013)
- The orexin/hypocretin system is involved in numerous physiological systems including sleep, arousal, and metabolism (Li, Hu, & de Lecea, 2014).
- Patients with narcolepsy are known to gain weight (Inocente et al., 2013), placing them at risk for developing OSAH.
    - Monitoring for weight gain and counselling on diet is required.

3.5 Obstructive Sleep Apnea/Hypopnea

- OSAH in older adults associated with clinical symptoms, particularly hypertension, cognitive dysfunction, nocturia, high levels of sleep disordered breathing (apnea/hypopnea index > 15 with oxygen desaturations), or cardiac disease, should be treated regardless of the age of the patient.
- Conservative management emphasizing weight loss may be appropriate in milder cases (apnea/hypopnea index < 15), but weight loss and maintaining a stable lower weight at any age is difficult.
- There are no large randomized controlled trials (RCTs) for drug therapy in OSAH; reduction in the apnea/hypopnea index has been shown with:
    - Donepezil in patients with Alzheimer's disease (AD) (Moraes et al., 2008)
    - Fluticasone in patients with allergic rhinitis (Lavigne et al., 2013)
- The treatment of choice is with CPAP but this may not be well tolerated, affecting compliance and outcome (Wickwire et al., 2013).
- Oral appliances fitted by dentists that advance the lower jaw up and forward can be effective in mild to moderate cases (apnea-hypopnea index < 30 events/hour) (Ngiam et al., 2013).
- There is a risk of a considerable financial outlay (> $1200) without benefit as response is variable.
- Weight gain after successful fitting will diminish the result, so continued attention to exercise and diet is required.
- Sedative sleep-promoting agents of any kind – including alcohol – are contraindicated in patients with OSAH, although, with varying effectiveness, the Z drugs have been used to improve compliance with CPAP (Glidewell, 2013).

3.6 Central Sleep Apnea and Sleep-Related Hypoventilation

- Patients with significant respiratory disease (e.g., COPD, severe asthma, or restrictive diseases, cardiac disease such as CHF, and complex OSAH patients [e.g, hypoventilation syndromes associated with obesity or impaired ventilation secondary to neuromuscular diseases]) should be referred to a respiratory sleep specialist for evaluation and treatment.

Therapy for CSA related to congestive heart failure includes (Aurora et al., 2012):

- CPAP therapy targeted to normalize the apnea-hypopnea index
- Oxygen therapy
- Adaptive servo-ventilation to normalize the apnea-hypopnea index

3.7 Circadian Rhythm Sleep-Wake Disorders

- Individualized sleep scheduling (based on diaries and/or actigraphy) is the cornerstone for managing circadian disruptions.
- Correcting the diminished circadian amplitude of the elderly (Zhou, Jung, & Richards, 2012) is effected by reinforcing relevant time cues (zeitgebers) through:

- – Timed light exposure
    - ▪ Bright light exposure is well tolerated and improves sleep performance and reduces sundowning (Zhou, Jung, & Richards, 2012).
  - – Melatonin supplementation
    - ▪ A recent RCT of 1-hour light treatment (> 2,500 lux) in the morning plus 5 mg of melatonin at bedtime for 10 weeks significantly increased wakefulness in the daytime and activity levels, and improved the rest activity rhythm (Dowling et al., 2008).
  - – Increased physical and social activity
- There are no studies of ramelteon – a melatonin receptor agonist – in dementia but a single case report notes a dramatic response to 8 mg given at 21:00 hours in a 79-year-old male (Asano et al., 2013).

3.8 Parasomnias

- The NREM parasomnias typically "burn out" in young adulthood; if they appear de novo in the elderly a full medical, psychiatric, and neurological work-up is required.
- Nonpharmacological management of parasomnias emphasizes the safety of the sleeper and his or her bed partner.
- The bedroom should be clear of dangerous objects, and the mattress should be on the floor.
- Exits should be alarmed and locked.
- Sleep deprivation from any cause should be avoided.
- Alcohol and substance use should be minimized, preferably eliminated.
- There are no RCTs in this patient population, but the long-acting benzodiazepines (diazepam, nitrazepam) have been used for many years.
- All first generation benzodiazepines probably work, but a non–evidence-based clinical consensus for using clonazepam (0.25 mg to 2 mg, if required) has developed.
- Nightmare disorder is managed by both verbal therapy and pharmacotherapy.
- A recent World Health Organization (WHO) guideline (Tol, Barbui, & van Ommeren, 2013) recommends stress management, cognitive behavioral therapy (CBT) with a trauma focus, and eye-movement desensitization reprocessing (EMDR) (van der Kolk et al., 2007).
- Unlike the APA guideline (Benedek et al., 2009), the WHO guideline does not recommend antidepressants unless psychological interventions are not available or have failed.
- Addressing sleep hygiene and sleep impairment is the first step in management (Bajor, Ticlea, & Osser, 2011).
- Imagery rehearsal – a CBT technique – is effective in treating nightmares (Germain & Nielsen, 2003), but nightmares may decrease in response to less focused therapies (Coelho et al., 2013).
- Prazosin – an inexpensive, generically available medication labelled for the treatment of hypertension, titrated to a maximum of 5 mg mid-morning and 20 mg at bedtime for men, and 2 mg and 10 mg, respectively, for women – decreases nightmare frequency and improves both sleep quality and global clinical status (Raskind et al., 2013).

3.9 REM Sleep Behaviour Disorder

- The safety measures for the NREM parasomnias (see section 3.8) apply for RBD; there is a serious risk of self-injury and bed-partner injury that must be discussed and addressed.
- Sleeping in separate beds is the safest for couples but may be unacceptable; treatment may improve the frequency and severity of nocturnal movements but breakthrough violent episodes can occur.
- If possible it is best to sleep on the mattress on the floor with no furniture or items within arm's length of the bed; liberal padding of sharp objects that cannot be removed is required.
- There is no known effective psychological therapy but events can emerge during stressful times, so general stress management and sleep hygiene principles should be followed.
- Level 4 evidence supports the use of clonazepam (0.25 titrated to effect and a maximum of 1 mg; 90% effective with benefit apparent in the first four days of use).
- Daytime sleepiness, sedation, dysphoria, and cognitive impairment may limit increasing the dose if required.
- Morning drowsiness may be relieved by taking the drug earlier.
- Temazepam, triazolam, and alprazolam have also been reported to be effective in a dozen patients (Aurora et al., 2010).
- Melatonin (3–12 mg qhs) has been reported to be effective in 31 of 38 subjects over 6 case series (Aurora et al., 2010).
- Donepezil (10–15 mg) and rivastigmine (4.5–6 mg) bid have been suggested for use in patients with synucleinopathies (Aurora et al., 2010).

3.10 Restless Legs Syndrome

- Good sleep hygiene practices should be followed as usual; some patients notice sensitivity to caffeine, alcohol, and other dietary triggers, and if present they should be avoided.
- A serum ferritin should be drawn and if < 50 µg/dl iron therapy should be started (Frauscher et al., 2009).
- The cornerstone of management is pharmacotherapy with the first-line drugs being the dopamine agonists ropinirole and pramipexole (Stiasny et al., 2000), as they lower the severity of RLS symptoms and reduce reoccurrence of symptoms or augmentation (worsening of symptoms after improvement with symptoms appearing earlier in the day).
- The risk of augmentation is reported to be less for ropinirole than for pramipexole (Yeh, Walters, & Tsuang, 2012).
- Second-line drugs include gabapentin (up to 1200 mg per day, given at night; Comella, 2014) and opioids (Schulte et al., 2013).
- It remains controversial if PLMs without RLS should be treated, and there is no guidance as to specific pharmacotherapy.
    - Options include masking treatment (benzodiazepines and gabapentin) or using the dopamine agonists ropinirole and pramipexole.

4. Key Points

- Insomnia symptoms are common in the elderly, and not all symptoms require treatment.
- Accurate diagnosis is crucial as diagnosis informs intervention.
- Untreated sleep disorders affect quality of life and risk the patient self-treating with alcohol, antihistamines, or sedative substances of abuse.
- Nocturnal sleep disruption (arousals and awakenings) has a bidirectional relationship with psychopathology and daytime impairment.
- Sleep loss, fatigue, and sleepiness adversely affect executive functioning.
- Most sleep disorders are chronic, and regular monitoring is required to ensure the appropriateness of interventions and to monitor for the development of new symptoms suggestive of psychiatric disorders.

QUESTIONS

1. List five common changes that occur in the sleep performance of older adults.
2. List three sleep disorders that either are only manifested during REM sleep or are more prominent during that sleep phase.
3. List the fundamentals of good sleep hygiene.
4. You are asked by the pharmacy committee at a local residential facility for seniors where you work to review the current pharmacy listing for hypnotic medications and to give your reasons for including or excluding the medications in an updated list.
   - Phenobarbital, 15 mg and 30 mg
   - Chloral hydrate, 500 mg and 1000 mg
   - Flurazepam, 15 mg and 30 mg
   - Nitrazepam, 2.5 mg and 5 mg
   - Triazolam, 0.125 mg
   - Oxazepam, 10 mg, 15 mg, and 30 mg
   - Lorazepam, 0.25 mg, 0.5 mg, and 1 mg
   - Zopiclone, 3.75 mg and 5 mg
   - Zolpidem, 5 mg and 10 mg
5. Sleep is divided into two physiologically distinct stages, NREM and REM sleep. What unique events occur in REM sleep, and what sleep disorders either worsen their expression in this sleep stage or occur exclusively within it?
6. When indicated, what strategies might be useful for reducing sleep-promoting medication use in older patients?

ANSWERS

1. Common changes that occur in the sleep performance of older adults include:
   - Relative advance of the sleep phase is experienced as difficulty in staying awake in the evening and waking earlier than younger subjects.
   - It may take longer to fall asleep.
   - Sleep is experienced as being lighter or more shallow.
   - Sleep is experienced as being interrupted (more awakenings).
   - Sleeper may wake earlier (without a phase advance).
   - Sleep is experienced as being less restorative.
   - Sleep duration may be shorter than when younger.
   - Dream content may be distressing.

- Sleeper may nap.
- Sleeper may snore.
- Prevalence of restless legs syndrome (Willis-Ekbom disease) with/without periodic limb movements increases with age.

2. Sleep disorders that either are only manifested during REM sleep or are more prominent during that sleep phase include:
   - Narcolepsy with cataplexy
   - Narcolepsy without cataplexy
   - REM sleep behaviour disorder
   - Obstructive sleep apnea
   - Nightmare disorder

3. The fundamentals of good sleep hygiene include:
   - Use the bed only for sleep and intimacy.
   - No visible time cues – always use an alarm.
   - If you cannot sleep, get out of bed and read or do other relaxing activity before attempting to sleep again.
   - Go to bed and get up at the same time every day; refrain from napping especially after 15:00 hours.
   - Have a comfortable bed in a cool, well-ventilated, sound-attenuated room that can be kept dark at all times of the year.
   - Develop a sleep routine: prepare for sleep with 20–30 minutes of relaxation (e.g., soft music, meditation, breathing exercises, yoga); take a warm bath; have a light snack of predominantly carbohydrates.
   - Avoid stimulating activities two hours before bedtime (including any screen-based activity).
   - If cognitive worries intrude at sleep onset or after awakening, distract and promote relaxation by focusing on regular breathing.
   - If unable to sleep within about 20 minutes (subjective sense; NOT clocked), get up and do something relaxing (non–screen based) until drowsy tired and then return to bed.

4. Regarding the medications on the listing:
   - Because of their abuse potential, long half-life (53 to 118 hours), rapid onset of tolerance, and safety, all barbiturates are contraindicated in managing sleep disorders.
   - Because of the rapid development of tolerance and low safety index, chloral hydrate is contraindicated in managing sleep disorders in any age group.
   - Flurazepam's major metabolite desalkyl-flurazepam has a very long half-life (47–100 hours), making it unsuitable for use in any age group due to accumulation, hangover effects, and risk of falling.
   - Nitrazepam also has a long half-life (mean half-life 26 hours) and is not indicated for managing sleep disturbances in any age group.
   - Triazolam is a high potency benzodiazepine with a very short half-life (1.5–5.5 hours), but in early recommended dosages (0.25–1 mg) was associated

with amnesia and unusual behavioural reactions. It is most effective in managing initial insomnia, and because of its short half-life it has been associated with increased daytime anxiety. There has been insufficient evaluation of it in the 0.125 mg dosage in the elderly to make a recommendation.

- Oxazepam is a low potency hypnotic with a relatively long time to Tmax that can be helpful in managing maintenance insomnia in the elderly. As for all hypnotics, the lowest dose should be used. It is used clinically but there are no adequate studies of the 10 mg dose in the elderly to direct usage, although clinical experience suggests it is useful.
- Lorazepam's half-life of 9–16 hours makes it less suitable as a sleep-promoting agent than shorter acting sedative-hypnotics but it is commonly used. As with all sleep-promoting medications, it should be started at the lowest dose (0.25 mg).
- Whether or not there are clinically significant differences between the Z drugs and the benzodiazepines is controversial, yet they are preferred to the traditional benzodiazepines because of a favourable side-effect profile, safety, and efficacy. The lowest effective dose of zopiclone (3.75 mg) in the elderly should be used; half of a 5 mg tablet (2.5 mg) has not been shown to be effective.
- Zolpidem: introduced to Canada initially as a sublingual 10 mg formulation, this dose is too high for most patients, especially the elderly. The 5 mg dosage may also be too high, and the short half-life (2–3 hours) means it may not be helpful in managing the more common maintenance insomnia associated with the sleep of the elderly.

5. Regarding REM sleep events and disorders:
   - Events in REM sleep include:
     – Dreaming
     – Rapid eye movements
     – Atonia of the antigravity/striated muscles
     – Erections/clitoral engorgement
     – Fluctuations in heart rate
     – Fluctuations in blood pressure (BP)
     – Changes in temperature regulation
   - Disorders that worsen or occur uniquely with REM sleep include:
     – Narcolepsy with cataplexy
     – Narcolepsy without cataplexy
     – REM sleep behaviour disorder
     – Obstructive sleep apnea
     – Nightmare disorder

6. Useful strategies for reducing sleep-promoting medication use in older patients include:
   - Review of history to ensure continued hypnotic use is not required.
   - Assess the patient's motivation to change; if low, suggest readings/websites (e.g., National Sleep Foundation) and monitor.
   - Institute good sleep hygiene practices prior to any attempt.
   - Simply recommend stopping.
   - Provide psychoeducation including bibliotherapy.

- Modify dosage (reduction).
  - Alternate night use
  - Specific night use (e.g., high stress nights [Sunday] or high fatigue days [mid-week])
  - Personal choice (2 pills a week for prn use)
- Institute tapering protocols including single blind dosage taper.
- Use cognitive behavioural therapy in person or web-based (e.g., sleepio.com, CBTforinsomnia.com).
- Institute sleep restriction (limiting time in bed to the average total sleep time from actigraphy somnologs or sleep diaries).
- Consider sedative hypnotic use replacement with pharmaceutical grade melatonin (3 mg or less).

CASE DISCUSSION

This is a partial arousal from sleep – a parasomnia. Unlike sleep walking or sleep terrors that usually first appear in childhood and adolescence, the presentation of this disorder is different as there is little confusion (Mr R. quickly assesses what has happened and acts appropriately), is not associated with previous parasomnias, and occurs in the last third of the night (sleep walking and sleep terrors most frequently emerge from deep or delta sleep that occurs in the first third of the night.)

Sleep walking and sleep terrors are NREM parasomnias, and usually the person has no recollection of the event, does not report narrative dreaming, and if awoken is confused and perplexed. They rarely occur in late life, especially in the absence of a childhood history. The presence of dream material and the timing suggests this might be a REM-associated parasomnia. Normally in REM sleep the only muscles working are the diaphragm, inner ear, and extraocular muscles, with the antigravity muscles being momentarily atonic during REM. Loss of REM atonia occurs with some drugs (e.g., antidepressants), idiopathically, and associated with the synucleinopathies (Parkinson's disease, dementia with Lewy bodies, etc.). This results in dream enactment, a key feature of REM sleep behaviour disorder. Mr R. did not form intent to harm his wife and pressing charges would be inappropriate, but psychoeducation and support is required. The disorder responds well to clonazepam in 0.25 to 2 mg dosages, and other medications can also be helpful (e.g., melatonin in high dosages). Nonetheless general safety measures are required, and co-sleeping is risky as there can be breakthrough events. The bedroom should be made safe around the bed (free from movable objects such as lamps, etc.), and as there is a risk of falling from the bed it should be lowered to prevent injury.

RECOMMENDED RESOURCES FOR REVIEW

Although these resources may not be specifically cited in the text, their approach informed the contents of the chapter, and they are recommended as useful further reading.

McMillan JM, Aitken E, Holroyd-Leduc JM. Management of insomnia and long-term use of sedative-hypnotic drugs in older patients. CMAJ. 2013;185(17):1499–505. http://dx.doi.org/10.1503/cmaj.130025. Medline:24062170

Wilson SJ, Nutt DJ, Alford C, et al. British Association for Psychopharmacology consensus statement on evidence-based treatment of insomnia, parasomnias and circadian rhythm disorders. J Psychopharmacol. 2010;24(11):1577–601. http://www.bap.org.uk/

pdfs/BAP_Sleep_Guidelines.pdf. http://dx.doi.org/10.1177/0269881110379307. Medline:20813762

Wolkove N, Elkholy O, Baltzan M, et al. Sleep and aging: 1. Sleep disorders commonly found in older people. CMAJ. 2007;176(9):1299–304. http://dx.doi.org/10.1503/cmaj.060792. Medline:17452665

– Sleep and aging: 2. Management of sleep disorders in older people. CMAJ. 2007;176(10):1449–54. http://dx.doi.org/10.1503/cmaj.070335. Medline:17485699

REFERENCES

Akintomide GS, Rickards H. Narcolepsy: a review. Neuropsychiatr Dis Treat. 2011;7:507–18. http://dx.doi.org/10.2147/NDT.S23624. Medline:21931493

Allen RE, Kirby KA. Nocturnal leg cramps. Am Fam Physician. 2012;86(4):350–5. Medline:22963024

Ancoli-Israel S, Kripke DF, Klauber MR, et al. Sleep-disordered breathing in community-dwelling elderly. Sleep. 1991;14(6):486–95. Medline:1798880

Anderson KN, Pilsworth S, Sharples LD, et al. Idiopathic hypersomnia: a study of 77 cases. Sleep. 2007;30(10):1274–81. Medline:17969461

Asano M, Ishitobi M, Tanaka Y, et al. Effects of ramelteon on refractory behavioral and psychological symptoms of dementia in Alzheimer disease. J Clin Psychopharmacol. 2013;33(4):579–81. http://dx.doi.org/10.1097/JCP.0b013e3182946702. Medline:23764686

Aurora RN, Chowdhuri S, Ramar K, et al. The treatment of central sleep apnea syndromes in adults: practice parameters with an evidence-based literature review and meta-analyses. Sleep. 2012;35(1):17–40. Medline:22215916

Aurora RN, Zak RS, Maganti RK, et al.; Standards of Practice Committee; American Academy of Sleep Medicine. Best practice guide for the treatment of REM sleep behavior disorder (RBD). J Clin Sleep Med. 2010;6(1):85–95. Medline:20191945

Babson KA, Boden MT, Harris AH, et al. Poor sleep quality as a risk factor for lapse following a cannabis quit attempt. J Subst Abuse Treat. 2013;44(4):438–43. http://dx.doi.org/10.1016/j.jsat.2012.08.224. Medline:23098380

Bajor LA, Ticlea AN, Osser DN. The Psychopharmacology Algorithm Project at the Harvard South Shore Program: an update on posttraumatic stress disorder. Harv Rev Psychiatry. 2011;19(5):240–58. http://dx.doi.org/10.3109/10673229.2011.614483. Medline:21916826

Baldwin DS, Aitchison K, Bateson A, et al. Benzodiazepines: risks and benefits. A reconsideration. J Psychopharmacol. 2013;27(11):967–71. http://dx.doi.org/10.1177/0269881113503509. Medline:24067791

Benedek DM, Friedman MJ, Zatzick D, et al. Guideline watch (March 2009): practice guideline for the treatment of patients with acute stress disorder and posttraumatic stress disorder. Arlington, VA: American Psychiatric Association; 2009. doi:10.1176/appi.books.9780890423479.156498 http://psychiatryonline.org/guidelines

Bloch F, Thibaud M, Dugué B, et al. Psychotropic drugs and falls in the elderly people: updated literature review and meta-analysis. J Aging Health. 2011;23(2):329–46. http://dx.doi.org/10.1177/0898264310381277. Medline:20947876

Bodkin CL, Manchanda S. Office evaluation of the "tired" or "sleepy" patient. Semin Neurol. 2011;31(1):42–53. http://dx.doi.org/10.1055/s-0031-1271311. Medline:21321832

Borja NL, Daniel KL. Ramelteon for the treatment of insomnia. Clin Ther. 2006;28(10):1540–55. http://dx.doi.org/10.1016/j.clinthera.2006.10.016. Medline:17157111

Brassington GS, King AC, Bliwise DL. Sleep problems as a risk factor for falls in a sample of community-dwelling adults aged 64-99 years. J Am Geriatr Soc. 2000;48(10):1234–40. http://dx.doi.org/10.1111/j.1532-5415.2000.tb02596.x. Medline:11037010

Broughton WA, Broughton RJ. Psychosocial impact of narcolepsy. Sleep. 1994;17(8 Suppl):S45–9. Medline:7701199

Brower KJ, Aldrich MS, Robinson EA, et al. Insomnia, self-medication, and relapse to alcoholism. Am J Psychiatry. 2001;158(3):399–404. http://dx.doi.org/10.1176/appi.ajp.158.3.399. Medline:11229980

Buysse DJ, Angst J, Gamma A, et al. Prevalence, course, and comorbidity of insomnia and depression in young adults. Sleep. 2008;31(4):473–80. Medline:18457234

Carrier J, Monk TH, Buysse DJ, et al. Sleep and morningness-eveningness in the 'middle' years of life (20-59 y). J Sleep Res. 1997;6(4):230–7. http://dx.doi.org/10.1111/j.1365-2869.1997.00230.x. Medline:9493522

Casey KR, Cantillo KO, Brown LK. Sleep-related hypoventilation/hypoxemic syndromes. Chest. 2007;131(6):1936–48. http://dx.doi.org/10.1378/chest.06-2334. Medline:17565028

Celle S, Roche F, Kerleroux J, et al. Prevalence and clinical correlates of restless legs syndrome in an elderly French population: the synapse study. J Gerontol A Biol Sci Med Sci. 2010;65A(2):167–73. http://dx.doi.org/10.1093/gerona/glp161. Medline:19914971

Chakravorty SS, Rye DB. Narcolepsy in the older adult: epidemiology, diagnosis and management. Drugs Aging. 2003;20(5):361–76. http://dx.doi.org/10.2165/00002512-200320050-00005. Medline:12696996

Chang WP, Liu ME, Chang WC, et al. Sleep apnea and the risk of dementia: a population-based 5-year follow-up study in Taiwan. PLoS One. 2013;8(10):e78655. http://dx.doi.org/10.1371/journal.pone.0078655. Medline:24205289

Claman DM, Ewing SK, Redline S, et al.; Study of Osteoporotic Fractures Research Group. Periodic leg movements are associated with reduced sleep quality in older men: the MrOS sleep study. J Clin Sleep Med. 2013;9(11):1109–17. Medline:24235891

Coelho GA, Rodrigues E, Andersen ML, et al. Psychotherapy improved the sleep quality in a patient who was a victim of child sexual abuse: a case report. J Sex Med. 2013;10(12):3146–50. http://dx.doi.org/10.1111/jsm.12323. Medline:24119035

Comella CL. Treatment of restless legs syndrome. Neurotherapeutics. 2014;11(1):177–87. http://dx.doi.org/10.1007/s13311-013-0247-9. Medline:24363103

Cuellar NG. The effects of periodic limb movements in sleep (PLMS) on cardiovascular disease. Heart Lung. 2013;42(5):353–60. http://dx.doi.org/10.1016/j.hrtlng.2013.07.006. Medline:23998383

Dauvilliers Y, Arnulf I, Mignot E. Narcolepsy with cataplexy. Lancet. 2007;369(9560):499–511. Medline:17292770

Dauvilliers Y, Lopez R, Ohayon M, et al. Hypersomnia and depressive symptoms: methodological and clinical aspects. BMC Med. 2013;11(1):78. http://dx.doi.org/10.1186/1741-7015-11-78. Medline:23514569

Dauvilliers Y, Winkelmann J. Restless legs syndrome: update on pathogenesis. Curr Opin Pulm Med. 2013;19(6):594–600. http://dx.doi.org/10.1097/MCP.0b013e328365ab07. Medline:24048084

De la Herrán-Arita AK, García-García F. Current and emerging options for the drug treatment of narcolepsy. Drugs. 2013;73(16):1771–81. http://dx.doi.org/10.1007/s40265-013-0127-y. Medline:24122734

DelRosso LM, Chesson AL Jr, Hoque R. Characterization of REM sleep without atonia in patients with narcolepsy and idiopathic hypersomnia using AASM scoring manual criteria. J Clin Sleep Med. 2013;9(7):675–80. Medline:23853561

Dowling GA, Burr RL, Van Someren EJW, et al. Melatonin and bright-light treatment for rest-activity disruption in institutionalized patients with Alzheimer's disease. J Am Geriatr Soc. 2008;56(2):239–46. http://dx.doi.org/10.1111/j.1532-5415.2007.01543.x. Medline:18070004

Fleming J. Dissociative episodes presenting as somnambulism: a case report. Sleep Res. 1987;16: 263.

Frauscher B, Gschliesser V, Brandauer E, et al. The severity range of restless legs syndrome (RLS) and augmentation in a prospective patient cohort: association with ferritin levels. Sleep Med. 2009;10(6):611–5. http://dx.doi.org/10.1016/j.sleep.2008.09.007. Medline:19200780

Fulda S, Szesny N, Ising M, et al. Further evidence for executive dysfunction in subjects with RLS from a non-clinical sample. Sleep Med. 2011;12(10):1003–7. http://dx.doi.org/10.1016/j.sleep.2011.04.013. Medline:22000419

Germain A, Nielsen T. Impact of imagery rehearsal treatment on distressing dreams, psychological distress, and sleep parameters in nightmare patients. Behav Sleep Med. 2003;1(3):140–54. http://dx.doi.org/10.1207/S15402010BSM0103_2. Medline:15600218

Glidewell RN. Comorbid insomnia and sleep disordered breathing. Curr Treat Options Neurol. 2013;15(6):692–703. http://dx.doi.org/10.1007/s11940-013-0259-0. Medline:24155146

Gunja N. In the Zzz zone: the effects of Z-drugs on human performance and driving. J Med Toxicol. 2013;9(2):163–71. http://dx.doi.org/10.1007/s13181-013-0294-y. Medline:23456542

Gupta R, Lahan V, Goel D. Restless legs syndrome: a common disorder, but rarely diagnosed and barely treated–an Indian experience. Sleep Med. 2012;13(7):838–41. http://dx.doi.org/10.1016/j.sleep.2012.03.018. Medline:22704403

– A study examining depression in restless legs syndrome. Asian J Psychiatr. 2013;6(4):308–12. http://dx.doi.org/10.1016/j.ajp.2013.01.011. Medline:23810138

Hoque R, Chesson AL Jr. Zolpidem-induced sleepwalking, sleep related eating disorder, and sleep-driving: fluorine-18-flourodeoxyglucose positron emission tomography analysis, and a literature review of other unexpected clinical effects of zolpidem. J Clin Sleep Med. 2009;5(5):471–6. Medline:19961034

Hornyak M, Kopasz M, Berger M, et al. Impact of sleep-related complaints on depressive symptoms in patients with restless legs syndrome. J Clin Psychiatry. 2005;66(9):1139–45. http://dx.doi.org/10.4088/JCP.v66n0909. Medline:16187772

Inocente CO, Lavault S, Lecendreux M, et al. Impact of obesity in children with narcolepsy. CNS Neurosci Ther. 2013;19(7):521–8. http://dx.doi.org/10.1111/cns.12105. Medline:23574649

Jaussent I, Dauvilliers Y, Ancelin M-L, et al. Insomnia symptoms in older adults: associated factors and gender differences. Am J Geriatr Psychiatry. 2011;19(1):88–97. http://dx.doi.org/10.1097/JGP.0b013e3181e049b6. Medline:20808113

Kalra MA, Hart LL. Gammahydroxybutyrate in narcolepsy. Ann Pharmacother. 1992;26(5):647–8. PMID:1591425

Kang SH, Yoon IY, Lee SD, et al. REM sleep behavior disorder in the Korean elderly population: prevalence and clinical characteristics. Sleep. 2013;36(8):1147–52. Medline:23904674

Kierlin L, Littner MR. Parasomnias and antidepressant therapy: a review of the literature. Front Psychiatry. 2011;2:71. http://dx.doi.org/10.3389/fpsyt.2011.00071. Medline:22180745

Kunz D, Bineau S, Maman K, et al. Benzodiazepine discontinuation with prolonged-release melatonin: hints from a German longitudinal prescription database. Expert Opin Pharmacother. 2012;13(1):9–16. http://dx.doi.org/10.1517/14656566.2012.638284. Medline:22107732

Lammers M, Ahmed AI. Melatonin for sundown syndrome and delirium in dementia: is it effective? J Am Geriatr Soc. 2013;61(6):1045–6. http://dx.doi.org/10.1111/jgs.12296. Medline:23772740

Lavigne F, Petrof BJ, Johnson JR, et al. Effect of topical corticosteroids on allergic airway inflammation and disease severity in obstructive sleep apnoea. Clin Exp Allergy. 2013;43(10):1124–33. Medline:24074330

Li J, Hu Z, de Lecea L. The hypocretins/orexins: integrators of multiple physiological functions. Br J Pharmacol. 2014;171(2):332–50. http://dx.doi.org/10.1111/bph.12415. Medline:24102345

Lichstein KL, Nau SD, Wilson NM, et al. Psychological treatment of hypnotic-dependent insomnia in a primarily older adult sample. Behav Res Ther. 2013;51(12):787–96. http://dx.doi.org/10.1016/j.brat.2013.09.006. Medline:24121096

Malhotra A, Owens RL. What is central sleep apnea? Respir Care. 2010;55(9):1168–78. Medline:20799999

Martin JL, Hakim AD. Wrist actigraphy. Chest. 2011;139(6):1514–27. http://dx.doi.org/10.1378/chest.10-1872. Medline:21652563

Meng L, Zheng Y, Hui R. The relationship of sleep duration and insomnia to risk of hypertension incidence: a meta-analysis of prospective cohort studies. Hypertens Res. 2013;36(11):985–95. http://dx.doi.org/10.1038/hr.2013.70. Medline:24005775

Mirza M, Shen WK, Sofi A, et al. Frequent periodic leg movement during sleep is an unrecognized risk factor for progression of atrial fibrillation. PLoS One. 2013;8(10):e78359. http://dx.doi.org/10.1371/journal.pone.0078359. Medline:24147132

Mishima K, Tozawa T, Satoh K, et al. Melatonin secretion rhythm disorders in patients with senile dementia of Alzheimer's type with disturbed sleep-waking. Biol Psychiatry. 1999;45(4):417–21. http://dx.doi.org/10.1016/S0006-3223(97)00510-6. Medline:10071710

Mitler MM, Browman CP, Menn SJ, et al. Nocturnal myoclonus: treatment efficacy of clonazepam and temazepam. Sleep. 1986;9(3):385–92. Medline:2876485

Monk TH. Aging human circadian rhythms: conventional wisdom may not always be right. J Biol Rhythms. 2005;20(4):366–74. http://dx.doi.org/10.1177/0748730405277378. Medline:16077155

Moraes W, Poyares D, Sukys-Claudino L, et al. Donepezil improves obstructive sleep apnea in Alzheimer disease: a double-blind, placebo-controlled study. Chest. 2008;133(3):677–83. http://dx.doi.org/10.1378/chest.07-1446. Medline:18198262

Morin CM, Bélanger L, LeBlanc M, et al. The natural history of insomnia: a population-based 3-year longitudinal study. Arch Intern Med. 2009;169(5):447–53. http://dx.doi.org/10.1001/archinternmed.2008.610. Medline:19273774

Morin CM, Colecchi C, Stone J, et al. Behavioral and pharmacological therapies for late-life insomnia: a randomized controlled trial. JAMA. 1999;281(11):991–9. http://dx.doi.org/10.1001/jama.281.11.991. Medline:10086433

Myers KA, Mrkobrada M, Simel DL. Does this patient have obstructive sleep apnea? The Rational Clinical Examination systematic review. JAMA. 2013;310(7):731–41. http://dx.doi.org/10.1001/jama.2013.276185. Medline:23989984

Ngiam J, Balasubramaniam R, Darendeliler MA, et al. Clinical guidelines for oral appliance therapy in the treatment of snoring and obstructive sleep apnoea. Aust Dent J. 2013;58(4):408–19. http://dx.doi.org/10.1111/adj.12111. Medline:24320895

Ohayon MM, Carskadon MA, Guilleminault C, et al. Meta-analysis of quantitative sleep parameters from childhood to old age in healthy individuals: developing normative sleep values across the human lifespan. Sleep. 2004;27(7):1255–73. Medline:15586779

Ohayon MM, Dauvilliers Y, Reynolds CF III. Operational definitions and algorithms for excessive sleepiness in the general population: implications for DSM-5 nosology. Arch Gen Psychiatry. 2012;69(1):71–9. http://dx.doi.org/10.1001/archgenpsychiatry.2011.1240. Medline:22213791

Ohayon MM, Ferini-Strambi L, Plazzi G, et al. How age influences the expression of narcolepsy. J Psychosom Res. 2005;59(6):399–405. http://dx.doi.org/10.1016/j.jpsychores.2005.06.065. Medline:16310022

Olde Rikkert MG, Rigaud AS. Melatonin in elderly patients with insomnia – a systematic review. Z Gerontol Geriatr. 2001;34(6):491–7. http://dx.doi.org/10.1007/s003910170025. Medline:11828891

Pearson VE, Allen RP, Dean T, et al. Cognitive deficits associated with restless legs syndrome (RLS). Sleep Med. 2006;7(1):25–30. http://dx.doi.org/10.1016/j.sleep.2005.05.006. Medline:16198145

Perez-Lloret S, Rey MV, Bondon-Guitton E, et al.; French Association of Regional Pharmacovigilance Centers. Drugs associated with restless legs syndrome: a case/noncase study in the French Pharmacovigilance Database. J Clin Psychopharmacol. 2012;32(6):824–7. http://dx.doi.org/10.1097/JCP.0b013e318272cdd8. Medline:23131889

Perlis M, Gehrman P, Riemann D. Intermittent and long-term use of sedative hypnotics. Curr Pharm Des. 2008;14(32):3456–65. http://dx.doi.org/10.2174/138161208786549290. Medline:19075721

Poryazova R, Oberholzer M, Baumann CR, et al. REM sleep behavior disorder in Parkinson's disease: a questionnaire-based survey. J Clin Sleep Med. 2013;9(1):55–9A. Medline:23319905

Punjabi NM. The epidemiology of adult obstructive sleep apnea. Proc Am Thorac Soc. 2008;5(2):136–43. http://dx.doi.org/10.1513/pats.200709-155MG. Medline:18250205

Raskind MA, Peterson K, Williams T, et al. A trial of prazosin for combat trauma PTSD with nightmares in active-duty soldiers returned from Iraq and Afghanistan. Am J Psychiatry. 2013;170(9):1003–10. http://dx.doi.org/10.1176/appi.ajp.2013.12081133. Medline:23846759

Reid KJ, Zee PC. Circadian disorders of the sleep-wake cycle. In: Kryger MH, Roth T, Dement WC, editors. Principles and practice of sleep medicine. 5th ed. St. Louis, MO: Elsevier Saunders; 2011. p. 470–482. http://dx.doi.org/10.1016/B978-1-4160-6645-3.00041-4

Rickels K. Should benzodiazepines be replaced by antidepressants in the treatment of anxiety disorders? Fact or fiction? Psychother Psychosom. 2013;82(6):351–2. http://dx.doi.org/10.1159/000353502. Medline:24061092

Robinson DM, Keating GM. Sodium oxybate: a review of its use in the management of narcolepsy. CNS Drugs. 2007;21(4):337–54. http://dx.doi.org/10.2165/00023210-200721040-00007. Medline:17381187

Roszkowska J, Geraci SA. Management of insomnia in the geriatric patient. Am J Med. 2010;123(12):1087–90. http://dx.doi.org/10.1016/j.amjmed.2010.04.006. Medline:20870196

Roth T, Dauvilliers Y, Mignot E, et al. Disrupted nighttime sleep in narcolepsy. J Clin Sleep Med. 2013;9(9):955–65. Medline:23997709

Roth T, Jaeger S, Jin R, et al. Sleep problems, comorbid mental disorders, and role functioning in the national comorbidity survey replication. Biol Psychiatry. 2006;60(12):1364–71. http://dx.doi.org/10.1016/j.biopsych.2006.05.039. Medline:16952333

Sack RL, Auckley D, Auger RR, et al.; American Academy of Sleep Medicine. Circadian rhythm sleep disorders: part II, advanced sleep phase disorder, delayed sleep phase disorder, free-running disorder, and irregular sleep-wake rhythm. An American Academy of Sleep Medicine review. Sleep. 2007;30(11):1484–501. Medline:18041481

Salvio MA, Wood JM, Schwartz J, et al. Nightmare prevalence in the healthy elderly. Psychol Aging. 1992;7(2):324–5. http://dx.doi.org/10.1037/0882-7974.7.2.324. Medline:1610522

Sasayama S, Izumi T, Seino Y, et al.; The CHF-HOT Study Group. Effects of nocturnal oxygen therapy on outcome measures in patients with chronic heart failure and Cheyne-Stokes respiration. Circ J. 2006;70(1):1–7. http://dx.doi.org/10.1253/circj.70.1. Medline:16377916

Scheltens P, Visscher F, Van Keimpema AR, et al. Sleep apnea syndrome presenting with cognitive impairment. Neurology. 1991;41(1):155–6. http://dx.doi.org/10.1212/WNL.41.1.155. PMID:1985284

Schenck CH, Boyd JL, Mahowald MW. A parasomnia overlap disorder involving sleepwalking, sleep terrors, and REM sleep behavior disorder in 33 polysomnographically confirmed cases. Sleep. 1997;20(11):972–81. Medline:9456462

Schenck CH, Bundlie SR, Patterson AL, et al. Rapid eye movement sleep behavior disorder. A treatable parasomnia affecting older adults. JAMA. 1987;257(13):1786–9. http://dx.doi.org/10.1001/jama.1987.03390130104038. Medline:3820495

Schenck CH, Mahowald MW. Subclinical REM sleep behavior disorder and its clinical and research implications. Sleep. 2008;31(12):1627. Medline:19090317

Schulte EC, Gross N, Slawik H, et al. When restless legs syndrome turns malignant. Sleep Med. 2013;14(6):575–7. http://dx.doi.org/10.1016/j.sleep.2013.02.012. Medline:23643657

Schutte-Rodin S, Broch L, Buysse D, et al. Clinical guideline for the evaluation and management of chronic insomnia in adults. J Clin Sleep Med. 2008;4(5):487–504. Medline:18853708

Skapinakis P, Rai D, Anagnostopoulos F, et al. Sleep disturbances and depressive symptoms: an investigation of their longitudinal association in a representative sample of the UK general population. Psychol Med. 2013;43(2):329–39. http://dx.doi.org/10.1017/S0033291712001055. Medline:22640482

Sofi F, Cesari F, Casini A, et al. Insomnia and risk of cardiovascular disease: a meta-analysis. Eur J Prev Cardiol. 2014;21(1):57–64. http://dx.doi.org/10.1177/2047487312460020. Medline:22942213

Stiasny K, Wetter TC, Trenkwalder C, et al. Restless legs syndrome and its treatment by dopamine agonists. Parkinsonism Relat Disord. 2000;7(1):21–5. http://dx.doi.org/10.1016/S1353-8020(00)00041-9. Medline:11008192

Tol WA, Barbui C, van Ommeren M. Management of acute stress, PTSD, and bereavement: WHO recommendations. JAMA. 2013;310(5):477–8. http://dx.doi.org/10.1001/jama.2013.166723. Medline:23925613

Trotti LM. REM sleep behaviour disorder in older individuals: epidemiology, pathophysiology and management. Drugs Aging. 2010;27(6):457–70. http://dx.doi.org/10.2165/11536260-000000000-00000. Medline:20524706

Tsunoda K, Uchida H, Suzuki T, et al. Effects of discontinuing benzodiazepine-derivative hypnotics on postural sway and cognitive functions in the elderly. Int J Geriatr Psychiatry. 2010;25(12):1259–65. http://dx.doi.org/10.1002/gps.2465. Medline:20054834

van der Kolk BA, Spinazzola J, Blaustein ME, et al. A randomized clinical trial of eye movement desensitization and reprocessing (EMDR), fluoxetine, and pill placebo in the treatment of posttraumatic stress disorder: treatment effects and long-term maintenance. J Clin Psychiatry. 2007;68(1):37–46. http://dx.doi.org/10.4088/JCP.v68n0105. Medline:17284128

Vernet C, Leu-Semenescu S, Buzare MA, et al. Subjective symptoms in idiopathic hypersomnia: beyond excessive sleepiness. J Sleep Res. 2010;19(4):525–34. http://dx.doi.org/10.1111/j.1365-2869.2010.00824.x. Medline:20408941

Vignatelli L, D'Alessandro R, Candelise L. Antidepressant drugs for narcolepsy. Cochrane Libr. 2006;4:1–11.

Wickwire EM, Lettieri CJ, Cairns AA, et al. Maximizing positive airway pressure adherence in adults: a common-sense approach. Chest. 2013;144(2):680–93. http://dx.doi.org/10.1378/chest.12-2681. Medline:23918114

Yaffe K, Laffan AM, Harrison SL, et al. Sleep-disordered breathing, hypoxia, and risk of mild cognitive impairment and dementia in older women. JAMA. 2011;306(6):613–9. http://dx.doi.org/10.1001/jama.2011.1115. Medline:21828324

Yeh P, Walters AS, Tsuang JW. Restless legs syndrome: a comprehensive overview on its epidemiology, risk factors, and treatment. Sleep Breath. 2012;16(4):987–1007. http://dx.doi.org/10.1007/s11325-011-0606-x. Medline:22038683

Zhang J, Lam SP, Li SX, et al. Restless legs symptoms in adolescents: epidemiology, heritability, and pubertal effects. J Psychosom Res. 2014;76(2):158–64. http://dx.doi.org/10.1016/j.jpsychores.2013.11.017. Medline:24439693

Zhou QP, Jung L, Richards KC. The management of sleep and circadian disturbance in patients with dementia. Curr Neurol Neurosci Rep. 2012;12(2):193–204. http://dx.doi.org/10.1007/s11910-012-0249-8. Medline:22314860

Zucconi M. Nocturnal frontal lobe epilepsy: a sleep disorder rather than an epileptic syndrome? Sleep Med. 2013;14(7):589–90. http://dx.doi.org/10.1016/j.sleep.2013.04.006. Medline:23746602

ADDITIONAL E-RESOURCES

American Sleep Apnea Association: http://sleepapnea.org/
Canadian Sleep Society: http://css-scs.ca/
Narcolepsy Network: http://narcolepsynetwork.org
National Sleep Foundation: https://sleepfoundation.org/
Restless Legs Syndrome Foundation (formerly Willis Ekbom Disease Foundation): http://rls.org/

3.4 Personality Disorders in Older Adults

Suzane Renaud, MD, CRCP(P), CSMQ, LDFAPA, FCPA-APC

INTRODUCTION

Personality disorders do not disappear in older adulthood, but rather remain significant sources of disability and comorbidity, particularly among clinical populations. Dr Renaud summarizes some of the changes in the way in which personality disorders present in older adulthood, and describes strategies for understanding and managing this disorder.

CASE SCENARIO

A 75-year-old woman is admitted to hospital with suicidal thoughts and complaints of severe depression. Upon admission, she is viewed to have a bright and reactive affect. She interacts actively and helpfully with co-patients and tends to idealize or devalue staff members. She threatens suicide if she is to be discharged, and would like to stay in hospital "until I feel better," which she estimates may take a year. The team is struggling to understand how much of her presentation may be related to a mood disorder.

What are some challenges in obtaining a proper personality disorder diagnosis in older adults?

OVERVIEW

1. Scientific Research Data on Personality Disorders in Older Adults

- Poorly documented topic with rare prospective studies on the evolution of personality traits and personality disorders in late life
- The current theoretical view suggests that personality evolves through developmental stages and is not just determined by biology. Thus inherited personality traits modulated by neurophysiological networks are also shaped by the social environment. Personality is constituted by the sum of previous experiences and the person's adaptation to them; this view is a more dynamic concept, as personality evolves and adapts to different contexts to which are added older age issues (Segal, Coolidge, & Rosowsky, 2006).
- General opinion is that personality disorders are stable during the adult stage and that some symptoms may decrease in older adults (DSM-IV).
- Yet personality disorders are known to show stable and extensive ongoing functional impairment in adults over 50 years (Abrams & Horowitz, 1999; Morey et al., 2007; Shiner, 2005; Weiss et al., 2009).

2. Alternatives to the DSM for Making Personality Disorder Diagnoses

2.1 Gerontological Personality Disorder Scale (GPS)

The GPS encompasses seventeen concepts of personality disorder, but is not linked to DSM criteria (van Alphen et al., 2006).

2.1.1 Habitual Behaviour

- Does not like growing older as less attractive
- Worries about health
- Concerned about memory
- Hopes others will solve problems
- Afraid of losing carers
- Feels being taken advantage of; difficult to fend for self

2.1.2 Biographical Information

- Vague physical complaints to doctor
- Expresses feeling no desire to live
- Admits having nerves
- Nerves, stress, and moodiness
- Psychiatric and psychological treatment in past
- Suicidal attempts
- Only one friend or acquaintance
- No interest in sexual contact
- Has taken tranquilizers and sleeping pills

2.2 Other Structured Interviews

- Hetero-Anamnestic Personality Questionnaire (Barendse et al., 2013)
- Hybrid Personality Disorder Scale (Balsis et al., 2007)

Also consider using:

- – Dimensional symptomatic criteria in DSM-5, section 3, chapter 3
- – Life narrative identity account story (McAdams & Olson, 2010)
- – Your own countertransference experience with patients who have a personality disorder (Betan et al., 2005; Gabbard, 1999; Malamud, 1996; Rosowsky, 1999; Rosowsky & Dougherty, 1998; Oltmanns & Balsis, 2011)

3. Potential Reasons for Poor Motivation and Low Interest among Clinicians in Studying Personality Disorder in Older Adults

- Fear that personality disorder is hard to treat, treatment resistant, and follows a chronic course
- Countertransferential reactions on the part of the medical team towards older people
- Psychiatrist's feelings about his or her own aging or that of his or her parents
- Dynamic response towards patients, with real behaviours provoking strong and non-neutral feelings, thoughts, and behaviours
- Family and institutions invested in the conflicts

Remember: intensity of conflict is proportional to psychological distress (Rosowsky, 1999; Rosowsky & Dougherty, 1998).

4. Treatment Objectives

Although at times not obvious, treatment objectives could include the following:
- Diminish suffering in patient/helpers/staff
- Improve understanding of personality disorder variable over other diagnoses (DSM-IV-TR, Axis I and III), its evolution and treatment
- Establish adequate personality disorder nosology in geriatric psychiatry

5. Evolution of Personality Disorder Traits with Age

In general:
- Obsessional-compulsive traits increase: older person becomes more obsessional, careful, and anxious.
- Schizoid and paranoid traits increase: older person becomes more eccentric and withdrawn.
- Borderline and antisocial personality disorders diminish: impulsive and aggressive traits decrease.
- Narcissistic personality disorder traits increase with loss of compensatory mechanisms.
- Passive-aggressive traits might increase.
- Passive-dependent personality disorder or traits could increase or diminish.

5.1 Study Findings

- Slight return of dramatic and anxious traits after 60 years (Reich, Nduaguba, & Yates, 1988)
- Impulsivity, novelty seeking exploration, and neuroticism decrease up to 70 years, and then increase slightly (Steunenberg et al., 2005).
- DSM-5 group B (borderline, antisocial, histrionic, and narcissistic) improved (impulsivity and interpersonal instability); groups A (paranoid, schizoid, and schizotypal) and C (avoidant, obsessional, and dependent) worsened (avoidance and rigidity) (Seivewright, Tyrer, & Johnson, 2002).
- Introversion, order, social conformity, and emotional stability augment with age, but hypochondriasis and suspiciousness may emerge (Solomon, 1981; van Alphen et al., 2006).
- Self-monitoring declines (seeking social feedback > personal feelings).
- Extraversion and conscientiousness protect against feelings of invalidity (Lautenschlager & Förstl, 2007).

6. Symptomatic and Behavioural Dimensions to Consider as a Potential Personality Disorder Presentation

- Psychiatric comorbidities such as cognitive decline
- Sedentariness/solitude, restricted over time or limited social circle
- Difficulty with new roles/identities
- Treatment refusal, non-compliance, or medication/alcohol abuse
- Dependency on medical staff
- Depressive withdrawal
- Increased narcissistic defenses

- Somatic preoccupations
- Interpersonal chaos

7. Personality Disorder Prevalence

- Personality disorder in general population: 2–17% (Samuels et al., 2002; Torgensen, 2005)
- Personality disorder in aging population: 6–13% (Ames & Molinari, 1994)
- Personality disorder in psychiatric outpatient clinic: 30–40% (Mezzich et al., 1987)
- Personality disorder in geriatric psychiatric outpatient clinic: 33–58% (Fogel & Westlake, 1990; Molinari & Marmion, 1993)
- Personality disorder in geriatric patients with depression: 26% (Zweig & Hinrichsen, 1992)
- Less antisocial and histrionic personality disorder
- In 1984, antisocial personality disorder incidence of 0.8% in > 65 years (Cohen et al., 1994)
- Personality disorder after 55 years in Epidemiological Catchment Area (ECA)/ Baltimore epidemiological catchment area study results (Pietrzak et al., 2007):
  - Bipolar disorder, generalized anxiety disorder more prominent if personality disorder present
  - Less alcohol intake and sexual disorders in older adults but more tobacco intake?
  - Rarer borderline and narcissistic personality disorder
  - There may be earlier mortality of patients with antisocial personality disorder or borderline personality disorder.

8. Medical Comorbidities

- Medical comorbidities, e.g., frequent obesity and diabetes in borderline personality disorder; people with this disorder also seek more healthcare (Frankenburg & Zanarini, 2006).
- Schizoid, avoidant, and obsessive-compulsive more prone to coronary heart disease (Pietrzak et al., 2007).

9. Adaptation Task Challenges in Older Adulthood

- Loss of stabilizing factors: functional, occupational, parental, and social roles; objects, accomplishments, autonomy, and liberty; but also failures of these:
  - Incongruity between self-perception and exterior self-image
  - Life in institutional communities forces intimacy and may provoke rage, primitive conflicts concerning dependency or anonymity, fear of abandonment and engulfment.

According to Sadavoy's 1996 psychodynamic model:

- Real or feared abandonment can provoke an intolerable anxiety in the context of solitude and aloneness.
- Interpersonal relationship failures may have pruned social support; less meaningful relations (see also Balsis et al., 2007).
- Increased marital aggression (O'Leary & Woodin, 2005; Vickerman & Margolin, 2008)

- Narcissistic failures
- Increased intolerance for dysphoric affects
- Inefficient rage modulation with more splitting
- Vulnerability towards loss of self-cohesion with temporary loss of reality evaluation and self-limitations
- Restriction of sexual or drug acting out to manage anxiety.
- Rigidity makes any required adaptation more difficult.

10. Potential Personality Disorder Complications

- Premature institutionalization
- Aggravation of physical illness, higher morbidity, and mortality in older patients with personality disorder; higher incidence of cardiovascular accidents
- Pathological grief
- Brief psychosis (vulnerability to losses of self-cohesion with temporary incapacity to evaluate reality and self-limitations)
- Cognition: cognitive-perceptual dysfunctions can be confused with aging; frontal lobe changes can present as disinhibition, impulsivity, affective lability, asocial behaviour, unpredictable rages.
- Biological deterioration can worsen or improve some personality traits.
- Intellectual deterioration linked to poor adaptation (Reichard, Livson, & Peterson, 1962)
- More vulnerability to end-of-life stresses
- Poorer perception of life quality and self-esteem, physical and cognitive functioning, autonomy in daily activities (Condello et al., 2003)
- Major depression and dysthymia in older patients, worse with personality disorder: personality disorder comorbidity associated with earlier age of onset and chronic depression, greater severity of dysthymic depression. Both personality disorder and depression have cumulative adverse effects (re longer course and less responsive to treatment) (Abrams et al., 1994; Camus et al., 1997; Devanand et al., 2000; Vine & Steingart, 1994; Weiss et al., 2009; Zweig & Hinrichsen, 1992)
- Hospital admission more likely (Rao, 2003)
- More hypochondria? (Agronin et Maletta, 2000)
- White matter hyperdensities? (Devanand et al., 2000)

11. Suicidal Risk in Older Adults with Personality Disorder

- More suicides without mental illness (Harwood et al., 2006)
- Increased suicidal risk in elderly can present with:
  - Previous self-injury, presence of suicidal ideation, mood disorders, and other psychopathology
  - Physical illness and physical impairment
  - Personality disorder traits including rigidity, emotional instability
  - Narcissistic personality or traits (Heisel et al., 2007)
  - Stressors, psychosocial problems, difficulty adjusting to life transition
  - Lack of family connectedness (Purcell et al., 2012)

12. Issues Particular to Personality Disorder Types

12.1 Narcissistic Personality Disorder

Narcissistic personality disorder can be exacerbated by:
- Decline in physical beauty, energy and capacities, professional achievements, loss of sources of narcissism and external admiration (Sadavoy, 1996)
- Humiliation and shame towards dependency on others
- Higher suicidal risk (Heisel et al., 2007)

Institutional strategies for narcissistic personality disorder:
- Identify most painful losses
- Understand previous dynamics
- Find social or personal validating experiences

12.2 Histrionic Personality Disorder

- This type of patient will try to charm and amuse, has a strong drive to seek attention, presents with affective instability and evasive cognitive style.
- Wants to have a relationship, responds to warmth and support, can drain resources when physically ill or seeking more attention (Schlesinger & Silk, 2005).

Institutional strategies for histrionic personality disorder:
- Identify precipitating factors
- Plan how to contain emotional explosions
- Find a role congruent with attention seeking

12.3 Borderline Personality Disorder

Some clinical presentations:
- Sense of void (resignation, disinterest, and drained feeling)
- Identity disorder (life choice regrets)
- Unstable interpersonal relations (frequent phone calls, despair messages, suicidal innuendos)
- Marked intolerance for dysphoric affects
- Inefficient rage modulation with more splitting
- Inappropriate anger (towards a caretaker or family; physical or verbal agitation)
- Restriction of sex or drug abuse to modulate anxiety can transform itself into somatization or hypochondria (Canuto, 2002)
- Impulsivity expressed in medication or alcohol abuse, chaotic help seeking, abrupt termination of help or medical care, hospital discharge against medical advice, refusal to respect health needs
- Suicidal threats without serious acting out or pseudo attempts, manipulative threats
- Suicidal anorexia

Institutional strategies for borderline or antisocial personality disorder:
- Consequences for unacceptable behaviour
- Analyse the context
- Find consensus/compromises
- But make judicial complaints if necessary

12.4 Other "Malignant" Personality Disorder Issues
(Sadavoy, 1996)

Possible clinical presentations:
- Unending demands, underlying rage, and fear of reprisal from the other
- Primitive defenses
- Stressed families with stronger children who got away and weaker ones caught up in emotionally intense demands as parent becomes emotionally and physically frail or cognitively disabled
- Rigid and inflexible stance
- Malignant interpersonal system that can be acted upon in dangerous ways

12.5 Institutional Strategies for Personality Disorder Group A

Possible clinical presentations:
- Need to create and maintain links in response to new dependency is threatening: avoids care
- Need for sustained caution and vigilance towards caretakers is draining for the paranoid: help or threat?

Institutional strategies:
- Limit number of contacts to what is essential; preserve intimacy
- Collaborative treatment for paranoid personality disorder

13. Older Personality Disorder Patients in an Institutional Context

Faced with the capacity of older personality disorder patients to create institutional chaos, ask the following questions:
- Where does the problem or ill feeling come from? Does it have to do with a specific task or systemic role, or is it connected to interpersonal relations, perhaps somebody from the staff?
- Has one changed variable (affect, cognition, behaviour) affected the whole presentation and other variables?
- How does the patient feel about being in an institution (Rosowsky, 2000)?

Consider:
- Patient wants his or her needs met
- Staff wants routine maintained
- Psychiatrist wants retroaction showing distress reduction and health promotion

Intervention techniques:
- Improve one variable (affect, cognition, behaviour) to change the whole presentation
- Facilitate verbalization
- Cognitive restructuring
- Behavioural technique or role modelling

QUESTIONS

1. List four developmental tasks of older adulthood.
2. List three countertransferential traps that can happen with patients who have borderline personality disorder which are particularly concerning in the frail elderly.

ANSWERS

1. Developmental tasks related to aging include:
   - Dealing with loss and grief in older age
   - Adjustment to physical decline (strength/health)
   - Adjustment to retirement/lower income
   - Adjustment to spouse's autonomy decline
   - Adjustment to new social roles, pruning of social network
   - Establishing links with peers
   - Securing appropriate living arrangements

2. Countertransferential traps with borderline personality disorder include:
   - Feeling coerced to feed, contain, and reassure
   - Smothering, pseudo-helping pulsion
   - Worn-out helper, no limits set
   - Idealization → devaluation, sense of abandonment cycle:
     – Escalation → withdrawal of the helping person
     – Improvement → withdrawal or abandonment → self-destructive escalation
   - Interpretations/hostile exchanges

CASE DISCUSSION

Some challenges in making a personality disorder diagnosis in older adults include the following:

- Challenge of obtaining a longitudinal and adequate history (over 6–9 decades) with or without collateral informant. Diagnostic interview is usually circumscribed over the last 5–10 years of life. Multiple factors to consider in history taking over 50–60 years/ hard to collect data: early development, previous psychopathology, comorbid physical illness, intimate interpersonal relations, anterior functioning, psychodynamic formulation
- Diagnostic methods and criteria poorly adapted to older age: psychopathology influences or in sync with older age? (Abrams & Bromberg, 2006)
- Personality disorder type can be mitigated with older age issues. For example: schizoid personality disorder DSM-IV criteria specify solitary activities choice, only one close or confident friend, no sexual interest in partner; but these symptoms can be experienced by many older persons.
- Attenuated presentations? With aging, many criteria are less obvious: neurological maturation and social experience might have attenuated the obvious symptomatic presentations of youthful prototypical personality disorder and behavioural acting out. Criteria do not take into account biopsychosocial changes related to older age, as prototypes are set for a young person (Kroessler, 1990, Balsis et al., 2007).

RECOMMENDED RESOURCES FOR REVIEW

Although these resources may not be specifically cited in the text, their approach informed the contents of the chapter, and they are recommended as useful further reading.

Abrams RC, Bromberg CE. Personality disorders in the elderly: a flagging field of inquiry. Int J Geriatr Psychiatry. 2006;21(11):1013–7. http://dx.doi.org/10.1002/gps.1614. Medline:17061248

Agronin ME, Maletta G. Personality disorders in late life. Understanding and overcoming the gap in research. Am J Geriatr Psychiatry. 2000;8(1):4–18. http://dx.doi.org/10.1097/00019442-200002000-00002. Medline:10648290

Oltmanns TF, Balsis S. Personality disorders in later life: questions about the measurement, course, and impact of disorders. Annu Rev Clin Psychol. 2011;7(1):321–49. http://dx.doi.org/10.1146/annurev-clinpsy-090310-120435. Medline:21219195

REFERENCES

Abrams RC, Horowitz SV. Personality disorders after age 50; a meta-analytic review of the literature. In: Rosowsky E, Abrams RC, Zweig R, editors. Personality disorders in older adults: emerging issues in diagnosis and treatment. Mahwah, NJ: Lawrence Erlbaum Associates; 1999. p. 55–68.

Abrams RC, Rosendahl E, Card C, et al. Personality disorder correlates of late and early onset depression. J Am Geriatr Soc. 1994;42(7):727–31. http://dx.doi.org/10.1111/j.1532-5415.1994.tb06532.x. Medline:8014347

Ames A, Molinari V. Prevalence of personality disorders in community-living elderly. J Geriatr Psychiatry Neurol. 1994;7(3):189–94. http://dx.doi.org/10.1177/089198879400700311. Medline:7916944

Balsis S, Woods CM, Gleason MEJ, et al. Overdiagnosis and underdiagnosis of personality disorders in older adults. Am J Geriatr Psychiatry. 2007;15(9):742–53. http://dx.doi.org/10.1097/JGP.0b013e31813c6b4e. Medline:17804828

Barendse HPJ, Thissen AJC, Rossi G, et al. Psychometric properties of an informant personality questionnaire (the HAP) in a sample of older adults in the Netherlands and Belgium. Aging Ment Health. 2013;17(5):623–9. http://dx.doi.org/10.1080/13607863.2012.756458. Medline:23323723

Betan E, Heim AK, Zittel Conklin C, et al. Countertransference phenomena and personality pathology in clinical practice: an empirical investigation. Am J Psychiatry. 2005;162(5):890–8. http://dx.doi.org/10.1176/appi.ajp.162.5.890. Medline:15863790

Camus V, de Mendonça Lima CA, Gaillard M, et al. Are personality disorders more frequent in early onset geriatric depression? J Affect Disord. 1997;46(3):297–302. http://dx.doi.org/10.1016/S0165-0327(97)00152-3. Medline:9547128

Canuto A. Personality disorders in the elderly: an entity to discover. Med Hyg (Geneve). 2002;60(2395):1161–3.

Cohen BJ, Nestadt G, Samuels JF, et al. Personality disorder in later life: a community study. Br J Psychiatry. 1994;165(4):493–9. http://dx.doi.org/10.1192/bjp.165.4.493. Medline:7804664

Condello C, Padoani W, Uguzzoni U, et al. Personality disorders and self-perceived quality of life in an elderly psychiatric outpatient population. Psychopathology. 2003;36(2):78–83. http://dx.doi.org/10.1159/000070362. Medline:12766317

Devanand DP, Turret N, Moody BJ, et al. Personality disorders in elderly patients with dysthymic disorder. Am J Geriatr Psychiatry. 2000;8(3):188–95. http://dx.doi.org/10.1097/00019442-200008000-00002. Medline:10910415

Fogel BS, Westlake R. Personality disorder diagnoses and age in inpatients with major depression. J Clin Psychiatry. 1990;51(6):232–5. Medline:2347860

Frankenburg FR, Zanarini MC. Personality disorders and medical comorbidity. CurrOpin Psychiatry. 2006;19(4):428–31. http://dx.doi.org/10.1097/01.yco.0000228766.33356.44. Medline:16721176

Gabbard GO, editor. Countertransference issues in psychiatric treatment. Review of Psychiatry Series; Oldham JM, Riba MB, series editors. Washington, DC: American Psychiatric Press; 1999.

Harwood DM, Hawton K, Hope T, et al. Life problems and physical illness as risk factors for suicide in older people: a descriptive and case-control study. Psychol Med. 2006;36(9):1265–74. http://dx.doi.org/10.1017/S0033291706007872. Medline:16734947

Heisel MJ, Links PS, Conn D, et al. Narcissistic personality and vulnerability to late-life suicidality. Am J Geriatr Psychiatry. 2007;15(9):734–41. http://dx.doi.org/10.1097/01.JGP.0000260853.63533.7d. Medline:17804827

Kroessler D. Personality disorder in the elderly. Hosp Community Psychiatry. 1990;41(12):1325–9. Medline:2276726

Lautenschlager NT, Förstl H. Personality change in old age. Curr Opin Psychiatry. 2007;20(1):62–6. http://dx.doi.org/10.1097/YCO.0b013e3280113d09. Medline:17143085

Malamud WI. Countertransference issues with elderly patients. J Geriatr Psychiatry. 1996;29:33–42.

McAdams DP, Olson BD. Personality development: continuity and change over the life course. Annu Rev Psychol. 2010;61(1):517–42. http://dx.doi.org/10.1146/annurev.psych.093008.100507. Medline:19534589

Mezzich JE, Fabrega H Jr, Coffman GA, et al. Comprehensively diagnosing geriatric patients. Compr Psychiatry. 1987;28(1):68–76. http://dx.doi.org/10.1016/0010-440X(87)90046-0. Medline:3802801

Molinari V, Marmion J. Personality disorders in geropsychiatric outpatients. Psychol Rep. 1993;73(1):256–8. http://dx.doi.org/10.2466/pr0.1993.73.1.256. Medline:8367565

Morey LC, Hopwood CJ, Gunderson JG, et al. Comparison of alternative models for personality disorders. Psychol Med. 2007;37(7):983–94. http://dx.doi.org/10.1017/S0033291706009482. Medline:17121690

O'Leary KD, Woodin EM. Partner aggression and problem drinking across the lifespan: how much do they decline? Clin Psychol Rev. 2005;25(7):877–94. http://dx.doi.org/10.1016/j.cpr.2005.03.004. Medline:15921837

Pietrzak RH, Morasco BJ, Blanco C, et al. Gambling level and psychiatric and medical disorders in older adults: results from the National Epidemiologic Survey on Alcohol and Related Conditions. Am J Geriatr Psychiatry. 2007;15(4):301–13. http://dx.doi.org/10.1097/01.JGP.0000239353.40880.cc. Medline:17095749

Purcell B, Heisel MJ, Speice J, et al. Family connectedness moderates the association between living alone and suicide ideation in a clinical sample of adults 50 years and older. Am J Geriatr Psychiatry. 2012;20(8):717–23. http://dx.doi.org/10.1097/JGP.0b013e31822ccd79. Medline:22048322

Rao R. Does personality disorder influence the likelihood of in-patient admission in late-life depression? Int J Geriatr Psychiatry. 2003;18(10):960–1. http://dx.doi.org/ 10.1002/gps.988. Medline:14533129

Reich J, Nduaguba M, Yates W. Age and sex distribution of DSM-III personality cluster traits in a community population. Compr Psychiatry. 1988;29(3):298–303. http://dx.doi.org/10.1016/0010-440X(88)90052-1. Medline:3378416

Reichard S, Livson F, Peterson PG. Aging and personality. New York: Wiley; 1962.

Rosowsky E. The patient-therapist relationship and the psychotherapy of the older adult with personality disorder. In: Rosowsky E, Abrams R, Zweig R, editors. Personality disorders in older adults: emerging issues in diagnosis and treatment. Mahwah, NJ, Lawrence Erlbaum Associates; 1999, p .153–74.

– Interventions for older adults with personality disorders. In: Molinari V., editor. Professional psychology in long term care. New York: Hatherleigh Press; 2000. p.161–77.

Rosowsky E, Dougherty LM. Personality disorders and clinician responses. Clin Gerontol. 1998;18(4):31–42. http://dx.doi.org/10.1300/J018v18n04_04.

Sadavoy J. Personality disorder in old age: symptom expression. Clin Gerontol. 1996;16(3):19–36. http://dx.doi.org/10.1300/J018v16n03_04

Samuels J, Eaton WW, Bienvenu OJ III, et al. Prevalence and correlates of personality disorders in a community sample. Br J Psychiatry. 2002;180(6):536–42. http://dx.doi.org/10.1192/bjp.180.6.536. Medline:12042233

Schlesinger A, Silk KR. Collaborative treatment. In: Oldham JM, Skodol AE, Bender DS, editors. The American Psychiatric Publishing textbook of personality disorders. Arlington, VA: American Psychiatric Publishing; 2005 . p. 431–446.

Segal D, Coolidge FL, Rosowsky E. Personality disorders and older adults: diagnosis, assessment, and treatment. Hoboken, NJ: John Wiley & Sons; 2006.

Seivewright H, Tyrer P, Johnson T. Change in personality status in neurotic disorders. Lancet. 2002;359(9325):2253–4. http://dx.doi.org/10.1016/S0140-6736(02)09266-8. Medline:12103293

Shiner RL. A developmental perspective on personality disorders: lessons from research on normal personality development in childhood and adolescence. J Pers Disord. 2005;19(2):202–10. http://dx.doi.org/10.1521/pedi.19.2.202.62630. Medline:15899716

Solomon K. Personality disorders in the elderly. In: Lion JR, editor. Personality disorders: diagnosis and management. 2nd ed. Baltimore: Williams and Wilkins; 1981. p. 310–38.

Steunenberg B, Twisk JW, Beekman AT, et al. Stability and change of neuroticism in aging. J Gerontol B Psychol Sci Soc Sci. 2005;60(1):27–33. http://dx.doi.org/10.1093/geronb/60.1.P27. Medline:15643035

Torgensen S. Epidemiology. In: Oldham JM, Skodol AE, Bender DS, editors. The American Psychiatric Publishing textbook of personality disorders. Arlington, VA: American Psychiatric Publishing; 2005. p. 129–41.

van Alphen SP, Engelen GJ. Reaction to 'personality disorder masquerading as dementia: a case of apparent Diogenes syndrome.' Int J Geriatr Psychiatry. 2005;20(2):189–90, author reply 190. http://dx.doi.org/10.1002/gps.1243. Medline:15696599 van Alphen SP, Engelen GJ, Kuin Y, et al. A preliminary study of the diagnostic accuracy of the Gerontological Personality disorders Scale (GPS). Int J Geriatr Psychiatry. 2006;21(9):862–8. http://dx.doi.org/10.1002/gps.1572. Medline:16955455

Vickerman KA, Margolin G. Trajectories of physical and emotional marital aggression in midlife couples. Violence Vict. 2008;23(1):18–34. http://dx.doi.org/10.1891/0886-6708.23.1.18. Medline:18396579

Vine RG, Steingart AB. Personality disorder in the elderly depressed. Can J Psychiatry. 1994;39(7):392–8. Medline:7987781

Weiss A, Sutin AR, Duberstein PR, et al. The personality domains and styles of the five-factor model are related to incident depression in Medicare recipients aged 65 to 100. Am J Geriatr Psychiatry. 2009;17(7):591–601. http://dx.doi.org/10.1097/JGP.0b013e31819d859d. Medline:19554673

Zweig R, Hinrichsen G. Impact of personality disorders on affective illness in older adults. Paper presented at the 45th Annual Scientific Meeting of the Gerontological Society of America, Washington, DC; 1992.

3.5 Neuropsychiatric Disorders in Older Adults

Mark Rapoport, MD, FRCPC

INTRODUCTION

There are numerous definitions of neuropsychiatry. Some geriatric psychiatrists contend that most of geriatric psychiatry is neuropsychiatry, given the evidence for neurobiological correlates of mental illness in later life. Cerebrovascular pathology is associated with late-onset mood disorders. Neuroimaging has highlighted structural and functional brain signatures of mood and psychotic disorders, and of behavioural disturbances in dementia. Alzheimer's disease itself is a quintessential neuropsychiatric disorder with clear-cut and well-known neuropathological substrates. For the purpose of this chapter, however, the focus is on psychiatric aspects of neurological disorders, which is the prevailing definition of the American Neuropsychiatric Association. Here, a modest three diagnoses are discussed. A general approach to the neurological patient with psychiatric symptoms is presented, followed by a discussion of mood and psychotic disorders in patients with stroke, brain injury, and Parkinson's disease. Discussion of cognitive impairment in neurological diseases is covered elsewhere in the book.

CASE SCENARIOS

Scenario 1. The wife of a 78-year-old man who sustained a mild traumatic brain injury (TBI) three months ago from a single motor vehicle crash tells you that he was perfectly well before the crash, but now has severe problems with his memory and needs a caregiver to help him with many basic activities of daily living (ADL). What is your approach to this issue?

Scenario 2. Consider a 75-year-old man with a history of hypertension and dyslipidemia who had a stroke about six months ago and presents to ER with florid manic symptoms. Describe your approach to determining whether or not the mania has anything to do with the stroke.

OVERVIEW

1. Neuropsychiatry Overview and Definitions

1.1 Psychiatric Manifestation of Neurological Disease

- The general definition of neuropsychiatry, as adapted by the American Neuropsychiatric Association: psychiatric care of adults with neurological disease; this overlaps significantly with behavioural or cognitive neurology
- Generally focal – stroke, tumour
- Generally diffuse – Parkinson's disease, multiple sclerosis, traumatic brain injury
- Behavioural neurology and neuropsychiatry is defined as "a medical specialty committed to better understanding links between neuroscience and behavior and to the care of individuals with neurologically based behavioral disturbances" (Silver, 2006).

1.2 Neurological Substrates of Psychiatric Illness

- Overlaps significantly with biological psychiatry (and not the focus of this chapter)
  - Major depression
  - Late-onset mania
  - Late-onset schizophrenia

1.3 Other Areas of Overlap

- Psychiatric precipitants and predictors of neurological events
  - Examples: stress and multiple sclerosis attacks, depression and stroke risk
- Dementia
  - Neurobiological changes associated with cognitive decline
  - Emotional and behavioural manifestations of cognitive decline
  - Neurological concomitants of the emotional and behavioural disturbances

1.4. Common Themes across Various Neuropsychiatric Conditions
(Lyketsos, Kozauer, & Rabins, 2007)

- Definable and recognizable groups of symptoms: mood, anxiety, cognitive, disinhibition, agitation, impulsivity and apathy
- Some consistent brain-behaviour links
- Little research, particularly on disease-specific therapy.

1.5 Three Dimensional Approach to Neuropsychiatric Assessments
(Marin, 2012)

Where is the lesion?
- Laterality – left/right
- Anteriority – front/back
- Verticality – cortical/subcortical

What are the brain-behaviour relationships in three dimensions?
- Laterality
    - Usually left – language, verbal memory
    - Usually right – nonverbal memory, praxis and gnosis
- Anteriority
    - Anterior
        - Personality (disinhibition, loss of empathy, stimulus bound)
        - Cognitive (dysexecutive, working memory, non-fluent aphasia if left, expressive aprosody if right)
        - Motivation (apathy, loss of initiative)
    - Posterior
        - Sparing of personality, executive cognition, and motivation
        - Fluent aphasia if left and receptive, aprosody if right
        - Visuospatial deficits, spatial disorientation, and hemineglect
- Verticality
    - Cortical
        - "Frontal" (i.e., anterior) behaviours and cognitive deficits
        - Aphasia, apraxia, agnosia, recall and retrieval deficit
        - Hemimotor or hemisensory symptoms
    - Subcortical
        - Executive deficits
        - Retrieval deficits
        - Slowing
        - Extrapyramidal symptoms

Understanding the frontal-subcortical paradox
- Patients with subcortical pathology often present with "frontal" symptoms as though they have anterior cortical pathology.
    - This is because of the parallel and distributed networks connecting the frontal lobes through the basal ganglia to the thalamus.

2. Neuropsychiatry of Stroke

2.1 Epidemiology

In Canada:
- Stroke is a leading cause of adult neurological disability with more than 50 000 strokes per year, and growing incidence, according to the Heart and Stroke Foundation.

In the United States:
- Prevalence of 2.8% in 2007–2010, with silent stroke 6–28%, affecting about 4 million (Go et al., 2014)

2.2 Post-Stroke Neuropsychiatric Disorders

Rough prevalence rates (Chemerinski & Robinson, 2000):
- Depression: 35%
- Anxiety: 25%
- Pathologic affect: 20%
- Catastrophic reaction: 20%

- Apathy: 20%
- Mania or psychosis: rare

- Delirium > 30%
- Dementia > 25%

2.3 Prevalence of Post-Stroke Depression (PSD)

- Prevalence in the literature ranges widely, from 20% to more than 65%.
- A recent meta-analysis showed a PSD prevalence of 33% (95% CI 29–36%) (Hackett et al., 2005).

2.3.1 Methodological Issues in Literature

- Depression measurement: self-administered scales vs structured interviews
- Population: prevalence in hospital 30–40% vs 10–20% in community samples
- Timing: rates higher in acute settings than rehab, which are higher than post-discharge months later

2.4 Post-Stroke Depression Risk Factors
(Starkstein & Manes, 2000)

- Severity of functional dependence
- Previous depression
- Social isolation

- Major events pre-stroke
- Female gender
- Previous stroke

2.5 Biological Mechanisms in Post-Stroke Depression

- Brain injury affects mood regulation
- Potential role for inflammation
- Depression after stroke > other illnesses
- Occurs even in "silent" stroke
- Lesion localization
  - Generally left > right, especially with proximity to frontal pole
  - Systematic review of 26 original articles (Bhogal et al., 2003)
    - Findings: left hemisphere lesions associated with PSD in hospital inpatient studies, but right hemisphere lesions associated with PSD in community studies; more standardized evidence required

2.6 Recovery and Survival in Post-Stroke Depression
(Starkstein & Manes, 2000; Whyte & Mulsant, 2002)

- Poor rehabilitation outcome
- Poor cognitive recovery
- Social withdrawal

- Worsened quality of life
- Increased caregiver burden
- Increased mortality

2.7 Identifying Post-Stroke Depression

- Some guidelines suggest that all patients with stroke should be screened for depression initially and at regular intervals or key stages of the rehabilitation process and after rehabilitation services have been discontinued.

- Challenges in diagnosis
  - Time
  - Communication difficulty
  - Cognitive impairment
  - Anosognosia or lack of awareness
  - Overlap of depression and medical illness
  - Stigma

2.8 Biological Treatment of Post-Stroke Depression

2.8.1 Antidepressants

- PSD poorly studied in randomized controlled trials (RCTs)
- Recruitment challenges, negative findings re: fatigue, major or minor depressive symptoms, possible longer-term benefit
- Caution re: drug interactions with warfarin, especially with fluoxetine, paroxetine, fluvoxamine (Fruehwald et al., 2003)

Effectiveness

- Sertraline vs placebo – no differences in main endpoint of Montgomery-Åsperg Depression Rating Scale (MADRS) score at 6 or 26 weeks (Murray et al., 2005)
- Fluoxetine vs placebo – small short-term trial; response rate of 62.5% vs 33.3% (NNT 3.4) (Wiart et al, 2000)
- Nortriptyline vs placebo – small short-term trial; improvement of mood and anxiety symptoms over placebo in stroke patients with comorbid major depression and generalized anxiety (Kimura, Tateno, & Robinson, 2003)

2.8.2 Stimulants

- No RCTs for patients with *major* depression in stroke
- Small RCT showing doses up to 30mg/d of methylphenidate improving mood scores (Hamilton Rating Scale for Depression [HAM-D]) and functional recovery in acute setting (Grade et al., 1998)
- Small retrospective study showing 53% remission with methylphenidate and 43% with nortriptyline in patients with major depression post-stroke (Lazarus et al., 1994)

2.8.3 ECT

- Case studies and case series only

2.9. Psychotherapy Themes in Post-Stroke Depression

- Loss of independence
- Physical limitations
- Identity and body image issues
- Loss of employment
- Financial strain
- Less access to social supports
- End-of-life issues
- Support, problem-solve, build coping skills
- Challenges regarding adaptation to language and physical limitations (Kneebone & Dunmore, 2000)

Antidepressant plus brief psychosocial behavioural intervention (47%, SD 26) is better than antidepressant plus usual care (32% SD 36) in reducing depressive symptoms (p = 0.02) (Mitchell et al., 2009).

2.10. Antidepressants for Non-Depressed Stroke Patients

1 year prevention studies:
- Antidepressants in the acute post-stroke period
    - Placebo (22.4%) vs escitalopram (8.5%), NNT 5 (Robinson et al., 2008)
    - Placebo (30%) vs sertraline (10%), NNT 5 (Rasmussen et al., 2003)
- Meta-analyses
    - Fluoxetine (4 studies) OR 0.25 (95% CI 0.11 to 0.56) (Yi, Liu, & Zhai, 2010)
    - Any antidepressant (10 studies) pooled rate difference = -0.17 (95% CI -0.26 to -0.08) (Chen et al., 2007)

2.11 Antidepressants and Disability in Stroke

- Large RCT of patients with stroke and significant motor deficits from France showed significant improvement in motor status scores among those randomized to fluoxetine (Chollet et al., 2011).
- Meta-analysis
    - Standardized mean difference 0.92 (95% CI 0.62–1.23) in 22 trials with 673 on selective serotonin reuptake inhibitor (SSRI) and 637 on placebo (Mead, Hsieh, & Hackett, 2013)

2.12 Antidepressants and Mortality in Stroke
(Jorge et al., 2003)

- Fluoxetine, nortriptyline or placebo x 12 weeks, n = 104, 9 years of follow-up
    - 68% survival antidepressant vs 36% placebo
- Antidepressants may modify pathophysiological processes associated with PSD and mortality.
- No guidelines currently recommend antidepressants for prevention.
    - Must weigh side effects and risk/benefit.
    - Recent epidemiological studies from the UK and Taiwan have reported associations between antidepressant use and subsequent risk of stroke (Coupland et al., 2011; Wu et al., 2011).

2.13 The Flip Side: Depression and Adversity as Risk Factors for Stroke

- Cohort study with 6095 stroke-free participants followed for on average 16 years (maximum 22 years)
    - High self-rated depression scores RR 1.73 (95% CI 1.30–2.31) (ns for white women) for stroke (Jonas & Mussolino, 2000)
    - Adjusted for age, sex, education, smoking, body mass index, alcohol, diabetes, coronary artery disease, systolic blood pressure, physical activity, and cholesterol

Adversity as a risk factor for stroke
- Large community sample, linked questionnaire on early childhood adversity to stroke on autopsy
    - Domains of adversity: emotional neglect, parental intimidation, parental violence, family turmoil, and financial need

- Adjusted for diabetes, physical activity, smoking, blood pressure, body mass index, and neuroticism
- Emotional neglect was associated with stroke at autopsy (OR 1.23, 95% CI 1.14–1.33), but not the other domains (Wilson et al., 2012)

3. Neuropsychiatry of Traumatic Brain Injury (TBI)

3.1 Epidemiology of TBI in Later Life

- TBI accounts for 80k emergency room visits per year in the Unites States.
- In 2003, the costs for TBI in the elderly exceeded 2.2 billion.
- Hospitalization rates for non-fatal TBI are more than twice as frequent in the elderly compared with the general population of younger adults (Thompson, McCormick, & Kagan, 2006).
- Falls are the #1 cause of TBI in the elderly.
- Fall-related TBI accounts for approximately half of unintentional fall deaths (Séguret et al., 2014).
- Rates of psychiatric disorders after TBI are variable (Silver, Hales, & Yudofsky, 2008); data are not specific for the elderly, in which rates may be lower, apart from dementia or delirium (Silver, Hales, & Yudofsky, 2008; Rapoport et al., 2003).
  - Prior psychiatric history ranges from 17–44%
  - Prior substance abuse from 22–30%
  - Prior psychiatric and substance histories increase the risk 1.3- to 4-fold
  - Depression described in section 3.6
  - Mania – few studies; 1.6% in Epidemiologic Catchment Area Study (ECA)
  - Psychotic disorders – few studies – range from 3.4–14%
  - Anxiety disorders – few studies – range from 6–24%, with general anxiety disorder (GAD) most common
  - Heterogeneity of findings vis-á-vis aggression and irritability from 5–70%!

3.2 Mortality and TBI in the Elderly

- Increased rates of mortality with increasing age following moderate or severe TBI
- Mortality with mild TBI approaches 9% (Flaada et al., 2007)

3.3 Other Catastrophic Outcomes of TBI in the Elderly
(Rapoport & Feinstein, 2000)

- Nursing home placement
- Neurological deterioration
- Slower rate of improvement
  - Although most of these studies are of severe TBI and short-term

3.4 Cognition and TBI in the Elderly

- Not well studied prospectively
- An older study showed high rates of dementia, but suffered from selection bias (Mazzucchi et al., 1992).

- More recent studies showed patients with moderate TBI (but not mild TBI) had greater cognitive impairment than a healthy comparison group, at one year. No differences were found at 2 years (Rapoport et al., 2006, 2008).
- Another study showed no differences compared with orthopedic in the acute period after injury (Aharon-Peretz et al., 1997).

3.5 TBI and Risk of Dementia
(Rapoport, Verhoeff, & van Reekum, 2004)

- Most of the studies conducted used case-control design.
- Meta-analysis showed increased risk for men OR 2.29, but not women (Fleminger et al., 2003).
- Cohort studies showed mixed findings.
- A bidirectional relationship exists.
- Apolipoprotein E epsilon 4 seems to increase the risk, although findings are inconsistent.
- Cholinesterase inhibitors showed mixed results in younger samples; an RCT of rivastigmine showed benefit in a subsample with memory impairment (Silver et al., 2006).

3.6 Depressive Disorders after TBI
(Jorge et al., 2004)

- 1 year prevalence rates are as high as 50%, and 80% of these meet criteria for major depressive episodes.
- Variable duration
- Risk factors: no association with severity, left frontal and left basal ganglia lesions, dysphoria at 1 week, and past depression
- Differential diagnosis includes grief reaction, post-traumatic stress disorder (PTSD), emotional lability, and apathy
- Commonly associated with anxiety, irritability, aggression, worsened cognition, and increased post-concussive symptoms
- Rates appear to be lower in elderly than younger adults, post–mild TBI (Rapoport et al., 2003)
- Treatment of depression in TBI: pharmacotherapy may reduce depressive symptoms as well as other post-concussive symptoms; off-label use; open-label studies only; caution re: more susceptible to adverse effects (Silver, McAllister, & Arciniegas, 2009)

4. Neuropsychiatry of Parkinson's Disease (PD)

4.1 Epidemiology of Parkinson's Disease

- Prevalence increases with age; onset is 40s–70s (mean early to mid-60s) (Weintraub & Burn, 2011).
- In Canada, using community surveys from 2010 to 2012, overall PD prevalence was 0.2% in the community, and 4.9% in residential care. The prevalence was higher in men than women, particularly in the elderly. The highest prevalence was for men aged 65–79 years living in institutions (9.3%, compared with 5.7% of women). Of those living at home, more than half reported often feeling either embarrassed about

their condition, left out of events, avoided or treated uncomfortably by others (Wong, Gilmour, & Ramage-Morin, 2014).

- A recent US study showed 7.7% prevalence in nursing homes in St. Louis (Hoegh et al., 2013).

4.2 Depression in Parkinson's Disease

- Rates of major depression of 5–20%, with an additional 10–30% with minor or subsyndromal depression; suicidal ideation is common, but suicide is rare (Weintraub & Burn, 2011)
- Risk factors: female, past or family psychiatric history, early onset, cognitive impairment
- Diagnosis challenging because of overlap of physical and mental symptoms
- In a recent study of diagnostic accuracy, the Geriatric Depression Scale (15) was compared to the use of two screening questions vis-á-vis depressed mood and anhedonia, with clinical diagnosis as a gold standard (Baillon et al., 2014). Both approaches were comparable – both had receiver operating characteristics (ROC) of above 0.90 and negative predictive values > 95%, but positive predictive value was low (< 60%), suggesting need for further diagnostic evaluation with positive responses.

4.3 Pharmacological Treatment of Depression in Parkinson's Disease

- Positive RCTs with nortriptyline and desipramine, although risks of falls
- SSRI studies negative
- Large recent SSRI/SNRI (serotonin norepinephrine reuptake inhibitor) study (Richard et al., 2012)
    - 12 week RCT: 115 subjects in 20 sites
    - Paroxetine, venlafaxine, or placebo for 12 weeks (6 for dose titration plus 6)
    - HAM-D antidepressants > placebo
    - But no statistically significant differences in response or remission, although likely underpowered for response and remission
        - Response: paroxetine 55%, venlafaxine 47%, placebo 38% (ns)
- Pramipexole as antidepressant vs SSRI (Barone et al., 2006)
    - RCT of 67 patients with major depression in Parkinson's disease
    - Mean dose of 3.24 mg/day vs sertraline 50mg/day for 14 weeks
    - NNT 3 of pramipexole over sertraline
- Pramipexole as antidepressant vs placebo (Barone et al., 2010)
    - 12 weeks; Europe and South Africa; entry based on depression scores rather than diagnosis of major depression
    - Pramipexole 0.125–1 mg TID (n = 139) vs placebo (n = 148)
    - Greater improvement in Beck Depression Inventory (BDI) scores (−5.9, SE 0.5) vs placebo (−4.0, SE 0.5), p < 0.01, and NNT 7 for Geriatric Depression Score < 5

4.4 Psychosis in Parkinson's Disease

(Weintraub & Burn, 2011; Seppi et al., 2011)

- Epidemiology data not limited to elderly, and focuses on cross-sectional point prevalence in clinic samples on dopaminergic treatment (Weintraub & Burn, 2011; Fénelon & Alves, 2010)

- Visual hallucinations 25–33% (lifetime 50%)
- Auditory hallucinations in 20%
- Illusions in 72%
- Delusions in 5%.
- Psychosis in < 10% of untreated patients with Parkinson's disease
- A complex and poorly understood area

Pharmacotherapy

- Antipsychotics have high propensity to worsen the Parkinsonian symptoms.
- Positive RCTs with clozapine, negative trial with olanzapine, and insufficient evidence with quetiapine
- Novel agent – pimavanserin (Cummings et al., 2014)
    - 5HT2a inverse agonist without dopaminergic activity
    - 6 week RCT with 2 week placebo lead-in, n = 185
    - Clinical Global Improvement (CGI) response: 49% vs 26% NNT 4

4.5 Impulse Control and Other Disorders
(Weintraub & Burn, 2011; Voon, Potenza, & Thomsen, 2007)

- Impulse control disorders (ICDs) 14%
- Repetitive actions (with or without urges) associated with negative consequences
- Thought to be a dopamine dysregulation syndrome
    - Examples: pathological gambling, hypersexuality, compulsive shopping, compulsive eating, compulsive medication use, punding syndrome

Management of ICD:

- D/c or decrease Da agonist (increase L-dopa if needed)
- Switch Da agnoist (esp if pramipexole)
- Low dose clozapine or quetiapine
- Family involvement to monitor Da intake
- Anti-androgens or antidepressants (libido)
- Cognitive behavioural therapy (CBT)
- Deep brain stimulation

Other disorders:

- Anxiety disorder symptoms up to 40%
- Sleep disorders 90%!
- Dementia – point prevalence 30%, cumulative prevalence 75% for those who survive about 10 years (Aarsland & Kurz, 2010)

5. Common Considerations

- Bidirectional relationship
- Avoid biological reductionism
- Consider psychiatric and motor sequelae of pharmacotherapy
- Need randomized controlled trials

QUESTIONS

1. List five factors associated with worse cognitive outcome following TBI in older adults.
2. What class of antidepressants has been consistently found to be useful in randomized placebo controlled trials among patients with depression secondary to PD?

3. List three adverse non-mood sequelae associated with major depression following stroke.

4. List three positive outcomes that have been associated with antidepressants in RCTs among patients with stroke.

5. Briefly outline in list form your clinical approach to the treatment of an otherwise healthy 78-year-old married woman with PD who presents for the first time ever with vivid and frightening visual hallucinations 10 years after initiation of treatment with levodopa/carbidopa and 3 years after initiation of treatment with pramipexole, in the absence of depression or cognitive impairment.

6. From a clinical point of view, how can we distinguish the neurovegetative symptoms associated with stroke, PD, and TBI from those associated with major depression?

7. Discuss the relationship between lesion location and post-stroke depression.

ANSWERS

1. Factors associated with worse cognitive outcome following TBI in older adults include:

   - Advanced age
   - Focal lesions
   - Other non-TBI injuries
   - History of cognitive impairment
   - History of functional impairment
   - Major depressive disorder
   - ApoE4 positive status
   - Delirium
   - Social isolation
   - Severity of TBI
   - Polypharmacy
   - Lower pre-morbid intelligence

2. Tricyclic antidepressants (TCAs) have been shown to be more efficacious, but are limited by side effects. SSRIs have been associated with improvements in Hamilton score, but have had no effect over placebo on response or remission. Others used commonly in clinical practice are mirtazapine, bupropion, and venlafaxine (all off-label).

3. Non-mood sequelae associated with major depression following stroke include:

   - Cognitive impairment
   - Increased mortality
   - Impairment in ADL
   - Apathy

4. Positive outcomes that have been associated with antidepressants in RCT among patients with stroke include:

   - Improvement in ADL if depression is treated within 1 month post-stroke
   - Cognitive improvement among patients responding to antidepressants
   - Reduced mortality
   - Improved outcomes with rehabilitation
   - Improved mood

5. The treatment of such a patient would involve:

   - Rule out underlying medical illnesses, medications, substances, and delirium.
   - Assess psychosocial stressors.
   - Reduce or eliminate dopamine agonists if possible.

- Reduce dose of levodopa/carbidopa if possible (or consider shorter acting formulation).
- Consider an antipsychotic, especially clozapine.
- Perform a cognitive examination (see chapter 1.2).
- Ensure that any sensory deficits (vision, hearing) are optimized.
- Discontinue anticholinergic medications.
- Carefully review medications.
- Eliminate medications using a well-established hierarchy (start with anticholinergics, finish with levodopa/carbidopa).

6. The neurovegetative symptoms associated with neurological disorders are difficult to distinguish from major depression, and there is no validated method:
   - Consider the "company they keep"
   - Temporal relationship between the depressed mood and/or anhedonia with the neurovegetative symptoms
   - Explore for psychological symptoms of depression
   - Review apathy vs depression
   - Language impairment makes this more challenging
   - Past and family history of mood disorder increases likelihood of same

7. The relationship between lesion location and post-stroke depression is controversial:
   - Classically, left frontal lesions are more likely to be associated with post-stroke depression, but refuted in recent meta-analyses.
   - Bhogal et al. (2003) meta-analysis
     – Right hemisphere community; left hemisphere hospital
     – Right hemisphere > 6 months post-stroke; left hemisphere if within 2 weeks of stroke

CASE DISCUSSION

1. The approach to this patient should include:
   - History, collateral, and mental status, including cognitive testing and neuroimaging
   - Rule out other medical conditions and psychiatric causes
   - Detailed record review of family medicine records and other health data prior to injury
   - Detailed interview with informants about pre-injury functional and cognitive status
   - Involve family other than wife as well
   - Occupational therapy assessment
   - If memory significantly impaired and no contraindications, can consider ChEI (a recent RCT [Silver et al., 2006] of rivastigmine post-TBI was negative, except for a subgroup with significant memory impairment)
   - Functional assessment
   - Assess for caregiver burden/stress
   - Determine if insurance claims or court actions are involved.

2. The approach to determining the relationship between the mania and the stroke should include:
   - History, collateral, mental status, physical (neurological) exam, record review including review of stroke-related imaging (right-sided lesions more common)
   - Careful delineation of past and family psychiatric history of mania, mood disorders, anxiety disorders, and substance-related disorders
   - Careful rule-out of other medical, medication, or substance causes
   - Careful review of temporal relationship between stroke and manic symptomatology

SUGGESTED RESOURCES FOR REVIEW

Although these resources may not be specifically cited in the text, their approach informed the contents of the chapter, and they are recommended as useful further reading.

Ashman TA, Cantor JB, Gordon WA, et al. A comparison of cognitive functioning in older adults with and without traumatic brain injury. J Head Trauma Rehabil. 2008;23(3):139–48. http://dx.doi.org/10.1097/01.HTR.0000319930.69343.64. Medline:18520426

Rapoport, MJ, Verhoeff, NP, van Reekum, R. Traumatic brain injury and dementia. Canadian Alzheimer Disease Review. Sept 2004;7(2):4–8.

Robinson RG, Spalletta G. Poststroke depression: a review. Can J Psychiatry. 2010;55(6):341–9. Medline:20540828

Weintraub D, Burn DJ. Parkinson's disease: the quintessential neuropsychiatric disorder. Mov Disord. 2011;26(6):1022–31. http://dx.doi.org/10.1002/mds.23664. Medline:21626547

REFERENCES

Aarsland D, Kurz MW. The epidemiology of dementia associated with Parkinson's disease. Brain Pathol. 2010;20(3):633–9. http://dx.doi.org/10.1111/j.1750-3639.2009.00369.x. Medline:20522088

Aharon-Peretz J, Kliot D, Amyel-Zvi E, et al. Neurobehavioral consequences of closed head injury in the elderly. Brain Inj. 1997;11(12):871–6. http://dx.doi.org/10.1080/026990597122945. PMID:9413621

Baillon S, Dennis M, Lo N, et al. Screening for depression in Parkinson's disease: the performance of two screening questions. Age Ageing. 2014;43(2):200–5. http://dx.doi.org/10.1093/ageing/aft152. Medline:24132854

Barone P, Poewe W, Albrecht S, et al. Pramipexole for the treatment of depressive symptoms in patients with Parkinson's disease: a randomised, double-blind, placebo-controlled trial. Lancet Neurol. 2010;9(6):573–80. http://dx.doi.org/10.1016/S1474-4422(10)70106-X. Medline:20452823

Barone P, Scarzella L, Marconi R, et al.; Depression/Parkinson Italian Study Group. Pramipexole versus sertraline in the treatment of depression in Parkinson's disease: a national multicenter parallel-group randomized study. J Neurol. 2006;253(5):601–7. http://dx.doi.org/10.1007/s00415-006-0067-5. Medline:16607468

Bhogal SK, Teasell RW, Foley NC, et al. Community reintegration after stroke. Top Stroke Rehabil. 2003;10(2):107–29. http://dx.doi.org/10.1310/F50L-WEWE-6AJ4-64FK. Medline:13680520

Chemerinski E, Robinson RG. The neuropsychiatry of stroke. Psychosomatics. 2000;41(1):5–14. http://dx.doi.org/10.1016/S0033-3182(00)71168-6. Medline:10665263

Chen Y, Patel NC, Guo JJ, et al. Antidepressant prophylaxis for poststroke depression: a meta-analysis. Int Clin Psychopharmacol. 2007;22(3):159–66. http://dx.doi.org/10.1097/YIC.0b013e32807fb028. Medline:17414742

Chollet F, Tardy J, Albucher JF, et al. Fluoxetine for motor recovery after acute ischaemic stroke (FLAME): a randomised placebo-controlled trial. Lancet Neurol. 2011;10(2):123–30. http://dx.doi.org/10.1016/S1474-4422(10)70314-8. Medline:21216670

Coupland C, Dhiman P, Morriss R, et al. Antidepressant use and risk of adverse outcomes in older people: population based cohort study. BMJ. 2011;343(aug02 1):d4551. http://dx.doi.org/10.1136/bmj.d4551. Medline:21810886

Cummings J, Isaacson S, Mills R, et al. Pimavanserin for patients with Parkinson's disease psychosis: a randomised, placebo-controlled phase 3 trial. Lancet. 2014;383(9916):533–40. http://dx.doi.org/10.1016/S0140-6736(13)62106-6. Medline:24183563

Fénelon G, Alves G. Epidemiology of psychosis in Parkinson's disease. J Neurol Sci. 2010;289(1-2):12–7. http://dx.doi.org/10.1016/j.jns.2009.08.014. Medline:19740486

Flaada JT, Leibson CL, Mandrekar JN, et al. Relative risk of mortality after traumatic brain injury: a population-based study of the role of age and injury severity. J Neurotrauma. 2007;24(3):435–45. http://dx.doi.org/10.1089/neu.2006.0119. Medline:17402850

Fleminger S, Oliver DL, Lovestone S, et al. Head injury as a risk factor for Alzheimer's disease: the evidence 10 years on; a partial replication. J Neurol Neurosurg Psychiatry. 2003;74(7):857–62. http://dx.doi.org/10.1136/jnnp.74.7.857. Medline:12810767

Fruehwald S, Gatterbauer E, Rehak P, et al. Early fluoxetine treatment of post-stroke depression--a three-month double-blind placebo-controlled study with an open-label long-term follow up. J Neurol. 2003;250(3):347–51. http://dx.doi.org/10.1007/s00415-003-1014-3. Medline:12638027

Go AS, Mozaffarian D, Roger VL, et al.; American Heart Association Statistics Committee and Stroke Statistics Subcommittee. Heart disease and stroke statistics–2014 update: a report from the American Heart Association. Circulation. 2014;129(3):e28–292. http://dx.doi.org/10.1161/01.cir.0000441139.02102.80. Medline:24352519

Grade C, Redford B, Chrostowski J, et al. Methylphenidate in early poststroke recovery: a double-blind, placebo-controlled study. Arch Phys Med Rehabil. 1998;79(9):1047–50. http://dx.doi.org/10.1016/S0003-9993(98)90169-1. Medline:9749682

Hackett ML, Yapa C, Parag V, et al. Frequency of depression after stroke: a systematic review of observational studies. Stroke. 2005;36(6):1330–40. http://dx.doi.org/10.1161/01.STR.0000165928.19135.35. Medline:15879342

Hoegh M, Ibrahim AK, Chibnall J, et al. Prevalence of Parkinson disease and Parkinson disease dementia in community nursing homes. Am J Geriatr Psychiatry. 2013;21(6):529–35. http://dx.doi.org/10.1016/j.jagp.2012.12.007. Medline:23567411

Jonas BS, Mussolino ME. Symptoms of depression as a prospective risk factor for stroke. Psychosom Med. 2000;62(4):463–71. http://dx.doi.org/10.1097/00006842-200007000-00001. Medline:10949089

Jorge RE, Robinson RG, Arndt S, et al. Mortality and poststroke depression: a placebo-controlled trial of antidepressants. Am J Psychiatry. 2003;160(10):1823–9. http://dx.doi.org/10.1176/appi.ajp.160.10.1823. Medline:14514497

Jorge RE, Robinson RG, Moser D, et al. Major depression following traumatic brain injury. Arch Gen Psychiatry. 2004;61(1):42–50. http://dx.doi.org/10.1001/archpsyc.61.1.42. Medline:14706943

Kimura M, Tateno A, Robinson RG. Treatment of poststroke generalized anxiety disorder comorbid with poststroke depression: merged analysis of nortriptyline trials. Am J Geriatr Psychiatry. 2003;11(3):320–7. http://dx.doi.org/10.1097/00019442-200305000-00009. Medline:12724111

Kneebone II, Dunmore E. Psychological management of post-stroke depression. Br J Clin Psychol. 2000;39(Pt 1):53–65. http://dx.doi.org/10.1348/014466500163103. Medline:10789028

Lazarus LW, Moberg PJ, Langsley PR, et al. Methylphenidate and nortriptyline in the treatment of poststroke depression: a retrospective comparison. Arch Phys Med Rehabil. 1994;75(4):403–6. http://dx.doi.org/10.1016/0003-9993(94)90163-5. Medline:8172499

Lyketsos CG, Kozauer N, Rabins PV. Psychiatric manifestations of neurologic disease: where are we headed? Dialogues Clin Neurosci. 2007;9(2):111–24. Medline:17726911

Marin RS. The three-dimensional approach to neuropsychiatric assessment. J Neuropsychiatry Clin Neurosci. 2012;24(4):384–93. http://dx.doi.org/10.1176/appi.neuropsych.11070148. Medline:23224445

Mazzucchi A, Cattelani R, Missale G, et al. Head-injured subjects aged over 50 years: correlations between variables of trauma and neuropsychological follow-up. J Neurol. 1992;239(5):256–60. Medline:1607886

Mead GE, Hsieh CF, Hackett M. Selective serotonin reuptake inhibitors for stroke recovery. JAMA. 2013;310(10):1066–7. http://dx.doi.org/10.1001/jama.2013.107828. Medline:24026602

Mitchell PH, Veith RC, Becker KJ, et al. Brief psychosocial-behavioral intervention with antidepressant reduces poststroke depression significantly more than usual care with antidepressant: living well with stroke: randomized, controlled trial. Stroke. 2009;40(9):3073–8. http://dx.doi.org/10.1161/STROKEAHA.109.549808. Medline:19661478

Murray V, von Arbin M, Bartfai A, et al. Double-blind comparison of sertraline and placebo in stroke patients with minor depression and less severe major depression. J Clin Psychiatry. 2005;66(6):708–16. http://dx.doi.org/10.4088/JCP.v66n0606. Medline:15960563

Rapoport MJ, Feinstein A. Outcome following traumatic brain injury in the elderly: a critical review. Brain Inj. 2000;14(8):749–61. http://dx.doi.org/10.1080/026990500413777. Medline:10969893

Rapoport MJ, Herrmann N, Shammi P, et al. Outcome after traumatic brain injury sustained in older adulthood: a one-year longitudinal study. Am J Geriatr Psychiatry. 2006;14(5):456–65. http://dx.doi.org/10.1097/01 .JGP.0000199339.79689.8a. Medline:16670250

Rapoport MJ, McCullagh S, Streiner D, et al. Age and major depression after mild traumatic brain injury. Am J Geriatr Psychiatry. 2003;11(3):365–9. http://dx.doi.org/10.1097/00019442-200305000-00015. Medline:12724117

Rapoport M, Wolf U, Herrmann N, et al. Traumatic brain injury, Apolipoprotein E-epsilon4, and cognition in older adults: a two-year longitudinal study. J Neuropsychiatry Clin Neurosci. 2008;20(1):68–73. http:// dx.doi.org/10.1176/jnp.2008.20.1.68. Medline:18305286

Rasmussen A, Lunde M, Poulsen DL, et al. A double-blind, placebo-controlled study of sertraline in the prevention of depression in stroke patients. Psychosomatics. 2003;44(3):216–21. http://dx.doi.org/10.1176/ appi.psy.44.3.216. Medline:12724503

Richard IH, McDermott MP, Kurlan R, et al.; SAD-PD Study Group. A randomized, double-blind, placebo-controlled trial of antidepressants in Parkinson disease. Neurology. 2012;78(16):1229–36. http://dx.doi.org/ 10.1212/WNL.0b013e3182516244. Medline:22496199

Robinson RG, Jorge RE, Moser DJ, et al. Escitalopram and problem-solving therapy for prevention of poststroke depression: a randomized controlled trial. JAMA. 2008;299(20):2391–400. http://dx.doi.org/ 10.1001/jama.299.20.2391. Medline:18505948

Séguret F, Ferreira C, Cambou JP, et al. Changes in hospitalization rates for acute coronary syndrome after a two-phase comprehensive smoking ban. Eur J Prev Cardiol. 2014;21(12):1575–82. Medline:23918841

Seppi K, Weintraub D, Coelho M, et al. The Movement Disorder Society Evidence-Based Medicine Review Update: treatments for the non-motor symptoms of Parkinson's disease. Mov Disord. 2011;26(S3 Suppl 3):S42–80. http://dx.doi.org/10.1002/mds.23884. Medline:22021174

Silver JM. Behavioral neurology and neuropsychiatry is a subspecialty. J Neuropsychiatry Clin Neurosci. 2006;18(2):146–8. http://dx.doi.org/10.1176/jnp.2006.18.2.146. Medline:16720790

Silver JM, Hales RE, Yudofsky SC. Neuropsychiatric aspects of traumatic brain injury. In: Yudofsky SC, Hales RE, editors. The American Psychiatric Publishing textbook of neuropsychiatry and behavioral neurosciences.5th ed. Arlington, VA: American Psychiatric Publishing; 2008. p. 595–648.

Silver JM, Koumaras B, Chen M, et al. Effects of rivastigmine on cognitive function in patients with traumatic brain injury. Neurology. 2006;67(5):748–55. http://dx.doi.org/10.1212/01.wnl.0000234062.98062.e9. Medline:16966534

Silver JM, McAllister TW, Arciniegas DB. Depression and cognitive complaints following mild traumatic brain injury. Am J Psychiatry. 2009;166(6):653–61. http://dx.doi.org/10.1176/appi.ajp.2009.08111676. Medline:19487401

Starkstein SE, Manes F. Apathy and depression following stroke. CNS Spectr. 2000;5(3):43–50. Medline:18277328

Thompson HJ, McCormick WC, Kagan SH. Traumatic brain injury in older adults: epidemiology, outcomes, and future implications. J Am Geriatr Soc. 2006;54(10):1590–5. http://dx.doi.org/10.1111/j.1532-5415.2006.00894.x. Medline:17038079

Voon V, Potenza MN, Thomsen T. Medication-related impulse control and repetitive behaviors in Parkinson's disease. Curr Opin Neurol. 2007;20(4):484–92. http://dx.doi.org/10.1097/WCO.0b013e32826fbc8f. Medline:17620886

Weintraub D, Burn DJ. Parkinson's disease: the quintessential neuropsychiatric disorder. Mov Disord. 2011;26(6):1022–31. http://dx.doi.org/10.1002/mds.23664. Medline:21626547

Whyte EM, Mulsant BH. Post stroke depression: epidemiology, pathophysiology, and biological treatment. Biol Psychiatry. 2002;52(3):253–64. http://dx.doi.org/10.1016/S0006-3223(02)01424-5. Medline:12182931

Wiart L, Petit H, Joseph PA, et al. Fluoxetine in early poststroke depression: a double-blind placebo-controlled study. Stroke. 2000;31(8):1829–32. http://dx.doi.org/10.1161/01.STR.31.8.1829. Medline:10926942

Wilson RS, Boyle PA, Levine SR, et al. Emotional neglect in childhood and cerebral infarction in older age. Neurology. 2012;79(15):1534–9. http://dx.doi.org/10.1212/WNL.0b013e31826e25bd. Medline:22993291

Wong SL, Gilmour H, Ramage-Morin PL. Parkinson's disease: prevalence, diagnosis and impact. Health Rep. 2014;25(11):10–4. Medline:25408491

Wu CS, Wang SC, Cheng YC, et al. Association of cerebrovascular events with antidepressant use: a case-crossover study. Am J Psychiatry. 2011;168(5):511–21. http://dx.doi.org/10.1176/appi.ajp.2010.10071064. Medline:21406464

Yi ZM, Liu F, Zhai SD. Fluoxetine for the prophylaxis of poststroke depression in patients with stroke: a meta-analysis. Int J Clin Pract. 2010;64(9):1310–7. http://dx.doi.org/10.1111/j.1742-1241.2010.02437.x. Medline:20653802

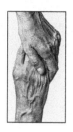

SECTION 4:
SPECIAL TOPICS

4.1 Epidemiology of Mental Illness in Older Adults

Mark Rapoport, MD, FRCPC

INTRODUCTION

Geriatric psychiatrists would ideally be perfect in their abilities to separate cases from non-cases and to make diagnoses with absolute certainty. Unfortunately, many older adults do not fit neatly into DSM classifications. Over the decades, epidemiology and psychiatric classification have evolved with more reliable methods, or at least more reproducible methodologies. However, reliability is still imperfect, and furthermore, the validity and predictive ability of these diagnoses remain questionable. In this chapter, the main findings of major epidemiological studies pertaining to late-life psychiatric disorders are summarized and critiqued. More details about epidemiology of individual disorders appear elsewhere in the respective chapters about psychiatric disorders, along with literature on comorbidity and risk factors for these disorders in older adults.

CASE SCENARIO

An 88-year-old man presents with a two-month history of delusions of persecution, jealousy, and theft, centring on his wife. The delusions change from day to day, and his affect is incongruous with the content, with no formal thought disorder. There are no hallucinations and no history of substances or alcohol. His Mini Mental State Examination (MMSE) score is 24/29 (repeat was not administered because English was not his first language, and he lost 2 points for recall, 1 point for date, and 1 point for serial 7s). Considering the epidemiology of mental disorders, what is the most likely diagnosis and what is your approach to diagnosis and management?

OVERVIEW

1. A Declining Prevalence of Disorders with Age?

1.1 Lower Prevalence of Disorders in Older Adults Compared with Younger Adults

- The Epidemiologic Catchment Area Study (ECA) (Regier et al., 1988) and National Comorbidity Study – Replication Study (NCS-R) (Gum, King-Kallimanis, & Kohn, 2009) show lower 1-year prevalence of mental disorder among those 65 plus compared with younger age groups, for any disorder, major depressive disorder, and any anxiety disorder. The same pattern was found for 6-month prevalence in the Edmonton Study (Bland, Newman, & Orn, 1988).

- See Table 4.1.1.

Table 4.1.1: Prevalence of Psychiatric Disorders in Older Adults
Compared with Younger Adults in Large Epidemiological Surveys

Study	Any Disorder (%)	MDE (%)	Anxiety (%)
ECA 1-year prevalence; n = 5702			
65+ years	12.3	0.7	5.5
45–64 years	13.3	2.0	6.5
25–44 years	17.3	3.0	8.3
Edmonton 6-month prevalence; n = 358			
65+ years	10.9	1.2	3.5
All adults	17.1	3.2	6.5
NCS-R 1-year prevalence; n = 1461			
65+ years	8.5	2.3	7.0
45–64 years	22.4	6.5	18.7

ECA = Epidemiologic Catchment Area Study; MDE = major depressive episode;
NCS-R = National Comorbidity Study – Replication Study

1.2 Why a Discrepancy between Young and Old?
(Streiner, et al., 2009; Corna et al., 2011)

1.2.1 If the Differences Are True, It Could Be:

- Different manifestation of illness
- More subsyndromal or minor symptoms with age
- Less likely to report
- More likely to express symptoms in somatic terms
- Cohort effect
  - Those born before a certain year are psychologically healthier.
- Cohort-period effect
  - Shared historical events have important impact on psychological resilience.
- Psychological differences between the groups
- Biological differences between the groups
- Note: The consistency of findings over a generation or more lends little credence to cohort or cohort-period effects.

1.2.2 If Differences Are an Artefact, It Could Be Issues Pertaining to:

- Sampling
- Mentally ill less likely to participate

- Mentally ill more likely to be institutionalized
- Healthy survivor effect
  - Mentally ill more likely to be deceased later in life
- Forgetting of symptoms
- Reframing or reattributing symptoms
- Differences in attitudes to surveys and approaches to questions

1.3 Problems with "Lifetime Prevalence"
(Patten et al., 2012)

- Recall drops significantly with time following illness.
- A recent study by Patten et al. demonstrated that less than half of participants with major depression recalled their most recent major depressive episode six or more years later.

2. Prevalence of Non-Cognitive Mental Disorders in Lay Interview Community Studies
(Regier et al., 1988; Gum, King-Kallimanis, & Kohn, 2009; Préville et al., 2010)

- These studies are based on lay interviews, conducted in the community.
- Semi-structured interview
- Variable response rates
- Not representative of clinic, hospitalized, or institutionalized samples
- Anxiety disorders consistently highest
- Women are much higher than men for prevalence of mood and anxiety disorders, but the reverse for alcohol-related disorders.
- Table 4.1.2 shows the 12-month prevalence ranges of the most common psychiatric disorders assessed across the ECA, NCS-R, and Enquête sur la Santé des Aînés (ESA) studies. The rows are organized by prevalence range for ease of study and memorization. Tables later in the chapter are organized by disorder in more detail.

3. Mood Disorders

3.1 Mood Disorders Seem to Decline with Age in Cross-Sectional Studies

- As shown in Table 4.1.3, the 1-year prevalence of major depressive episode (MDE) declined in women but not men in the Canadian Community Health Survey (CCHS) 1.2 Study (Streiner, Cairney, & Veldhuizen, 2006).

3.2 Summary of Cross-Sectional Prevalence Data for Mood Disorders in Community-Dwelling Elderly (Semi-Structured Lay Interviews)

- Table 4.1.4 summarizes cross-sectional prevalence data (based on semi-structured lay interviews) for mood disorders in community-dwelling elderly.

3.3 Antidepressant Use Is Common
(Streiner, Cairney, & Veldhuizen, 2006; Mamdani et al., 2005; Parabiaghi et al., 2011)

- Although community rates of major depression are low, this should be contrasted with higher community antidepressant prevalence rates.
  - 12-month prevalence of antidepressants: 4.1% in age 65 years plus (CCHS 1.2)
  - Current antidepressant use in Ontario and Lombardy, Italy, 2002: 10% in age 65 plus

Table 4.1.2: Overview of the 12-Month Prevalence of Major Psychiatric Disorders in Older Adults in Large Epidemiological Surveys

Prevalence Ranges (%) (12 months)	ECA (12 months; n = 5702)	NCS-R (12 months; n = 1461)	ESA (12 months; n = 2798)
5.0–7.0	• Any anxiety disorder	• Any anxiety disorder	• Any anxiety disorder
4.0–4.9	• Phobia	• Phobia	–
3.0–3.9	–	–	–
2.0–2.9	–	• MDE • Social phobia	• Phobia • "Psychotropic dependency"
1.0–1.9	• Dysthymia	• GAD	• GAD • MDE
0–0.9	• Panic • Manic • Substance • OCD • MDE • Schizophrenia	• Panic • Bipolar disorder • Dysthymia • Substance	• Panic • Manic • Social phobia

ECA = Epidemiologic Catchment Area Study; ESA = Enquête sur la Santé des Aînés; GAD = generalized anxiety disorder; MDE = major depressive episode; NCS-R = National Comorbidity Study – Replication Study; OCD = obsessive-compulsive disorder

Table 4.1.3: 1-Year Prevalence of Major Depressive Episode in Cross-Sectional Surveys

1-Year Prevalence MDE (n = 12 729; 55+ years)	65–69 years (%)	70–74 years (%)	75+ years (%)
Male	2.0	1.7	2.4
Female	2.8	1.6	1.3

MDE = major depressive episode

3.4 Prospective Longitudinal Studies Do Not Show Reduction in Depression with Age

- Evaluations by psychiatrists using semi-structured schedule
- Sweden (Pálsson, Östling, & Skoog, 2001):
  - Clinically significant mood disorder (included community and institutionalized)
  - Age 70 to 79
    - Incidence 17/1000 person-years

Table 4.1.4: Cross-Sectional Prevalence of Dysthymia, Major Depressive Episode, and Mania

Study	Age/Time	N	Dysthymia (%)	MDE (%)	Mania (%)
ECA (*Regier et al., 1988*)	65+ years/ 1 month	18 571	1.8	0.7	0
Edmonton (*Bland, Newman, & Orn, 1988*)	65+ years/ 6 months	358	3.3	1.2	0
NCS-R (*Gum, King-Kallimanis, & Kohn, 2009*)	65+ years/ 12 months	1461	0.5	2.3	0.2 (bipolar disorder)
Quebec, ESA (*Préville et al., 2010*)	65+ years/ 12 months	2798	5.7 (minor depression)	1.1	0.6
CCHS 1.2 (*Streiner, Cairney, & Veldhuizen, 2006*)	55+ years/ 12 months	12 792	–	2.9	0.2 (bipolar disorder)
LASA (*Beekman et al., 1998*)	55–85 years/ Current	3056	–	2.0	–

CCHS = Canadian Community Health Survey; ECA = Epidemiologic Catchment Area Study; ESA = Enquête sur la Santé des Aînés Study; LASA = Longitudinal Aging Study Amsterdam; MDE = major depressive episode; NCS-R = National Comorbidity Study – Replication Study

- – Age 83 to 85
  - ▪ Incidence 38/1000 person-years
- – One month prevalence
  - ▪ 5.6% age 70
  - ▪ 13.0% age 85
- Rotterdam, Netherlands (Luijendijk et al., 2008)
  - – Incidence of clinically relevant depressive syndromes
  - – Age 55 years plus
    - ▪ Incidence 7.0/1000 person-years

3.5 Subthreshold Depression

- Among those age 55 years and over, approximate point prevalence rates (Meeks et al., 2011):
  - – Community – 10%
  - – Primary care – 25%
  - – Medical inpatients – 30%+
  - – Long-term care – 45–50%
- Rates vary depending on definition
- Conversion rate approximately 10%/year to major depressive disorder (MDD) in primary care
- Higher conversion rate to MDD if prior MDE
- Correlates: cognitive impairment, poor physical healthy, functional disability, increased health care utilization and cost
- Diagnostic stability – 6-year remission rate of 26% vs 5% for MDD

3.6 Major Depression and Depressive Symptoms Are Very Common in Long-Term Care
(Seitz, Purandare, & Conn, 2010)

- Table 4.1.5 shows the prevalence of major depression and depression symptoms among older adults in long-term care.

Table 4.1.5: Point Prevalence of Major Depression and Depressive Symptoms in Long-Term Care

Symptoms	# Studies	Median (%)	Range (%)
Major depression	26	10	2–25
Depression or depressive symptoms	26	29	14–82

3.7 Mood Disorders Common among Older Psychiatric Inpatients
(Seitz et al., 2012)

- Major depression accounts for 32% of admissions in Ontario to acute psychiatric units.
- Bipolar disorder accounts for 11%.

3.8 Recent Meta-Analysis of Depression in the Elderly
(Luppa et al., 2012)

- A recent meta-analysis examined 24 studies in which age- and gender-specific prevalence of depression in adults age 75 years and older were found.
  - The point prevalence of major depression ranged from 4.6–9.3% in eight of these studies.
  - The pooled point prevalence for major depression was 7.2% (95% CI 4.4–10.6) in the three studies that used DSM criteria, although the results were very heterogeneous ($I^2 = 94.3\%$).
  - The ratio of men to women was 1:1.4–1.8.
  - Lowest rates were found in North America and highest in the UK.
  - The point prevalence of "depressive disorders" categorized by rating scales ranged from 4.5–37.4% in fourteen of these studies.
    - The pooled prevalence rate was rate was 17.1% (95% CI 9.7–26.1%), again with significant heterogeneity ($I^2 = 99.8\%$).
    - Prevalence increased with age.
    - Studies of lower methodological quality reported the lowest prevalence rates.

4. Anxiety Disorders

4.1 Prevalence Varies by Study

Any anxiety disorder
- LASA (Amsterdam) had highest rate of "all anxiety disorders" at 10.2% 6-month prevalence, but age was 55 plus (Beekman et al., 1998).

65 years plus

- ECA: 1-month prevalence 5.5% (Regier et al., 1988)
- Edmonton: 6-month prevalence 3.5% (Bland, Newman, & Orn, 1988)
- NCS-R: 12-month prevalence 7.0% (Gum, King-Kallimanis, & Kohn, 2009)

Most common anxiety disorder

- Phobic disorder in ECA (Préville et al., 2010), Edmonton, and NCS-R (ranging from 3.0–4.8%)
- General anxiety disorder (GAD) according to LASA (7.3% 6-month prevalence, age 55 years plus)

Rare in the community-based studies

- Panic and obsessive-compulsive disorder (OCD)
    - 1% or less, except 1.5% for OCD in Edmonton Study, 6-month prevalence
- Social phobia
    - 2.3% 1-year prevalence in NCS-R, age 65 years plus
    - 1.3% 1-year prevalence in CCHS 1.2, age 55 years plus (Streiner, Cairney, & Veldhuizen, 2006)

4.2 Self-Reported "Feelings of Anxiety" May Be Important

- In a Swedish study, 5% of 966 participants age 65 years and over reported being "anxious most of the time" (Forsell & Winblad, 1998).
    - Half of those had anxiety disorder vs none for those who reported being "calm most of the time."

4.3 Hospitalizations and Comorbidity

(Lenze et al., 2000)

- Older adults, especially women, have much higher rates of hospitalizations for anxiety disorders compared with younger adults.
- Among patients with major depression in clinical populations, anxiety disorders are very common.
- 30% had at least one current anxiety disorder, and 14% had more than one.
    - Most commonly, GAD, panic disorder, specific or social phobia

5. Substance-Related Disorders

5.1 Large-Scale Lay Interview–Based Epidemiological Studies Report Low Rates of Substance-Related Disorders for the Elderly

- Large-scale lay interview–based epidemiological studies show that substance-related disorders in the elderly are low (Table 4.1.6).

5.2 Alcohol Consumption Patterns in the Elderly

- Large sample of patients age 65 years and over in Liverpool family practices (n = 1070) (Saunders et al., 1989)
    - 10% drank daily, 20% drank weekly
        - Among those who drank at least weekly:

Table 4.1.6: Prevalence of Substance-Related Disorders in Older Adults

Study	Prevalence (%)
ECA – 1-month prevalence (Regier et al., 1988)	0.9
Edmonton – 6-month prevalence (Bland, Newman, & Orn, 1988)	1.7
NCS-R – 1-year prevalence (Gum, King-Kallimanis, & Kohn, 2009)	1.0
ESA – 1-year prevalence (Préville et al., 2010)	2.3 (psychotropic)

ECA = Epidemiologic Catchment Area Study; ESA = Enquête sur la Santé des Aînés Study; NCS-R = National Comorbidity Study – Replication Study

- Rates for men were more than double those for women.
- Rates for men declined with age, and the same applied for women, but to a lesser extent.
  - Mean weekly alcohol consumption (standard drinks) among regular drinkers:
    - Men – 13.9
    - Women – 8.3
- Self-reported "problem with alcohol" 0.94% (very similar to ECA)

5.3 The Rate of Alcohol Dependence Is Higher among "Past Year Users," and Subthreshold Dependence Is Common

- Table 4.1.7 shows the rates of alcohol abuse, dependence, and subthreshold dependence in elderly subjects reported in the US National Survey of Drug Use and Health (2011) (Blazer & Wu, 2011).

Table 4.1.7: Point Prevalence of Alcohol Dependence, Abuse, and Subthreshold Dependence in Older Adults in the US National Survey of Drug Use and Health (2011)*

Diagnosis	65+ (%)	65+ "Past Year Users" (i.e., abstainers excluded) (%)
Alcohol dependence	0.6	1.3
Alcohol abuse	0.9	2.1
Subthreshold dependence	5.2	12.0

*N = 6289 over the age of 65

5.4 The Rate of Alcohol Abuse Is Higher When Physician Examination, Informant Interview, and MCV Test Done
(Thomas & Rockwood, 2001)

- In the Canadian Study of Health and Aging (CSHA), 8.9% current alcohol abuse, plus additional 3.7% possible alcohol abuse

6. Psychotic Disorders

6.1 Rates Are Almost Non-Existent in Large-Scale, Structured Interview Studies

- 0.1% ECA 1-month prevalence
- 0% Edmonton 6-month prevalence
- Liverpool family practice registry (Copeland et al., 1998)
  - Nursing screen plus DSM-III-R examination by psychiatrist
    - Schizophrenia 0.12% prevalence
    - Delusional disorder 0.04% prevalence

6.1.1 Theories

- Selective mortality
- Burnout
- Studies not capturing homeless
- Diagnostic instability

6.2 Psychotic Symptoms Are Common in Community-Dwelling Elderly
(Christenson & Blazer, 1984; Henderson et al., 1998; Östling, Pálsson, & Skoog, 2007)

- 4% generalized persecutory ideation in North Carolina
- 5.7% auditory hallucinations or paranoid delusions in community-dwelling older adults in Australia, although the rate was 3.8% in cognitively intact community-dwelling older adults
- 20% cumulative incidence of psychotic symptoms by age 85 in a prospective Swedish study of those 70 years and over followed prospectively over time

7. Dementia

7.1 Rates Were Low in the Large-Scale Epidemiological Studies of Psychiatric Illness
(Regier et al., 1988; Bland, Newman, & Orn, 1988)

- 4.9% 1-month prevalence in ECA
- 3.3% 6-month prevalence in Edmonton Study
- Dementia not addressed in the NCS-R, CCHS 1.2, or ESA studies

7.2 Rates Were Higher in Large-Scale Community Studies Involving Examination
(CSHA Working Group, 1994; Brookmeyer et al., 2011; Ferri et al., 2005)

- CSHA: 8% prevalence, age 65+
- US Aging, Demographics, and Memory Study (ADAMS): 14% prevalence, age 71+
- Delphi study:
  - 6.4% prevalence, age 60+ North American studies
  - 3.9% prevalence, age 60+ international studies

7.3 Age and Setting Matter in Predicting Dementia Prevalence
(CSHA Working Group, 1994; Brookmeyer et al., 2011; Ebly et al., 1994)

CSHA
- 85–89 years – 23%
- 90–94 years – 40%
- 95+ years – 58%

ADAMS (US)
- 71–79 years – 5%
- 80–89 years - 24%
- 90+ years – 37%

Table 4.1.8 shows the prevalence of dementia in community and institutional settings for older adults in Canada.

Table 4.1.8: Point Prevalence of Dementia in the Canadian Study of Health and Aging (CSHA)

CSHA	Community (%)	Institution (%)
65 years +	4	57
85 years +	13	69

7.4 Dementia and BPSD Are Very Common in Long-Term Care
(Seitz, Purandare, & Conn, 2010)

- Studies show that dementia, behavioural and psychological symptoms of dementia (BPSD), and depression are very common in older adults in long-term care settings (Table 4.1.9).

Table 4.1.9: Prevalence of Dementia and BPSD in Long-Term Care

Disorder	# Studies	Median Prevalence (%)	Prevalence Range (%)
Dementia	30	58	12–95
BPSD	9	78	38–92
Major depression	26	10	2–25
Depression or depressive symptoms	26	29	14–82

BPSD = behavioural and psychological symptoms of dementia

7.5 Dementia and Cognitive Impairment Are Common among Older Patients on Acute Psychiatric Units
(Seitz et al., 2012)

- In Ontario, prevalence in acute psychiatric units for those patients age 65 years plus are as follows:
    - Dementia – 20%
    - Moderate or severe cognitive impairment – 47%
    - Moderate or severe functional impairment – 22%

7.6 Less Severe Forms of Cognitive Impairment Are Even More Common Than Dementia
(CSHA Working Group, 1994; Brookmeyer et al., 2011)

- Cognitive impairment no dementia (CIND)
    - 16.8% in CSHA (age 65 years plus)
    - 22% in ADAMS (age 71 years plus)
        - 71–79 years – 16%
        - 80–89 years – 29%
        - 90+ years – 39%
- Prevalence of minor cognitive impairment (MCI) depends on criteria used.
    - In one study, rates ranged from < 5% for "amnestic MCI" using traditional criteria to 25% using Clinical Dementia Rating Scale 0.5, or 33% using a cognitive classification on psychometric testing (Ganguli et al., 2010).

8. Final Points and Interpretive Tips

- The main limitations of the epidemiological data are:
    - Selective participation
    - Arbitrary age cut-off of 65 years, and in some cases 55 years
    - Retrospective ratings subject to memory problems, reframing
    - Few exceptional studies with prospective clinical exams, chart reviews, and informant histories
    - Most studies largely cross-sectional and lay administered
- When interpreting primary epidemiological studies, consider:
    - Who is being studied? Who is not captured?
    - How are the disorders being measured, and who is making the measurements and decisions?
    - What are the thresholds for illness?

QUESTIONS

1. List five possible reasons why cross-sectional studies show a reduced prevalence of major depression in community-dwelling older adults compared with younger adults.
2. List the two most common anxiety disorders in late life.
3. List four factors affecting the prevalence of cognitive impairment in community studies.
4. Subthreshold symptoms of which four disorders have been found to be associated with adverse outcomes in older adults in community samples?

5. List four settings in which mood disorders in older adults are more common as compared with the low rates in community-dwelling samples.

6. Should we be moving away from categorical studies of prevalence of mental illness in late life towards a more dimensional approach?

7. Describe ways of improving accurate detection of mental illness in epidemiological studies in older populations.

ANSWERS

1. Reasons for the reduced prevalence of major depression in cross-sectional studies of community-dwelling older adults compared with younger adults include:
   - Different manifestation of illness
   - Psychological differences compared with younger adults
   - Limited recall, especially in studies of lifetime prevalence
   - Reframing
   - Different attitudes to surveys
   - More depressed less likely to participate (sampling error)
   - Cohort and cohort-period effect acceptable answers (but less likely)

2. The two most common anxiety disorders in late life are:
   - Phobia
   - Generalized anxiety disorder

(Note: Social phobia and panic disorder are also common in clinic samples with comorbid late-life depression, but rare in "all-comers" in community studies.)

3. Factors affecting the prevalence of cognitive impairment in community studies include:
   - Age
   - Setting (long-term care > community)
   - Country (see Ferri's 2005 Delphi study)
   - Diagnostic criteria
   - Cognitive tests used
   - Functional measures used
   - Sampling procedures

4. Subthreshold symptoms of these disorders are associated with adverse outcomes in older adults in community samples:
   - Depression
   - Delirium
   - Dementia
   - Substance-related disorders

5. Settings in which mood disorders in older adults are more common as compared with the low rates in community-dwelling samples include:
   - Psychiatry inpatients
   - Long-term care
   - Medical inpatients
   - Family practice

6. There are disadvantages and advantages to the categorical approach:
   - Problems with the categorical approach
     - Ignores the fact that those who meet more criteria may have a more serious form of the disorder requiring more intensive intervention
     - Ignores the fact that those who do not meet all criteria ("subthreshold" cases) may still have a disabling and treatable condition
     - Exclusion criteria often leads to an artefactual increase in "co-morbidities"
   - Advantages of the categorical approach
     - Improves communication among clinicians
     - Facilitates treatment decisions

7. Ways of improving accurate detection of mental illness in epidemiological studies in older populations include:
   - Using proxy respondents
   - Using age-appropriate instruments (e.g., those that separate symptoms of depression from changes that accompany normal aging and common medical conditions)
   - Using facilitated recall (e.g., calendars; headlines from newspapers to remind people what was happening in different years)
   - Supplementing with data from administrative databases (e.g., hospitalizations, medications)
   - In the future – technology

CASE DISCUSSION

Knowledge of epidemiology can help guide diagnosis. The most likely diagnosis is dementia, given the vastly higher prevalence of dementia than depression or primary psychotic disorders in the ninth decade of life, and the high prevalence of delusions in dementia. Delirium is also a possible consideration. The approach to the work-up would include a careful history and mental status, collateral history, safety assessment, and consideration of a cholinesterase inhibitor and atypical antipsychotic (further discussion of assessment and management appears in section 1).

RECOMMENDED RESOURCES FOR REVIEW

Although these resources may not be specifically cited in the text, their approach informed the contents of the chapter, and they are recommended as useful further reading.

Meeks TW, Vahia IV, Lavretsky H, et al. A tune in "a minor" can "b major": a review of epidemiology, illness course, and public health implications of subthreshold depression in older adults. J Affect Disord. 2011;129(1-3):126–42. http://www.ncbi .nlm.nih.gov/pubmed/20926139. http://dx.doi.org/10.1016/j.jad.2010.09.015. Medline:20926139

Streiner DL, Patten SB, Anthony JC, et al. Has 'lifetime prevalence' reached the end of its life? An examination of the concept. Int J Methods Psychiatr Res. 2009;18(4):221–8. http://www.ncbi.nlm.nih.gov/pubmed/20052690. http://dx.doi.org/ 10.1002/mpr.296. PMID:20052690

REFERENCES

Beekman AT, Bremmer MA, Deeg DJ, et al. Anxiety disorders in later life: a report from the Longitudinal Aging Study Amsterdam. Int J Geriatr Psychiatry. 1998;13(10):717–26. http://dx.doi.org/10.1002/(SICI)1099-1166(1998100)13:10<717::AID-GPS857>3.0.CO;2-M. Medline:9818308

Bland RC, Newman SC, Orn H. Prevalence of psychiatric disorders in the elderly in Edmonton. Acta Psychiatr Scand Suppl. 1988;77(S338):57–63. http://dx.doi.org/10.1111/j.1600-0447.1988.tb08548.x. PMID:3165596

Blazer DG, Wu LT. The epidemiology of alcohol use disorders and subthreshold dependence in a middle-aged and elderly community sample. Am J Geriatr Psychiatry. 2011;19(8):685–94. http://dx.doi.org/10.1097/JGP.0b013e3182006a96. Medline:21785289

Brookmeyer R, Evans DA, Hebert L, et al. National estimates of the prevalence of Alzheimer's disease in the United States. Alzheimers Dement. 2011;7(1):61–73. http://dx.doi.org/10.1016/j.jalz.2010.11.007. Medline:21255744

Canadian Study of Health and Aging (CSHA) Working Group. Canadian study of health and aging: study methods and prevalence of dementia. CMAJ. 1994;150(6):899–913. Medline:8131123

Christenson R, Blazer D. Epidemiology of persecutory ideation in an elderly population in the community. Am J Psychiatry. 1984;141(9):1088–91. http://dx.doi.org/10.1176/ajp.141.9.1088. PMID:6235752

Copeland JR, Dewey ME, Scott A, et al. Schizophrenia and delusional disorder in older age: community prevalence, incidence, comorbidity, and outcome. Schizophr Bull. 1998;24(1):153–61. http://dx.doi.org/10.1093/oxfordjournals.schbul.a033307. Medline:9502553

Corna LM, Gage L, Cairney J, et al. Psychiatric disorder in later life: a Canadian perspective. In: Cairney J, Streiner DL, editors. Mental disorder in Canada: an epidemiological perspective. Toronto: University of Toronto Press; 2011.

Ebly EM, Parhad IM, Hogan DB, et al. Prevalence and types of dementia in the very old: results from the Canadian Study of Health and Aging. Neurology. 1994;44(9):1593–600. http://dx.doi.org/10.1212/WNL.44.9.1593. Medline:7936280

Ferri CP, Prince M, Brayne C, et al.; Alzheimer's Disease International. Global prevalence of dementia: a Delphi consensus study. Lancet. 2005;366(9503):2112–7. http://dx.doi.org/10.1016/S0140-6736(05)67889-0. Medline:16360788

Forsell Y, Winblad B. Feelings of anxiety and associated variables in a very elderly population. Int J Geriatr Psychiatry. 1998;13(7):454–8. http://dx.doi.org/10.1002/(SICI)1099-1166(199807)13:7<454::AID-GPS795>3.0.CO;2-D. Medline:9695033

Ganguli M, Chang CC, Snitz BE, et al. Prevalence of mild cognitive impairment by multiple classifications: the Monongahela-Youghiogheny Healthy Aging Team (MYHAT) project. Am J Geriatr Psychiatry. 2010;18(8):674–83. http://dx.doi.org/10.1097/JGP.0b013e3181cdee4f. Medline:20220597

Gum AM, King-Kallimanis B, Kohn R. Prevalence of mood, anxiety, and substance-abuse disorders for older Americans in the national comorbidity survey-replication. Am J Geriatr Psychiatry. 2009;17(9):769–81. http://dx.doi.org/10.1097/JGP.0b013e3181ad4f5a. Medline:19700949

Henderson AS, Korten AE, Levings C, et al. Psychotic symptoms in the elderly: a prospective study in a population sample. Int J Geriatr Psychiatry. 1998;13(7):484–92. http://dx.doi.org/10.1002/(SICI)1099-1166(199807)13:7<484::AID-GPS808>3.0.CO;2-7. Medline:9695039

Lenze EJ, Mulsant BH, Shear MK, et al. Comorbid anxiety disorders in depressed elderly patients. Am J Psychiatry. 2000;157(5):722–8. http://dx.doi.org/10.1176/appi.ajp.157.5.722. Medline:10784464

Luijendijk HJ, van den Berg JF, Dekker MJ, et al. Incidence and recurrence of late-life depression. Arch Gen Psychiatry. 2008;65(12):1394–401. http://dx.doi.org/10.1001/archpsyc.65.12.1394. Medline:19047526

Luppa M, Sikorski C, Luck T, et al. Age- and gender-specific prevalence of depression in latest-life – systematic review and meta-analysis. J Affect Disord. 2012;136(3):212–21. http://dx.doi.org/10.1016/j.jad.2010.11.033. Medline:21194754

Mamdani M, Rapoport M, Shulman KI, et al. Mental health-related drug utilization among older adults: prevalence, trends, and costs. Am J Geriatr Psychiatry. 2005;13(10):892–900. http://dx.doi.org/10.1097/00019442-200510000-00009. Medline:16223968

Östling S, Pálsson SP, Skoog I. The incidence of first-onset psychotic symptoms and paranoid ideation in a representative population sample followed from age 70-90 years. Relation to mortality and later development of dementia. Int J Geriatr Psychiatry. 2007;22(6):520–8. http://dx.doi.org/10.1002/gps.1696. Medline:17117394

Pálsson SP, Östling S, Skoog I. The incidence of first-onset depression in a population followed from the age of 70 to 85. Psychol Med. 2001;31(7):1159–68. http://dx.doi.org/10.1017/S0033291701004524. Medline:11681542

Parabiaghi A, Franchi C, Tettamanti M, et al. Antidepressants utilization among elderly in Lombardy from 2000 to 2007: dispensing trends and appropriateness. Eur J Clin Pharmacol. 2011;67(10):1077–83. http://dx.doi .org/10.1007/s00228-011-1054-z. Medline:21553002

Patten SB, Williams JV, Lavorato DH, et al. Recall of recent and more remote depressive episodes in a prospective cohort study. Soc Psychiatry Psychiatr Epidemiol. 2012;47(5):691–6. http://dx.doi.org/10.1007/ s00127-011-0385-5. Medline:21533819

Préville M, Boyer R, Vasiliadis HM, et al.; Scientific Committee of the ESA Study. Persistence and remission of psychiatric disorders in the Quebec older adult population. Can J Psychiatry. 2010;55(8):514–22. Medline:20723279

Regier DA, Boyd JH, Burke JD Jr, et al. One-month prevalence of mental disorders in the United States. Based on five Epidemiologic Catchment Area sites. Arch Gen Psychiatry. 1988;45(11):977–86. http://dx.doi .org/10.1001/archpsyc.1988.01800350011002. Medline:3263101

Saunders PA, Copeland JRM, Dewey ME, et al. Alcohol use and abuse in the elderly: findings from the Liverpool longitudinal study of continuing health in the community. Int J Geriatr Psychiatry. 1989;4(2):103– 8. http://dx.doi.org/10.1002/gps.930040208

Seitz D, Purandare N, Conn D. Prevalence of psychiatric disorders among older adults in long-term care homes: a systematic review. Int Psychogeriatr. 2010;22(7):1025–39. http://dx.doi.org/10.1017/S1041610210000608. Medline:20522279

Seitz DP, Vigod SN, Lin E, et al. Characteristics of older adults hospitalized in acute psychiatric units in Ontario: a population-based study. Can J Psychiatry. 2012;57(9):554–63. Medline:23073033

Streiner DL, Cairney J, Veldhuizen S. The epidemiology of psychological problems in the elderly. Can J Psychiatry. 2006;51(3):185–91. Medline:16618010

Thomas VS, Rockwood KJ. Alcohol abuse, cognitive impairment, and mortality among older people. J Am Geriatr Soc. 2001;49(4):415–20. http://dx.doi.org/10.1046/j.1532-5415.2001.49085.x. Medline:11347785

4.2 Aging and Psychopharmacology

Nathan Herrmann, MD, FRCPC

INTRODUCTION

The ability to safely prescribe medications in an older adult population is a fundamental skill of the geriatric psychiatrist. Prescribing medications to this population is made more difficult and challenging by the variability imposed by the physical effects of age, which can alter both the effect of medications on the patient as well as how the medications are metabolized by the body. Further challenges are the additional effect that disease creates on these processes, and finally, the additional complications posed by medications added to help with these diseases. This chapter provides a succinct review and helps the clinician understand and deal with these many complex interactions.

CASE SCENARIO

Mrs G. is a 78-year-old woman referred by her family physician for the assessment and management of depression. She had a major depressive episode following the birth of her first child at the age of 25, but has been well and without psychiatric treatment since that time. She has a history of diabetes, coronary artery disease (CAD) with stent placement five years ago, and had a left-sided stroke six months ago, leaving her with mild right hemiparesis and dysarthria. Her mood began to decline shortly after the stroke, and she has become increasingly resistive to doing her physiotherapy. She has terminal insomnia and has lost five pounds over the past month. Her medications include metoprolol, hydrochlorothiazide, tolterodine, clopidogrel, glyburide, metformin, and ranitidine. On mental status exam, she is weepy, dysphoric, and hopeless. She scores 25/30 on the Mini Mental State Examination (MMSE).

1. Considering pharmacokinetics and pharmacodynamics, what would you think about before prescribing an antidepressant for this woman?
2. Are medications affecting her clinical presentation in any way?
3. How would you go about ensuring you would not cause a drug-drug interaction (DDI)?

OVERVIEW

1. Some Definitions

- Pharmacodynamics – what a drug does to the body

- Pharmacokinetics – what the body does to the drug
- Pharmacogenetics – how genetic predisposition affects pharmacodynamics and pharmacokinetics

2. Pharmacokinetic Changes

2.1 Drug Absorption and Aging

- Decreased gastric acids and mesenteric blood flow impair absorption.
- Anticholinergic drugs delay absorption.
- Antacids containing Al, Mg, Ca delay absorption.

2.2 Volume of Distribution and the Elderly

- Total body water decreases with age.
- Total body fat increases with age.
- Elimination half-life is directly proportional to volume of distribution (Vd).
- Lipid soluble drugs have large Vd in the elderly.

2.3 Other Pharmacokinetic Facts

- Most psychotropic drugs are highly protein bound (not lithium [Li]).
- Plasma albumin decreases with age.
- Hepatic metabolism decreases with age.
- Congestive heart failure (CHF) impairs hepatic metabolism.

2.4 Renal Clearance with Age

- Glomerular filtration rate (GFR) decreases by 10% per decade > 40 years.
- Half-life of Li in elderly is 36 hours, compared to 24 hours in young.
- Renal clearance plays a significant role in the metabolism of risperidone.
- Thiazide diuretics, some non-steroidal anti-inflammatory drugs (NSAIDs), and angiotensin-converting enzyme inhibitors (ACEIs) decrease Li clearance.

3. Pharmacodynamic Changes

3.1 More Aging Facts

- Decreased baroreceptor responsivity/sensitivity with age
- Decreased acetylcholine (Ach) with age
- Decreased dopamine type 2 (D2) receptors with age
- Increased monoamine oxidase (MAO) with age

3.2 Common Anticholinergic Side Effects

- Common anticholinergic side effects include all of the following:
    - Dry mouth
    - Urinary retention
    - Constipation
    - Exacerbation of closed-angle glaucoma
    - Delirium
    - Tachycardia

3.3 Neurotransmitters and Aging

3.3.1 Norepinephrine (NE)

- NE important for mood, arousal, cognition
- Fewer neurons in locus ceruleus (major brainstem nucleus of NE neurons projecting to cortex)
- Less tyrosine hydroxylase and dihydroxyphenylalanine (DOPA) decarboxylase (decreased synthesis of NE)
- Increased MAOB (greater NE metabolism)
- Some evidence of age-related reductions in NE activity
- But, more NE in plasma and cerebrospinal fluid (CSF) (older men)!

3.3.2 Dopamine (DA)

- Nigrostriatal (movement/posture), tuberoinfundibular (prolactin), mesolimbic and mesocortical (psychosis, mood, cognition)
- Decreased tyrosine hydroxylase and DOPA decarboxylase (decreased synthesis)
- Decreased DA neurons in nigrostriatal tract
- 40–50% reduction in D2 receptors with aging
- Increased MAO increases DA metabolism (more homovanillic acid [HVA] in CSF)
- Increased sensitivity to extrapyramidal symptoms (EPS) from antipsychotics

3.3.3 Serotonin (5-HT)

- Important for mood, appetite, sleep, aggression
- Midbrain raphe nuclei
- Conflicting data on changes in enzymatic synthesis
- Some 5-HT receptors decline with aging (e.g., 5-HT1, 5-HT2), and decreased sensitivity.
    - ? Responsible for changes in sleep, appetite, mood, and/or serotonergic drugs

3.3.4 Acetylcholine (Ach)

- Important for memory, attention, sleep (and muscle movement!)
- Reduced Ach synthesis (choline acetyltransferase [CAT])
- Reduced Ach neurons in basal forebrain nucleus (nucleus basalis of Meynert [NbM])
- Changes in cognition, sleep, and susceptibility to anticholinergic effects

3.4 Some Other Aging Tidbits

- Increased blood-brain barrier (BBB) permeability
- Reduced baroreceptor sensitivity
- Syndrome of inappropriate antidiuretic hormone secretion (SIADH) and hyponatremia with selective serotonin reuptake inhibitors (SSRIs) most common in the elderly
- Decline in P450 activity with some isoenzymes (CYP2C19) but not others (CYP2D6)

4. Drug-Drug Interactions (DDIs)

- More than 2 million adverse drug reactions (ADRs) annually, including 100 000 deaths, in the United States
- 5% of hospital admissions due to ADRs (10–17% of admissions for the elderly)
- 10–30% of ADRs attributable to DDIs

4.1 Pharmacodynamic Interactions

- Determined by drug mechanism of action
- Should therefore be anticipated by clinician
- Some examples:
    - SSRI + L-tryptophan = serotonin syndrome
    - SSRI + ASA = bleeding
    - L-dopa + antipsychotic = Parkinson's disease worsening
    - Cholinesterase inhibitor (ChEI) + oxybutynin = loss of anticipated benefits

4.2 Pharmacokinetic Interactions

- Absorption
    - Antacids, anticholinergics
- Distribution
    - Altered protein binding
    - Diazepam + phenytoin
- Metabolism (see section 4.3)
- Elimination
    - Lithium + diuretics
- P-glycoprotein

4.3 Metabolism

- Most psychotropics metabolized in the liver (not Li and some others).
- Enzymatic transformations:
    - Demethylation
        - Phase 1 (CYP450)
        - Phase 2
- Cytochrome P450 (CYP450) enzymes
    - Enzymes are responsible for oxidation of xenobiotics and drugs.
    - Located in liver, gut, lungs, kidney, brain, skin
    - Influenced by genetic, constitutional, and environmental factors
    - Drugs can be CYP450 substrates, inhibitors, inducers (and combinations of substrates/inducers, substrates/inhibitors).
    - There are genetic polymorphisms for some CYP450.

4.3.1 CYP2D6

- Clinically important, accounts for 30% of oxidative metabolism
- Substrates
  - Psychotropics: tricyclic antidepressants (TCAs), SSRIs (paroxetine, fluoxetine, fluvoxamine), venlafaxine, mirtazapine, antipsychotics (haloperidol, perphenazine, risperidone), ChEIs (galantamine, donepezil)
  - Others: beta-blockers, codeine, dextromethorphan, mexiletine
- Inhibitors
  - Quinidine, fluoxetine, paroxetine, cimetidine
- Inducers – none
- Important polymorphisms
  - Poor metabolizers, extensive metabolizers, ultra-rapid metabolizers
- Consequences of CYP2D6 polymorphisms
  - Unanticipated – we don't genotype (yet!)
  - Clinically important for poor metabolizers – high drug concentrations
    - Cardiotoxicity with venlafaxine; ADRs with TCAs, metoprolol; poor response to codeine
  - Clinically important for ultra-rapid metabolizers – lack of efficacy
    - But … morphine-like reactions with codeine!
- Phenocopying with potent CYP2D6 inhibitors

4.3.2 CYP3A4

- Clinically important, accounts for 50% of oxidative metabolism
- Substrates
  - Psychotropics: TCAs, sertraline, venlafaxine, mirtazapine, alprazolam, antipsychotics (quetiapine, risperidone), ChEIs (galantamine, donepezil)
  - Other: corticobasilar degeneration syndrome, steroids, cyclosporine, protease inhibitors, atorvastatin, clarithromycin, sildenafil
- Inhibitors
  - Fluvoxamine, erythromycin, ketoconazole, amiodarone
- Inducers
  - Carbamazepine, rifampin, phenobarbital, Saint John's Wort
- Grapefruit juice is a potent inhibitor of CYP3A4.

4.3.3 CYP1A2

- Substrates
  - Psychotropics: TCAs, mirtazapine, clozapine, olanzapine
  - Others: theophylline, caffeine, warfarin
- Inhibitors
  - Fluvoxamine, cimetidine, ciprofloxacin
- Inducers
  - Cigarette smoke, cabbage and Brussels sprouts, omeprazole, rifampin

4.3.4 CYP2C9/19

- Substrates
    - Psychotropics: TCAs, citalopram, diazepam, valproic acid
    - Others: NSAIDs, warfarin, proton pump inhibitors (PPIs), losartan
- Inhibitors
    - Fluvoxamine, fluoxetine, amiodarone, cimetidine, fluconazole, omeprazole
- Inducers
    - Carbamazepine, rifampin

4.3.5 Should We Worry about CYP450 DDIs?

- World literature search for DDIs with antidepressants suggests that the most problematic drugs are monoamine oxidase inhibitors (MAOIs) leading to hypertensive crises and serotonin syndrome.
- Most common DDIs with psychotropics that lead to serious problems are pharmacodynamic and not pharmacokinetic.
- Elderly, female, most at risk

4.3.6 When to Worry

- Older age, medically ill, polypharmacy
- Drugs known to cause serious toxicity
    - Antithrombotics, hypoglycemics
- Powerful inhibitors/inducers
- Two or more inhibitors of the same CYP
- Recent discontinuation of CYP450 inducer/inhibitor

4.3.7 How to Avoid DDIs

- Avoid polypharmacy.
- Know the bad guys.
- Develop a personal formulary.
- Use resources.
    - Examples:
        - Epocrates Multicheck (https://online.epocrates.com)
        - Lexicomp (http://online.lexi.com)
- Trust your local pharmacist.

4.3.8 The "Bad Guys"

- Antidepressants
    - Fluoxetine, fluvoxamine, paroxetine
- Others
    - Inhibitors
        - Quinidine, amiodarone, cimetidine, clarithromycin, itraconazole, ketoconazole, verapamil (and grapefruit juice!)
    - Inducers
        - Carbamazepine, phenobarbital, phenytoin, rifampin, St. John's Wort

4.3.9 Some "Good Guy" Suggestions

- Antidepressants
  - Citalopram, escitalopram, sertraline, mirtazapine, desvenlafaxine
- Antipsychotics
  - Loxapine, quetiapine, paliperidone
- Anxiolytics
  - Lorazepam, oxazepam, temazepam
- Cognitive enhancers
  - Rivastigmine, memantine

QUESTIONS

1. List three age-related changes that might affect the pharmacodynamic effects of psychotropic drugs in the elderly.
2. List three potential pharmacodynamic DDIs that might arise in elderly patients prescribed psychotropics.
3. List three age-related changes and three non–age-related factors that might affect the pharmacokinetics of psychotropic drugs in the elderly.
4. List three CYP450 enzymes that could potentially lead to DDIs in elderly patients prescribed psychotropics.
5. Describe three strategies for avoiding DDIs in elderly patients prescribed psychotropics.
6. How concerned should clinicians really be about DDIs in the elderly?
7. Is the safe prescribing of psychotropics really any different for elderly patients compared to younger adults?

ANSWERS

1. Age-related changes that might affect the *pharmacodynamic* effects of psychotropic drugs in older patients include:
   - Decreased baroreceptor responsivity/sensitivity with age (more orthostatic hypotension)
   - Decreased dopamine D2 receptors (increased sensitivity to EPS)
   - Increased monoamine oxidase
   - Decreased acetylcholine (greater sensitivity to anticholinergic effects)
   - Increased permeability of BBB

2. Pharmacodynamic DDIs that might arise in older patients prescribed psychotropics include:
   - ChEI and anticholinergic overactive bladder drugs (e.g., oxybutynin, tolterodine) resulting in less therapeutic benefit from both drugs
   - L-dopa and an antipsychotic, leading to worsening of Parkinsonism
   - SSRI and an antiplatelet drug (e.g., aspirin, clopidogrel), leading to increased bleeding

- SSRI and L-tryptophan, leading to serotonin syndrome
- SSRI and an MAOI leading to serotonin syndrome
- ChEI and beta-blockers, leading to bradycardia
- SSRI and hydrochlorothiazide, leading to increased risk of hyponatremia

3. Factors that might affect the *pharmacokinetics* of psychotropic drugs in older patients include:
   - Age-related
     - Changes in volume of distribution
     - Decreased gastric acid
     - Decreased mesenteric blood flow
     - Decline in renal function
   - Non–age-related
     - Genetic polymorphisms in CYP450 isoenzymes
     - Polypharmacy leading to DDI
     - Diet (e.g., grapefruit juice, cabbage, Brussels sprouts)
     - Smoking and alcohol use
     - Medical comorbidities
     - Race
     - CYP450 interactions (e.g., induction or inhibition)

4. CYP450 enzymes that could potentially lead to DDIs in older patients prescribed psychotropics include:
   - CYP 2D6 (e.g., paroxetine inhibits tamoxifen metabolism)
   - CYP 3A4 (e.g., erythromycin inhibits alprazolam metabolism)
   - CYP 1A2 (e.g., fluvoxamine inhibits theophylline metabolism)
   - CYP 2C9 (e.g., fluvoxamine inhibits warfarin metabolism)
   - CYP 2C19 (e.g., fluoxetine inhibits phenytoin metabolism)

5. Strategies for avoiding DDIs in older patients prescribed psychotropics include:
   - Avoid polypharmacy.
   - Medication reconciliation
   - Avoid drugs with significant potential DDIs (e.g., fluoxetine, fluvoxamine, carbamazepine).
   - Choose drugs with few potential DDIs (e.g., escitalopram, sertraline, lorazepam, quetiapine).
   - Develop a "personal pharmacy" and memorize the metabolic pathways.
   - Work with a good pharmacist.
   - Use online resources and Smartphone apps (e.g., Epocrates, Lexicomp).
   - Obtain blood levels of measurable drugs.
   - Start low, go slow.
   - Patient education

- Select medications that are less likely to accumulate in patients if the context is hepatic or renal impairment.
- Take a full medication history that includes prescribed, over-the-counter (OTC), and herbal medications.

6. The literature suggests that the most concerning DDIs are the pharmacodynamic interactions, which should be predictable based on knowledge of the mechanisms of action of the drugs prescribed. Extra care should be taken with drugs that have narrow therapeutic windows and severe potential toxicity such as warfarin, insulin, antiplatelets, oral hypoglycemics, and anti-epileptic drugs. It is important to keep in mind that most DDIs are not life-threatening.

7. The process of prescribing is the same as in younger adults, but more challenging. Due to age-related pharmacokinetic and pharmacodynamic changes, concomitant medical conditions, and concomitant medications, elderly patients are much more susceptible to adverse drug events and the consequences of DDIs, and do not tolerate them as well as younger patients. Some adverse events are more concerning in elderly patients (e.g., falls, hyponatremia, EPS), while others (e.g., sexual side effects) may be less of a concern.

CASE DISCUSSION

1. Regarding pharmacokinetics and pharmacodynamics, the following concepts should be considered when providing an antidepressant prescription:
   - With history of vascular disease, this patient may also have some renal dysfunction and/or CHF.
   - She is taking multiple medications that have narrow therapeutic windows and may interact with psychotropics.
   - Remember to start low and go slow, but to aim for a therapeutic dosage.

2. Her current medications may be affecting her mental status:
   - Large anticholinergic load with tolterodine and ranitidine
   - β-blockers could impair cognition, and mimic depressive symptoms.
   - Glyburide can cause severe and prolonged hypoglycemia.
   - Diuretic (hydrochlorothiazide) may cause hypokalemia, increase risk of cardiac events, and may contribute to insomnia if patient has nocturia.

3. In order to minimize DDI risk:
   - Choose an antidepressant that is least likely to interact with her medications.
     - Particular concerns with clopidogrel (SSRI may slightly increase risk of gastrointestinal bleed, but potent inhibitors of CYP 2C19 might reduce effects of clopidogrel)
   - Would probably consider escitalopram, which has an excellent safety profile in the studies of its use in post-stroke depression.
   - Obtain a complete list of prescription and OTC medications.
   - Patient education about DDIs and symptoms to look for
   - Ensure that only one pharmacy is involved.
   - Ensure primary care MD aware of new antidepressant.

RECOMMENDED RESOURCES FOR REVIEW

Although these resources may not be specifically cited in the text, their approach informed the contents of the chapter, and they are recommended as useful further reading.

Pollock B, Forsyth C, Bies R. The critical role of clinical pharmacology in geriatric psychopharmacology. Clin Pharmacol Ther. 2009;85(1):89–93. http://dx.doi. org/10.1038/clpt.2008.229. Medline:19037202

Wilkinson GR. Drug metabolism and variability among patients in drug response. N Engl J Med. 2005;352(21):2211–21. http://dx.doi.org/10.1056/NEJMra032424. Medline:15917386

REFERENCES

American Geriatrics Society 2012 Beers Criteria Update Expert Panel. American Geriatrics Society updated Beers Criteria for potentially inappropriate medication use in older adults. J Am Geriatr Soc. 2012;60(4):616–31. http://dx.doi.org/10.1111/j.1532-5415.2012.03923.x. Medline:22376048

Budnitz DS, Lovegrove MC, Shehab N, et al. Emergency hospitalizations for adverse drug events in older Americans. N Engl J Med. 2011;365(21):2002–12. http://dx.doi.org/10.1056/NEJMsa1103053. Medline:22111719

Montastruc F, Sommet A, Bondon-Guitton E, et al. The importance of drug-drug interactions as a cause of adverse drug reactions: a pharmacovigilance study of serotoninergic reuptake inhibitors in France. Eur J Clin Pharmacol. 2012;68(5):767–75. http://dx.doi.org/10.1007/s00228-011-1156-7. Medline:22116460

Nieuwstraten C, Labiris NR, Holbrook A. Systematic overview of drug interactions with antidepressant medications. Can J Psychiatry. 2006;51(5):300–16. Medline:16986820

Spina E, Trifirò G, Caraci F. Clinically significant drug interactions with newer antidepressants. CNS Drugs. 2012;26(1):39–67. http://dx.doi.org/10.2165/11594710-000000000-00000. Medline:22171584

4.3 Antipsychotics in Older Adults

Nathan Herrmann, MD, FRCPC

INTRODUCTION

The use of antipsychotics has been under intense scrutiny, especially when prescribed to patients who also suffer from dementia. Despite these concerns, this class of medications remains an important tool in the arsenal of treatments that geriatric psychiatrists draw upon. In this chapter, Dr Herrmann deals with specific safety concerns. He also presents an evidence-based overview of the literature in the geriatric population, addressing efficacy both in psychotic disorders and other illnesses where these agents are often used, as well as highlighting differences that can affect a clinician's choice for individual antipsychotics.

CASE SCENARIO

Mrs L. is a 78-year-old woman living in a retirement residence who has been referred for the management of her moderate dementia. The family physician at the residence has been treating her with donepezil 10 mg, and with trazodone 100 mg hs for the management of sundowning. She has become progressively more aggressive with the staff, and recently hit another resident following accusation of theft. The home is threatening to discharge her. On mental status exam she is irritable and paranoid. She scores 18/30 on the Mini Mental State Examination (MMSE).

1. What are your therapeutic options for this patient?
2. If you decide to recommend an antipsychotic, which would you choose?
3. If you recommend an antipsychotic, how would you discuss the risks and benefits of therapy with the substitute decision maker (SDM)?

OVERVIEW

1. Antipsychotic Indications

- Delirium
- Dementia
- Delusional disorder
- Schizophrenia, schizoaffective disorder
- Psychotic disorder due to a general medical condition

- Substance/alcohol-induced psychotic disorder
- Major affective disorder with psychosis
- Major affective disorder without psychosis

1.1 Antipsychotic Effectiveness in Delirium

- Flaherty, Gonzales, & Dong, 2011 review:
    - 13 studies, 1 randomized controlled trial (RCT), "severe" limitations
    - Open label studies suggested improvement in delirium severity scores
    - RCT (Tahir et al., 2010) showed no benefit with quetiapine
- Devlin et al., 2010
    - RCT quetiapine vs placebo (added to prn haloperidol), n = 36
    - Faster resolution of delirium, less concomitant haloperidol required

1.2. Evidence of Antipsychotic Effectiveness for Behavioural and Psychological Symptoms of Dementia (BPSD)

- Lanctôt et al., 1998
    - Meta-analysis of 16 RCTs
        - Pooled response: 61% neuroleptic vs 34% placebo (p < .001)
        - Equal drop-out rates, more adverse events with antipsychotics
- Sink, Holden, & Yaffe, 2005
    - Qualitative review: 3 risperidone RCTs, 3 olanzapine RCTs
        - "Doses of 5–10 mg of olanzapine, or 1 mg risperidone appear to be at least modestly effective for treating neuropsychiatric symptoms."
        - "Among the many drugs in use … only the atypical antipsychotics, risperidone and olanzapine, have convincing evidence of efficacy."
- Schneider, Dagerman, & Insel, 2006
    - Meta-analysis 15 RCTs
        - Statistically significant effect sizes for improvement with risperidone and aripiprazole

1.3 Antipsychotic Effectiveness for Schizophrenia

- Few RCTs for schizophrenia
    - Typical antipsychotics
        - Honigfeld et al., 1965: trifluoperazine better than placebo
        - Tsuang et al., 1971: thioridazine = haloperidol
        - Branchey et al., 1978: fluphenazine = thioridazine
    - Atypical antipsychotics
        - Howanitz et al., 1999: clozapine = chlorpromazine
        - Barak et al., 2002: olanzapine better efficacy and less extrapyramidal symptoms (EPS) compared with haloperidol
        - Jeste et al., 2003: risperidone = olanzapine
        - Tzimos et al., 2008: paliperidone = placebo

1.4 Antipsychotic Effectiveness in Affective Disorders

- No RCTs in mania
  - Some "elderly" included in adult RCTs
- No RCTs in acute non-psychotic major depressive episode (MDE)
- Alexopoulos et al., 2008 (very young "elderly")
  - RCT: risperidone augmentation not statistically better than placebo augmentation for depression relapse prevention
- Meyers et al., 2009 (incl. large elderly group)
  - RCT: sertraline + olanzapine better than olanzapine monotherapy for psychotic depression
- Katila et al., 2013
  - RCT of quetiapine (50–300 mg/day) in 338 elderly MDE; significant, rapid improvement in depression compared to placebo, with reasonable tolerability

2. Antipsychotics: Some Details

2.1 Typical/Conventional Antipsychotics

- Chlorpromazine
- Thioridazine
- Haloperidol
- Perphenazine
- Loxapine
- Pimozide
- Methotrimeprazine
- Trifluoperazine

2.2 Typical Antipsychotic Side Effects

- Sedation
- Confusion
- Orthostatic hypotension
- Anticholinergic effects
- Extrapyramidal effects:
  - Annual incidence of tardive dyskinesia (TD) in the elderly is 26% (Jeste et al., 1995)

2.3 Atypical Antipsychotics

- Clozapine
- Risperidone
- Olanzapine
- Quetiapine
- Ziprasidone
- Aripiprazole
- Paliperidone
- Asenapine

2.4 Clozapine

- Least likely to cause/exacerbate EPS
- Risk of agranulocytosis (.5–2%)
  - Likely higher in the elderly
- Cholinergic effects: potent M1 (confusion) receptor blockade and M4 agonist (hypersalivation)
- Blocks α1 (orthostatic hypotension) and H1 (sedation) receptors

- Age-related decreases in clearance (women)
- Partial metabolism by CYP3A4
- 2 RCTs in Parkinson's disease/psychosis
    - Recommended for Parkinson's disease psychosis by American Academy of Neurology (AAN) Practice Parameter (Miyasaki et al., 2006)
    - Recommended for Parkinson's disease psychosis by Movement Disorders Society (Seppi et al., 2011)

2.5 Risperidone

- Potent D2 and α1 receptor blockade, little M1 receptor blockade
- Metabolized by CYP2D6 to 9-OH-risperidone, eliminated primarily by renal excretion
- Minimal sedation, moderate dose-dependent EPS, swelling of ankles (!)
- Multiple RCTs for BPSD, RCT for schizophrenia
    - Recommended for BPSD by the 3rd Canadian Consensus Conference on the Diagnosis and Treatment of Dementia (CCCDTD3), 9–11 March 2006, Montreal (Herrmann & Gauthier, 2008)

2.6 Olanzapine

- High or low M1 receptor blockade?
- Lowest coefficient of inhibition (K1) for H1 blockade (sedation and weight gain?)
- Little α1 blockade
- ? Reduced clearance in the elderly
- Metabolized by CYP1A2 (some CYP2D6)
- Multiple RCTs for BPSD, 1 RCT for schizophrenia, 1 RCT for depression with psychosis (STOP PD) (Meyers et al., 2009)
    - Recommended by CCCDTD3 for BPSD (Herrmann & Gauthier, 2008)

2.7 Quetiapine

- Closest to clozapine in receptor-binding profile
- Low EPS over whole dose range
- Little M1 blockade, modest α1, significant H1 blockade (sedation)
- Clearance reduced by 30–50% in the elderly
- Metabolized by CYP3A4 (some CYP2D6)
- Multiple RCTs in BPSD, multiple RCTs in Parkinson's disease dementia (PDD)
    - Recommended for Parkinson's disease psychosis by AAN Practice Parameter (Miyasaki et al., 2006)
    - Not recommended for Parkinson's disease psychosis by Movement Disorders Society (Seppi et al., 2011)

2.8 Ziprasidone

- 5-HT1A agonist (and a SNRI at higher concentrations)
- Moderate α1 and H1 blockade
- Better metabolic profile?
- Clearance unchanged in older adults

- Metabolized by CYP3A4
- No published RCTs in older adults

2.9 Aripiprazole

- D2 partial agonist, 5-HT1A partial agonist (AD effects?), 5-HT2A antagonist
- Better metabolic profile?
- 3 RCTs with dementia patients (n = 951)
    - Dosages:
        - Start 2 mg/day, max 15 mg/day
        - Usual effective doses 5–10 mg/day
    - Efficacy for agitation, irritability, psychosis
    - Mild excess sedation
- Recommended for BPSD by 4th Canadian Consensus Conference on the Diagnosis and Treatment of Dementia (CCCDTD4) (Herrmann, Lanctôt, & Hogan, 2013)

2.10 Paliperidone

- Active metabolite of risperidone
- No significant hepatic metabolism
- RCT in schizphrenia (Tzimos et al., 2008)
    - N = 114 (not powered for efficacy), average age 70
    - More tachycardia and hyperprolactinemia
    - Greater improvement on Positive and Negative Syndrome Scale (PANSS)

2.11 Asenapine

- High affinity for 5-HT, D3,4, α2, moderate affinity for H1, minimal M1
- Predominant CYP 1A2 metabolism
- No placebo-controlled or comparator RCTs in the elderly
- Dubovsky et al., 2012:
    - RCT of 2 dose escalation regimens, n = 122
    - Decreased clearance in the elderly
        - Reasonably well tolerated with low EPS

3. Antipsychotic Safety Issues

- EPS
- Negative effects on cognition
- Weight gain
- Diabetes mellitus
- Hyperlipidemia
- QTc prolongation
- Cerebrovascular adverse events (CVAEs)
- Mortality

3.1 Extrapyramidal Symptoms (EPS)

- Schneider, Dagerman, & Insel, 2006; meta-analysis of 15 BPSD RCTs
    - Increased risk of EPS: 13% vs 8%: OR 1.51 (95% CIs 1.20–1.91)
        - Accounted for by risperidone alone
    - Increased gait abnormalities: 10% vs 2%: OR 3.42 (95% CIs 1.78–6.56)

- Atypical antipsychotics and Parkinsonism (Rochon et al., 2005)
  - Retrospective cohort study, n = 25 000, dementia, average age 82
  - Risk of incident Parkinsonism compared to atypical antipsychotics (HR, 95%CIs)
    - Typicals 1.30 (1.04–1.58)
    - Untreated 0.40 (0.29–0.43)

3.2 Antipsychotics and Risk of Hip Fracture
(Liperoti et al., 2007)

- Case control study of nursing home residents
- Results: OR for users vs non-users
  - Typicals: 1.35 (95% CI: 1.06–1.71)
  - Atypicals: 1.37 (95% CI 1.11–1.69)

3.3 Antipsychotics and Cognition

- Schneider, Dagerman, & Insel, 2006; meta-analysis
  - MMSE scores reported in 7/15 trials
    - Weighted mean difference 0.73 ($p < .0001$) favouring placebo; greater worsening of cognition in 6/7 studies
- Ballard et al., 2005; RCT with quetiapine
  - Mean worsening on Severe Impairment Battery (SIB) score of 14.6 ($p = 0.009$) (6/52) and 15.4 ($p = 0.01$) (26/52) compared to placebo

3.4 Antipsychotic Metabolic Effects

- May be less of a concern in older adults
- Weight gain in Clinical Antipsychotic Trials of Intervention Effectiveness – Alzheimer's Disease (CATIE-AD) trial (Zheng et al., 2009)
  - Average weight gain 0.08 lbs/week
  - Females demonstrated a statistically significant weight gain of 0.14 lbs/week and a significant effect of duration of use
  - Significant weight gain (7%) noted in 7% placebo-treated patients vs 10% (up to 12 weeks), 17% (12–24 weeks), vs 20% (> 24 weeks) of antipsychotic use
- Glucose and lipids in BPSD RCTs
  - No significant changes from baseline or compared with placebo in risperidone trials or olanzapine trials
  - CATIE-AD 2006 – no significant differences compared with placebo (Zheng et al., 2009)
- Antipsychotics in elderly with diabetes mellitus (DM) (Lipscombe et al., 2009)
  - Nested case control study using administrative health databases including a diabetes registry
  - Subjects > 65 with DM; 13 817 followed for 2 years
  - Cases: hospitalization for hyperglycemia; matched with 10 controls
  - Results:
    - Risk significantly increased with typical and atypical antipsychotics
    - 70% events occur within 14 days of treatment initiation

- ▪ Number needed to harm (NNH) 21 for insulin-treated patients, 42 for oral hypoglycemic-treated patients
- Antipsychotics in non-DM elderly (Lipscombe et al., 2011)
  - Nested case control study of elderly patients hospitalized for hyperglycemia
  - N = 44 121, age = 78, cases = 220
  - Current antipsychotic use significantly associated with hyperglycemia: aOR 1.52 (95%CI 1.07–2.17)
    - ▪ Atypical antipsychotic: aOR 1.44 (95%CI 1.01–2.07)
    - ▪ Typical antipsychotic: aOR 2.86 (95%CI 1.46–5.59)

3.5 *Antipsychotics and QTc*

- QTc > 500 ms increases risk of arrhythmias
- All antipsychotics can lengthen QTc (dose dependent)
- Many risk factors for lengthened QTc
- Not all QTc lengthening leads to arrhythmias
- Significant problem with some typicals (thioridazine, pimozide, etc.)
- Atypicals and QTc changes (msec)

(from ziprasidone FDA submission; Glassman & Bigger, 2001)

– Haloperidol – 4.7	– Quetiapine – 14.5
– Olanzapine – 6.8	– Ziprasidone – 20.3
– Risperidone – 11.6	– Thioridazine – 35.6

3.6 *Antipsychotics and Risk of Ventricular Arrhythmias or Cardiac Arrest*
(Liperoti et al., 2005)

- Case control study, n = 649, 2962 controls, age > 65, various diagnoses
- Risk of hospitalization (adjusted OR, 95% CIs):
  - Atypical vs no use – .87 (.58–1.32)
  - Typical vs no use – 1.86 (1.27–2.74)
  - Typical vs atypical – 2.13 (1.27–3.60)

3.7 *Antipsychotics and Cerebrovascular Adverse Events (CVAEs)*

- UK Committee on Safety of Medicines (CSM, n.d., 9 March 2009; reviewed in Herrmann & Lanctôt, 2005)
  - Calculation of CVAE numbers needed to treat – to harm (NNT[H]) from RCT data (CSM, n.d.):
    - ▪ 6.3 for 1 year of exposure
    - ▪ 37 for 8–12 weeks of exposure
  - Advice: "There is clear evidence of an increased risk of stroke in older patients with dementia who are treated with risperidone or olanzapine. The magnitude of this risk is sufficient to outweigh likely benefits in the treatment of behavioural disturbances." (CSM, 9 March 2004)
- Meta-analysis of BPSD RCTs with risperidone and olanzapine (Herrmann & Lanctôt, 2005)
  - Risperidone (6 studies)

- Total CVAEs: 33/1009 vs 8/712 with placebo
  - RR 3.2 (1.4–7.2)
- Serious CVAEs: 15/1009 vs 4/712 with placebo
  - RR 2.3 (0.5–10.7)
  - Olanzapine (5 studies)
    - Total CVAEs: 15/1179 vs 2/478 with placebo
      - RR 1.8 (0.5–6.3)
- Antipsychotic and stroke risk (Gill et al., 2005)
  - Retrospective cohort study, dementia patients > 65
  - 5-year observation hospitalization for stroke
  - Adjusted hazard ratio comparing atypicals to typicals: no significant difference
  - No difference in subgroups at high risk for stroke

3.8 Antipsychotics and Mortality

- June 2005 Health Canada (Health Canada, 2005)
  - "Of total of 13 placebo-controlled studies performed with risperidone, quetiapine, and olanzapine in elderly demented patients with behavioural disorders, 10 showed numerical increases in all-cause mortality compared to the placebo-treated groups ... [There was] a mean 1.6 fold increase in death rate ... [and] most deaths [were] due to heart-related events or infections." (Health Canada, 2005)
- Risk of death with atypical antipsychotic drug treatment for dementia (Schneider, Dagerman, & Insel, 2005)
  - Meta-analysis of 15 RCTs (9 unpublished)
  - Aripiprazole (3), olanzapine (5), quetiapine (3), risperidone (5)
  - N = 3353 drug treated, n = 1757 placebo
  - Mortality
    - 118 (3.5%) drug treated
    - 40 (2.3%) placebo
  - OR – 1.54 (95% CI 1.06–2.23)
  - 2 trials with haloperidol had similar ORs
- Antipsychotics, BPSD, and mortality (Gill et al., 2007)
  - Retrospective population-based cohort study
  - Age > 65, dementia (n = 20 700)
  - Atypical antipsychotics vs typical antipsychotics vs untreated
  - Results:
    - Typicals > atypicals (e.g., 4.0% vs 2.6%)
    - Atypicals > untreated (e.g., 2.1% vs 1.7%)
- Dementia Antipsychotic Withdrawal Trial (DART-AD) (Ballard et al., 2009)
  - Follow-up of 165 patients who had completed an RCT of antipsychotic withdrawal
  - 12-month survival 70% treated with continued antipsychotic vs 77% treated with placebo
  - HR 0.58 (95% CIs .35-.95)
- Long-term effects of conventional and atypical antipsychotic in patients with probable Alzheimer's disease (Lopez et al., 2013)

- Observational study of 957 AD patients
- Average follow-up 4.3 years for death or institutionalization
- Results:
  - Use of antipsychotics not associated with time to death or institutionalization after controlling for covariates
  - Presence of BPSD (including psychosis and agitation) strongly associated with time to death and institutionalization
- Mortality associated with antipsychotics in patients with Parkinson's disease (Marras et al., 2012)
  - Nested case control study of deaths within 30 days of starting an antipsychotic in elderly with Parkinsonism
  - N = 25 000; cases = 5300
  - Exposure to antipsychotics significantly associated with risk of death: aOR = 2.0 (95% CI 1.4–2.7)
    - Quetiapine aOR = 1.8 (95% CI 1.1–3.0)
    - Typical antipsychotic aOR = 2.4 (95% CI 1.1–5.7)

4. Recommendations for Antipsychotic Prescribing for the Elderly

- Consider evidence for efficacy.
- Consider patients at particular risk for adverse events (AEs): Parkinson's disease, dementia, DM, cerebrovascular risk factors.
- Consider specific drug based on efficacy (?), AE profile, DDI potential.
- Baseline work-up:
  - ECG(?)
  - American Diabetes Association/American Psychiatric Association 2004 guidelines:
    - Weight and height for BMI, BP, fasting blood glucose, fasting lipids
- Monitor for AEs (EPS, metabolic).
- Discontinue when appropriate.

5. Summary

- While there are numerous RCTs of antipsychotics for BPSD, their efficacy is modest and there are many negative studies.
- There are few RCTs of antipsychotics for other indications in the elderly.
- Antipsychotic-treated patients experience more adverse events including EPS, cognitive decline, weight gain, and worsening of some metabolic parameters.
- Antipsychotic-treated patients are more likely to suffer from CVAEs and die with treatment.
- Significant attention should be paid to patients with pre-existing DM and Parkinsonism.
- Antipsychotics continue to be used frequently despite safety concerns.

QUESTIONS

1. List three potential advantages for using atypical antipsychotics over typical antipsychotics in older adults.

2. List three potential adverse effects associated with atypical antipsychotics that are more common in older adults than in younger adults.

3. List three potential adverse effects associated with atypical antipsychotics that are less common in older adults than in younger adults.

4. What is the evidence for the efficacy and safety of antipsychotics for the treatment of schizophrenia in late life?

5. Describe the steps you would take to initiate treatment with an antipsychotic in an older patient with depression and psychotic features.

6. Given the risk of excess mortality, should antipsychotic ever be used to treat patients with dementia?

7. Describe your approach for discussing the risks and benefits of antipsychotic use with the caregiver of a patient with dementia.

ANSWERS

1. Potential advantages for using atypical antipsychotics over typical antipsychotics in older adults include:
   - A more robust evidence base for efficacy and safety
   - Less Parkinsonism
   - Less TD
   - Lower risk of neuroleptic malignant syndrome (NMS)
   - Potential antidepressant effects
   - Fewer EPS
   - Fewer anticholinergic, anti-adrenergic, and antihistaminic side effects (but depends on medication)
   - Less prolactin increase and lower risk of osteoporosis (but depends on medication)

2. Potential adverse effects associated with atypical antipsychotics that are more common in older adults than in younger adults include:
   - Drug-induced Parkinsonism
   - TD
   - Falls/hip fractures
   - Orthostatic hypotension
   - Ankle swelling (especially risperidone)
   - Sedation
   - Confusion
   - Infections/pneumonia
   - Sudden death and other cardiac events (e.g., QTc prolongation, arrhythmias)
   - Cerebrovascular adverse events (elderly patients with dementia)
   - Cognitive decline

3. Potential adverse effects associated with atypical antipsychotics that are less common in older adults than in younger adults include:
   - Metabolic side effects: weight gain, hyperglycemia/diabetes, and hyperlipidemia
   - Acute dystonic reactions

4. Regarding the efficacy and safety of antipsychotics for the treatment of schizophrenia in late life:
   - Overall, evidence is scarce and mostly extrapolated from studies on younger patients

- Efficacy
  - Expert consensus opinion
  - Small number of very old RCTs study typical antipsychotics, and a couple more recent comparator trials (e.g., olanzapine vs risperidone [Jeste et al., 2003])
  - The only recent placebo-controlled trial studied paliperidone vs placebo in 114 patients for 6 weeks (Tzimos et al., 2008), and showed remarkably low efficacy
- Safety
  - Very little data on long-term safety (except for follow-up studies looking at TD that demonstrate extremely high rates in the elderly – up to 60% at 3 years, 4–5 times the rate of younger populations)
  - Evidence from their use in dementia may provide information on safety and side effects

5. In initiating an antipsychotic in an older patient with depression and psychotic features, consider:
   - Discussion with patient and family about risks, benefits, and alternative therapies
   - Review medical history (and family history) of diabetes mellitus, hypertension, hyperlipidemia, heart disease, stroke, concomitant medications, and allergies
   - Past psychiatric history, especially previous treatments
   - Physical exam including BMI, sitting and standing blood pressure, and waist circumference
   - Neurological exam, especially EPS, gait, and postural stability
   - Labs: CBC, electrolytes, TSH, liver function tests, fasting blood glucose, fasting lipids, urinalysis, renal function, prolactin levels if hyperprolactinemia has been a problem in the past
   - Electrocardiogram (ECG)
   - Cognitive assessment
   - Discuss specific adverse effects to report immediately
   - Book timely follow-up to monitor efficacy, adverse effects, and make dose adjustments

6. If behaviour still represents a risk to patient and others after appropriate assessment, use of nonpharmacological approaches, and pharmacotherapy with other agents, using an antipsychotic is an appropriate intervention (assuming informed consent with caregiver); this has been reaffirmed by the 4th Canadian Consensus Conference on the Diagnosis and Treatment of Dementia (Herrmann, Lanctôt, & Hogan, 2013), as well as the most recent American Psychiatric Association (2007) guidelines.

7. An approach for discussing antipsychotic risks and benefits with a caregiver of a patient with dementia would include:
   - Review what has been tried and why you need to consider a change in therapy.
   - Present the option of antipsychotic use in the context of safety as well as quality of life for the patient and caregiver.
   - Emphasize that antipsychotics are the class of drugs with the best evidence of efficacy for managing severe agitation and aggression, and this has been carefully studied in thousands of patients.

- Be specific about safety concerns – start with EPS, then discuss cerebrovascular adverse events and mortality; you may mention the number needed to harm of 100 (i.e., for every 100 patients treated with an antipsychotic, 1 is potentially at risk of dying based on exposure to the drug).
- End by stating that even though there are clearly important potential side effects, you (and the caregiver) will monitor the patient closely for these, and will hopefully plan to discontinue the drug as soon as possible once there has been a reasonable period of stability.

CASE DISCUSSION

1. For this patient:
   - Assessment – rule out delirium.
   - Nonpharmacological approaches (including staff education): recreational therapy, exercise, opportunities to socialize one-on-one or individually, music, etc.
   - Consider increasing the trazodone (adding another daytime dose), trying memantine, or trying an SSRI such as citalopram.
   - Given the risk of harm, an antipsychotic would certainly be indicated.

2. For antipsychotic choice:
   - A low dose of risperidone (most evidence and least sedating), olanzapine or aripiprazole (less likely to produce EPS)
   - If sleep was an issue and/or the aggression occurred in the evening as part of her sundowning, consider quetiapine.

3. See question #2 above in the question and answer section.

RECOMMENDED RESOURCES FOR REVIEW

Although these resources may not be specifically cited in the text, their approach informed the contents of the chapter, and they are recommended as useful further reading.

Chahine LM, Acar D, Chemali Z. The elderly safety imperative and antipsychotic usage. Harv Rev Psychiatry. 2010;18(3):158–72. http://dx.doi.org/10.3109/10673221003747690. Medline:20415632

Leon C, Gerretsen P, Uchida H, et al. Sensitivity to antipsychotic drugs in older adults. Curr Psychiatry Rep. 2010;12(1):28–33. http://dx.doi.org/10.1007/s11920-009-0080-3. Medline:20425307

REFERENCES

Alexopoulos GS, Canuso CM, Gharabawi GM, et al. Placebo-controlled study of relapse prevention with risperidone augmentation in older patients with resistant depression. Am J Geriatr Psychiatry. 2008;16(1):21–30. http://dx.doi.org/10.1097/JGP.0b013e31813546f2. Medline:17928573

American Diabetes Association, American Psychiatric Association, American Association of Clinical Endocrinologists, North American Association for the Study of Obesity. Consensus development conference on antipsychotic drugs and obesity and diabetes. Diabetes Care. 2004;27(2):596–601. http://dx.doi.org/10.2337/diacare.27.2.596. Medline:14747245

American Psychiatric Association. Practice guideline for the treatment of patients with Alzheimer's disease and other dementias. 2nd ed. Am J Psychiatry. 2007;164 (12 Suppl):5–56. Medline:18340692

Ballard C, Hanney ML, Theodoulou M, et al.; DART-AD investigators. The dementia antipsychotic withdrawal trial (DART-AD): long-term follow-up of a randomised placebo-controlled trial. Lancet Neurol. 2009;8(2):151–7. http://dx.doi.org/10.1016/S1474-4422(08)70295-3. Medline:19138567

Ballard C, Margallo-Lana M, Juszczak E, et al. Quetiapine and rivastigmine and cognitive decline in Alzheimer's disease: randomised double blind placebo controlled trial. BMJ. 2005;330(7496):874. http://dx.doi.org/10.1136/bmj.38369.459988.8F. Medline:15722369

Barak Y, Shamir E, Zemishlani H, et al. Olanzapine vs. haloperidol in the treatment of elderly chronic schizophrenia patients. Progr Neuropsychopharmacol Biol Psychiatry. 2002;26(6):1199–202. http://dx.doi.org/10.1016/S0278-5846(01)00322-0. Medline:12452546

Branchey MH, Lee JH, Amin R, et al. High- and low-potency neuroleptics in elderly psychiatric patients. JAMA. 1978;239(18):1860–2. http://dx.doi.org/10.1001/jama.1978.03280450032019. Medline:347110

Cheung G, Stapelberg J. Quetiapine for the treatment of behavioural and psychological symptoms of dementia (BPSD): a meta-analysis of randomised placebo-controlled trials. N Z Med J. 2011;124(1336):39–50. Medline:21946743

Committee on Safety of Medicines (CSM). Atypical antipsychotic drugs and stroke. Letter from CSM Chairman Gordon Duff to medical contacts, 9 March 2004. http://webarchive.nationalarchives.gov.uk/20040628050631/info.doh.gov.uk/doh/embroadcast.nsf/vwDiscussionAll/3D8DBB48B26FF90280256E520045977Af

– Summary of clinical trial data on cerebrovascular adverse events (CVAEs) in randomised clinical trials of risperidone conducted in patients with dementia. n.d. http://www.mhra.gov.uk/home/groups/pl-p/documents/websiteresources/con019490.pdf

Devlin JW, Roberts RJ, Fong JJ, et al. Efficacy and safety of quetiapine in critically ill patients with delirium: a prospective, multicentre randomized double-blind placebo-controlled pilot study. Crit Care Med. 2010;38(2):419–27. http://dx.doi.org/10.1097/CCM.0b013e3181b9e302

Dubovsky SL, Frobose C, Phiri P, et al. Short-term safety and pharmacokinetic profile of asenapine in older patients with psychosis. Int J Geriatr Psychiatry. 2012;27(5):472–82. http://dx.doi.org/10.1002/gps.2737. Medline:21755540

Flaherty JH, Gonzales JP, Dong B. Antipsychotics in the treatment of delirium in older hospitalized adults: a systematic review. J Am Geriatr Soc. 2011;59(Suppl 2):S269–76. http://dx.doi.org/10.1111/j.1532-5415.2011.03675.x. Medline:22091572

Gill SS, Bronskill SE, Normand SL, et al. Antipsychotic drug use and mortality in older adults with dementia. Ann Intern Med. 2007;146(11):775–86. http://dx.doi.org/10.7326/0003-4819-146-11-200706050-00006. Medline:17548409

Gill SS, Rochon PA, Herrmann N, et al. Atypical antipsychotic drugs and risk of ischaemic stroke: population based retrospective cohort study. BMJ. 2005;330(7489):445. http://dx.doi.org/10.1136/bmj.38330.470486.8F. Medline:15668211

Glassman AH, Bigger JT Jr. Antipsychotic drugs: prolonged QTc interval, torsade de pointes, and sudden death. Am J Psychiatry. 2001;158(11):1774–82. Medline:11691681

Health Canada. Atypical antipsychotic drugs and dementia – advisories, warnings and recalls for health professionals. 2005. http://www.healthycanadians.gc.ca/recall-alert-rappel-avis/hc-sc/2005/14307a-eng.php

Herrmann N, Gauthier S. Diagnosis and treatment of dementia: 6. Management of severe Alzheimer disease. CMAJ. 2008; 179(12): 1279–87. http://dx.doi.org/10.1503/cmaj.070804. Medline:19047609

Herrmann N, Lanctôt KL. Do atypical antipsychotics cause stroke? CNS Drugs. 2005;19(2):91–103. http://dx.doi.org/10.2165/00023210-200519020-00001. Medline:15697324

Herrmann N, Lanctôt KL, Hogan DB. Pharmacological recommendations for the symptomatic treatment of dementia: the Canadian Consensus Conference on the Diagnosis and Treatment of Dementia 2012. Alzheimers Res Ther. 2013;5(Suppl 1):S5. http://dx.doi.org/10.1186/alzrt201. PMID:24565367

Honigfeld G, Rosenblum MP, Blumenthal IJ, et al. Behavioral improvement in the older schizophrenic patient: drug and social therapies. J Am Geriatr Soc. 1965;13(1):57–72. http://dx.doi.org/10.1111/j.1532-5415.1965.tb00574.x. PMID:14256223

Howanitz E, Pardo M, Smelson DA, et al. The efficacy and safety of clozapine versus chlorpromazine in geriatric schizophrenia. J Clin Psychiatry. 1999;60(1):41–4. Medline:10074877

Jeste DV, Barak Y, Madhusoodanan S, et al. International multisite double-blind trial of the atypical antipsychotics risperidone and olanzapine in 175 elderly patients with chronic schizophrenia. Am J Geriatr Psychiatry. 2003;11(6):638-47. Medline:14609804

Jeste DV, Caligiuri MP, Paulsen JS, et al. Risk of tardive dyskinesia in older patients. A prospective longitudinal study of 266 outpatients. Arch Gen Psychiatry. 1995;52(9):756–65. http://dx.doi.org/10.1001/archpsyc.1995.03950210050010. Medline:7654127

Katila H, Mezhebovsky I, Mulroy A, et al. Randomized, double-blind study of the efficacy and tolerability of extended release quetiapine fumarate (quetiapine XR) monotherapy in elderly patients with major depressive disorder. Am J Geriatr Psychiatry. 2013;21(8):769–84. http://dx.doi.org/10.1016/j.jagp.2013.01.010. Medline:23567397

Lanctôt KL, Best TS, Mittmann N, et al. Efficacy and safety of neuroleptics in behavioral disorders associated with dementia. J Clin Psychiatry. 1998;59(10):550–61, quiz 562–3. http://dx.doi.org/10.4088/JCP.v59n1010. Medline:9818639

Liperoti R, Gambassi G, Lapane KL, et al. Conventional and atypical antipsychotics and the risk of hospitalization for ventricular arrhythmias or cardiac arrest. Arch Intern Med. 2005;165(6):696–701. http://dx.doi.org/10.1001/archinte.165.6.696. Medline:15795349

Liperoti R, Onder G, Lapane KL, et al. Conventional or atypical antipsychotics and the risk of femur fracture among elderly patients: results of a case-control study. J Clin Psychiatry. 2007;68(6):929–34. http://dx.doi.org/10.4088/JCP.v68n0616. Medline:17592919

Lipscombe LL, Lévesque L, Gruneir A, et al. Antipsychotic drugs and hyperglycemia in older patients with diabetes. Arch Intern Med. 2009;169(14):1282–9. http://dx.doi.org/10.1001/archinternmed.2009.207. Medline:19636029

– Antipsychotic drugs and the risk of hyperglycemia in older adults without diabetes: a population-based observational study. Am J Geriatr Psychiatry. 2011;19(12):1026–33. http://dx.doi.org/10.1097/JGP.0b013e318209dd24. Medline:22123274

Lopez OL, Becker JT, Chang YF, et al. The long-term effects of conventional and atypical antipsychotics in patients with probable Alzheimer's disease. Am J Psychiatry. 2013;170(9):1051–8. http://dx.doi.org/10.1176/appi.ajp.2013.12081046. Medline:23896958

Marras C, Gruneir A, Wang X, et al. Antipsychotics and mortality in Parkinsonism. Am J Geriatr Psychiatry. 2012;20(2):149–58. http://dx.doi.org/10.1097/JGP.0b013e3182051bd6. Medline:22273735

Meyers BS, Flint AJ, Rothschild AJ, et al.; STOP-PD Group. A double-blind randomized controlled trial of olanzapine plus sertraline vs olanzapine plus placebo for psychotic depression: the study of pharmacotherapy of psychotic depression (STOP-PD). Arch Gen Psychiatry. 2009;66(8):838–47. http://dx.doi.org/10.1001/archgenpsychiatry.2009.79. Medline:19652123

Miyasaki JM, Shannon K, Voon V, et al.; Quality Standards Subcommittee of the American Academy of Neurology. Practice parameter: evaluation and treatment of depression, psychosis, and dementia in Parkinson disease (an evidence-based review): report of the Quality Standards Subcommittee of the American Academy of Neurology. Neurology. 2006;66(7):996–1002. http://dx.doi.org/10.1212/01.wnl.0000215428.46057.3d. Medline:16606910

Rochon PA, Stukel TA, Sykora K, et al. Atypical antipsychotics and Parkinsonism. Arch Intern Med. 2005;165(16):1882–8. http://dx.doi.org/10.1001/archinte.165.16.1882. Medline:16157833

Schneider LS, Dagerman KS, Insel P. Risk of death with atypical antipsychotic drug treatment for dementia: meta-analysis of randomized placebo-controlled trials. JAMA. 2005;294(15):1934–43. http://dx.doi.org/10.1001/jama.294.15.1934. Medline:16234500

– Efficacy and adverse effects of atypical antipsychotics for dementia: meta-analysis of randomized, placebo-controlled trials. Am J Geriatr Psychiatry. 2006;14(3):191–210. http://dx.doi.org/10.1097/01.JGP.0000200589.01396.6d. Medline:16505124

Seppi K, Weintraub D, Coelho M, et al. The Movement Disorder Society Evidence-Based Medicine Review Update: treatments for non-motor symptoms of Parkinson's disease. Mov Disord. 2011;26(Suppl S3):S42–80. http://dx.doi.org/10.1002/mds.23884. Medline:22021174

Sink KM, Holden KF, Yaffe K. Pharmacological treatment of neuropsychiatric symptoms of dementia: a review of the evidence. JAMA. 2005;293(5):596–608. http://dx.doi.org/10.1001/jama.293.5.596. Medline:15687315

Tahir TA, Eeles E, Karapareddy V, et al. A randomized controlled trial of quetiapine versus placebo in the treatment of delirium. J Psychosom Res. 2010;69(5):485–90. http://dx.doi.org/10.1016/j.jpsychores.2010.05.006. Medline:20955868

Tsuang MM, Lu LM, Stotsky BA, et al. Haloperidol versus thioridazine for hospitalized psychogeriatric patients: double-blind study. J Am Geriatr Soc. 1971;19(7):593–600. http://dx.doi.org/10.1111/j.1532-5415.1971.tb02580.x. PMID:4937658

Tzimos A, Samokhvalov V, Kramer M, et al. Safety and tolerability of oral paliperidone extended-release tablets in elderly patients with schizophrenia: a double-blind, placebo-controlled study with six-month open-label extension. Am J Geriatr Psychiatry. 2008;16(1):31–43. http://dx.doi.org/10.1097/JGP.0b013e31815a3e7a. Medline:18165460

Zheng L, Mack WJ, Dagerman KS, et al. Metabolic changes associated with second-generation antipsychotic use in Alzheimer's disease patients: the CATIE-AD study. Am J Psychiatry. 2009;166(5):583–90. http://dx.doi.org/10.1176/appi.ajp.2008.08081218. Medline:19369318

4.4 Anticholinergic Drugs and Inappropriate Medications in Older Adults

Maria Hussain, MD, FRCPC
Sudeep S. Gill, MD, MSc, FRCPC

INTRODUCTION

The population of older adults is increasing worldwide, and consequently the number of medical comorbidities in this population is also on the rise. The use of potentially inappropriate medications is common in older adults, and some potent anticholinergic medications may be inappropriate as they can provoke adverse events in the elderly, including delirium, falls, and fractures. It is important for geriatric psychiatrists to be knowledgeable about anticholinergic medications and other inappropriate medication use in the elderly, as well as be able to recognize the impact of these medications on this vulnerable population.

CASE SCENARIO

Mrs E. is a 76-year-old woman whom you are seeing for the first time in consultation at the request of her family physician. The reason for referral is memory complaints on a background of depression and chronic pain related to osteoarthritis (OA) and neuropathic pain. Her other medical conditions include urinary urge incontinence, diabetes mellitus, dyslipidemia, gastroesophageal reflux disease, and hypothyroidism. Her Montreal Cognitive Assessment (MoCA) score is 20/30 and her attention is poor, but there are no major functional deficits. At the present time she has no complaints or symptoms aside from her cognition, and bloodwork and other screening investigations are normal. Her current prescribed medications include metformin 500 mg po bid, oxybutynin 5 mg po od, atorvastatin 20 mg po od, mirtazapine 30 mg po od, amitriptyline 25 mg po qhs, Tylenol #3 po tid, and levothyroxine 0.1 mg po od.

You suspect that her cognitive complaints may be partially attributable to anticholinergic medications. What are some potential medication and non-medication recommendations that may be helpful to reduce her current overall anticholinergic burden?

OVERVIEW

1. Classification of Anticholinergic Drugs and Inappropriate Medications in the Elderly

(American Geriatrics Society 2015 Beers Criteria Update Expert Panel, 2015; Carnahan et al., 2002; Carnahan et al., 2006)

- According to the Beers criteria, certain medications are classified as potentially inappropriate medications (PIMs) if the risk of adverse drug events associated with the medication outweighs its potential benefits.

1.1 Anticholinergic Agents

- Anticholinergic agents block the neurotransmitter acetylcholine typically at its muscarinic receptors, and this muscarinic receptor blockade can take place in the central nervous system as well as the peripheral target organs (e.g., respiratory system, cardiovascular system, gastrointestinal tract, genitourinary tract).
- This mechanism is responsible for the therapeutic action of certain anticholinergic agents such as antispasmodic agents for overactive bladder and urge urinary incontinence (e.g., oxybutynin, tolterodine), as well as bronchodilating medications (e.g., ipratropium, tiotropium). Inhaled anticholinergic medications used as bronchodilating medications are thought to have relatively limited systemic absorption.
- There are also many medications whose main mechanism of action may not be recognized as the blockade of acetylcholine, but which still have significant anticholinergic activity. Example of these would be antidepressants (e.g., tricyclic antidepressants), antipsychotics (e.g., low potency typical antipsychotics), and gastrointestinal agents (e.g., Belladonna alkaloids).
- Many medications with significant anticholinergic activity do not require a prescription and are available as over-the-counter medications. Examples of over-the-counter medications with strong anticholinergic activity include diphenhydramine, dimenhydrinate and loratidine.
- The anticholinergic burden carried by each agent is different, and is referred to as its anticholinergic activity (AA).
- The AA of anticholinergic agents is determined by the particular agent as well as the dose at which it is administered.
- Serum AA represents the binding of all of the compounds in a person's body, including medications and endogenous substances, to muscarinic receptors. Serum AA is measured using a radio receptor competitive binding assay.
- The Anticholinergic Drug Scale (ADS) is a tool that allows estimation of the cumulative anticholinergic burden in a clinical setting, and some studies have shown that its total scores are significantly associated with serum AA assays. Several cumulative anticholinergic drug burden scales have been developed; some are designed primarily for research purposes and may be too cumbersome for use in clinical settings.

1.2 Other Inappropriate Medications in the Elderly

(American Geriatrics Society 2015 Beers Criteria Update Expert Panel, 2015)

- Apart from anticholinergic medications, the Beers criteria also incorporates a number of other medications that are deemed potentially inappropriate and can result in adverse effects, especially when used in the elderly.

- Some of the reasons older adults are more vulnerable to these medications are changes in drug metabolism with aging, drug-disease interactions, and drug-drug interactions.
- These medications include cardiovascular medications (e.g., clonidine, methyldopa), pain medications (e.g., meperidine), as well as medications used to treat diabetes (e.g., long-duration sulfonylureas).
- Although these medications may cause adverse effects in any individual, these effects are accentuated in the elderly, potentially due to multiple medical comorbidities as well as alterations in drug metabolism in this population.
- Some examples of commonly used psychotropic medications that would fall in this category according to the Beers criteria are:
    - Benzodiazepines: recommended that these be avoided for the use of insomnia and delirium in the elderly due to the risk of decreased metabolism, risk of cognitive impairment and delirium, as well as risk of falls, accidents, and fractures
    - Non-benzodiazepine hypnotics (e.g., zolpidem, zaleplon): chronic use exceeding 3 months should be avoided, due to similar risks with use as for benzodiazepines
- It should also be noted that sliding scale insulin, which is commonly used in hospital settings, should be avoided due to higher risk of hypoglycemia without benefit for control of hyperglycemia.

2. Drug Metabolism in the Elderly

(Bressler & Bahl, 2003; Klotz, 2009):

(See also chapter 4.2)

- Numerous age-related physiological changes that have a direct impact on drug metabolism occur in the body.
- These changes include, but are not restricted to, increased gastric pH, increased body fat, decreased total body water, decreased serum albumin, decreased hepatic mass and blood flow, and decreased renal blood flow and creatinine clearance.
- Absorption, for most drugs, remains unchanged in the elderly.
- The volume of distribution of water soluble drugs appears to decrease, while the volume of distribution and half-life of lipophilic drugs may increase.
- Hepatic drug clearance can be reduced significantly; phase I metabolism is more likely to be impaired, whereas phase II metabolism is preserved.
- Renal clearance of drugs, especially those that are primarily excreted renally, decreases.

3. Side Effects of Anticholinergic Medications in the Elderly

- Anticholinergic medications can potentially have numerous side effects, particularly in older adults.
- One way of categorizing these side effects is to classify them as cognitive and non-cognitive side effects (Table 4.4.1).

3.1 Cognitive Side Effects of Anticholinergic Medications

(Mintzer & Burns, 2000; Chew et al., 2008; Campbell et al., 2009)

- Acetylcholine modulates higher functions of the brain like attention, learning, and memory.
- Cholinergic function decreases with age, but cholinergic deficits are especially prominent in people with cognitive dysfunction.

Table 4.4.1: Side Effects of Anticholinergic Medications

Cognitive Side Effects	Non-Cognitive Side Effects
• Decreased attention	• Dry mouth
• Decreased concentration	• Speech difficulties
• Memory impairment	• Swallowing difficulties
• Delirium	• Vision disturbances
• Global cognitive decline with prolonged use (possibly MCI and worsening of pre-existing cognitive dysfunction)	• Conduction abnormalities
	• Hyperthermia
	• Urinary retention
	• Constipation
	• Falls

MCI = mild cognitive impairment

- Therefore older adults, particularly those with pre-existing cognitive impairment, are vulnerable to the anticholinergic side effects of medications (Table 4.4.1).

3.1.1 Delirium

- Delirium is an acute adverse cognitive effect of anticholinergic medications.
- Anticholinergic medications are the most common cause of drug-induced delirium.
- The Confusion Assessment Method (CAM) and DSM criteria for delirium have been used in many studies investigating the impact of anticholinergic medications on delirium, and most identify a positive relationship.
- Some studies have shown that the serum AA is positively correlated with the development of delirium, whereas others do not support this association.

3.1.2 Other Cognitive Deficits

- Anticholinergic medications affect attention and concentration; these may or may not be part of an episode of delirium.
- Memory is affected as well, and a long-term consequence of anticholinergic use may be mild cognitive impairment, or a worsening of cognitive impairment in those who have pre-existing dementia.
- It has been shown that acute administration of scopolamine produces a cognitive presentation that is similar to Alzheimer's disease.
- It has also been demonstrated that serum AA correlates with global cognitive decline in older adults who are taking anticholinergic medications.

3.2 Non-Cognitive Side Effects of Anticholinergic Medications
(Mintzer & Burns, 2000)

- There are a number of non-cognitive side effects of anticholinergic medications that can impact the quality of life for older adults, and can cause significant morbidity (Table 4.4.1).
- Some of these side effects include dry mouth, which in more severe cases can cause speech and swallowing difficulties; urinary retention; constipation; fatigue; cardiovascular side effects including conduction disturbances and exacerbation of

angina; vision disturbances secondary to pupillary dilatation, which can produce blurry vision and lead to falls and subsequent morbidity from fractures and other injuries.

- Falls can also be a consequence of drowsiness secondary to anticholinergic medications, as well as due to the cognitive sequelae of anticholinergic medications, e.g., delirium.

4. Developing an Approach to Limiting the Use of Anticholinergic and Other Inappropriate Medication Use in the Elderly

(Mintzer & Burns, 2000; Garfinkel, Zur-Gil, & Ben-Israel, 2007; Hajjar, Cafiero, & Hanlon, 2007; Chew et al., 2008)

4.1 Pharmacology in Older Adults

- As described earlier, it is imperative that clinicians recognize the changes in drug metabolism that occur as a part of normal aging.
- Recognize that a number of medications that may not be primarily appreciated as having anticholinergic activity can cause muscarinic receptor blockade.
- Older adults are more vulnerable to side effects caused by the same medications as compared to when these agents are administered to younger adults.

4.2 Polypharmacy

- Older adults may have multiple medical comorbidities, including mental health and medical conditions, which require treatment and therefore result in polypharmacy.
- Studies have also found that many elderly patients may be taking medications without indication, and/or at subtherapeutic doses, as well as with therapeutic duplication.
- It has been shown that unnecessary medications can be safely reduced and/or discontinued, following a systematic approach, and this leads to decreased mortality, decrease in referrals to acute-care facilities, lowered costs, and improvement of quality of life.

4.3 Psychotropic Medications

- Psychotropic medications are some of the commonest medications prescribed to older adults.
- Many antidepressants and antipsychotics (typical and atypical) carry a high anticholinergic burden, and sedative hypnotics are also classified as inappropriate when prescribed to older adults.

4.3.1 Decreasing Anticholinergic Load, and Other Side Effects Due to Antidepressants in Older Adults

- Avoid the use of tricyclic antidepressants (TCAs).
- In the case where there is a strong need for use of TCAs (e.g., due to failed adequate trials of other medications like selective serotonin reuptake inhibitors [SSRIs]), the physician should be aware that within this class of medications each carries a different anticholinergic burden (e.g., nortriptyline is less anticholinergic than amitriptyline).
- Certain SSRIs, like paroxetine, have significant anticholinergic activity.
- Other SSRIs like fluoxetine have very long half-lives, which may potentiate adverse effects.

- Paroxetine and fluoxetine also have significant propensity for drug-drug interactions.
- Use the minimum effective dose of antidepressant, and review progress and adverse effects periodically.

4.3.2 Decreasing Anticholinergic Burden and Other Side Effects Due to Use of Antipsychotic Medication in Older Adults

- Antipsychotics are another class of psychotropic medications with a high anticholinergic load.
- Clinicians must remain aware that these medications have a spectrum of neurotransmitter activity, which can result in different adverse effects.
- For example, some antipsychotics (e.g., haloperidol, risperidone) have low anticholinergic activity, but are potent dopamine antagonists and therefore have a high propensity to cause extrapyramidal adverse effects in older adults.
- Examples of antipsychotics with high anticholinergic activity include the low potency typical antipsychotic chlorpromazine, and the atypical antipsychotics clozapine and olanzapine.
- These medications should be used in their minimal effective doses as well, and the patient closely observed for the range of adverse effects.

QUESTIONS

1. List five strategies to decrease the likelihood of inappropriate prescribing to older adults.
2. List five highly anticholinergic medications.
3. List four anticholinergic medications used in the treatment of urinary incontinence.
4. List five consequences of adverse drug events in older adults.

ANSWERS

1. To decrease the likelihood of inappropriate prescribing:
   - Ascertain all current medications.
   - Identify high-risk patients.
   - Estimate life expectancy.
   - Define care goals in light of life expectancy.
   - Define indications for ongoing treatment.
   - Estimate the magnitude of benefit or harm.
   - Review the relative utility of drugs.
   - Identify drugs to be discontinued.
   - Implement and monitor drug minimization strategies.
2. Highly anticholinergic medications include:
   - Tricyclic antidepressants: doxepin, amitriptyline, imipramine
   - Antipsychotics: clozapine, olanzapine, and low potency typical antipsychotics (chlorpromazine, methotrimeprazine)
   - Anti-Parkinsonian drugs: benztropine
   - First-generation antihistamines: diphenhydramine
   - Bladder anticholinergics: oxybutynin, tolterodine (see also #3 below)
   - Atropine (including eye drops)

3. Anticholinergic medications used in the treatment of incontinence include:
   - Oxybutynin
   - Tolterodine
   - Darifenacin, solifenacin
   - Trospium
4. Consequences of adverse drug effects in older adults include:
   - Cognitive impairment (acute = delirium, or chronic = MCI or new/worsened dementia)
   - Dry mouth, urinary retention, constipation
   - Falls, fall-related injuries such as fractures
   - Hospitalization
   - Death

CASE DISCUSSION

Non-medication recommendations:
- Timed toileting
- Caffeine restriction and substitution with non-caffeinated fluids
- Incontinence pads/undergarments
- Physiotherapy and/or occupational therapy if patient is having trouble getting to bathroom on time
- Referral to continence advisor to teach pelvic floor muscle (Kegel) exercises
- Bladder scan or in-and-out urinary catheterization to measure post-void residual urine volume in order to rule out urinary retention and resultant overflow incontinence as a contributor to this patient's urinary incontinence
- Rule out urinary tract infection, atrophic vaginitis, and urinary retention.
- Exercise and weight loss to decrease reliance on metformin for glycemic control
- Sleep assessment (initially by diary, followed by polysomnography if necessary/indicated)
- Increased social engagement
- Evaluate symptoms of depression as it may be suboptimally controlled.
- Repeat MoCA 4 weeks after medication discontinuation is implemented.
- Check thyroid function to ensure that it is not contributing to the clinical picture.

Medication recommendations:
- Discontinue amitriptyline and consider substituting with another medication to manage the condition for which the amitriptyline was being used, e.g., for neuropathic pain consider either gabapentin or pregabalin, or for nighttime sedation, consider nonpharmacological approaches (e.g., warm glass of milk, sleep hygiene measures).
- Discontinue oxybutynin.
- Taper and discontinue Tylenol #3; replace with acetaminophen for OA pain and consider topical anti-inflammatory agent (e.g., topical diclofenac) for breakthrough pain.
- Refer to pain clinic for specialty management if pain persists despite above recommendations.

RECOMMENDED RESOURCES FOR REVIEW

Although these resources may not be specifically cited in the text, their approach informed the contents of the chapter, and they are recommended as useful further reading.

Carrière I, Fourrier-Reglat A, Dartigues JF, et al. Drugs with anticholinergic properties, cognitive decline, and dementia in an elderly general population: the 3-city study. Arch Intern Med. 2009;169(14):1317–24. http://dx.doi.org/10.1001/archinternmed .2009.229. Medline:19636034

Guaraldo L, Cano FG, Damasceno GS, et al. Inappropriate medication use among the elderly: a systematic review of administrative databases. BMC Geriatr. 2011;11(1):79.

Rudolph JL, Salow MJ, Angelini MC, et al. The anticholinergic risk scale and anticholinergic adverse effects in older persons. Arch Intern Med. 2008;168(5):508–13. http:// dx.doi.org/10.1001/archinternmed.2007.106. Medline:18332297

REFERENCES

American Geriatrics Society 2015 Beers Criteria Update Expert Panel. American Geriatrics Society 2015 updated Beers Criteria for potentially inappropriate medication use in older adults. J Am Geriatr Soc. 2015;63(11):2227–46. http://dx.doi.org/10.1111/jgs.13702. Medline:26446832

Bressler R, Bahl JJ. Principles of drug therapy for the elderly patient. Mayo Clin Proc. 2003;78(12):1564–77. http://dx.doi.org/10.4065/78.12.1564

Campbell N, Boustani M, Limbil T, et al. The cognitive impact of anticholinergics: a clinical review. Clin Interv Aging. 2009;4:225–33. Medline:19554093

Carnahan RM, Lund BC, Perry PJ, Pollock BG. A critical appraisal of the utility of the serum anticholinergic activity assay in research and clinical practice. Psychopharmacol Bull. 2002;36(2):24–39. Medline:12397838

Carnahan RM, Lund BC, Perry PJ, Pollock BG, Culp KR. The Anticholinergic Drug Scale as a measure of drug-related anticholinergic burden: associations with serum anticholinergic activity. J Clin Pharmacol. 2006;46(12):1481–6. http://dx.doi.org/10.1177/0091270006292126. Medline:17101747

Chew ML, Mulsant BH, Pollock BG, et al. Anticholinergic activity of 107 medications commonly used by older adults. J Am Geriatr Soc. 2008;56(7):1333–41. http://dx.doi.org/10.1111/j.1532-5415.2008.01737.x. Medline:18510583

Garfinkel D, Zur-Gil S, Ben-Israel J. The war against polypharmacy: a new cost-effective geriatric-palliative approach for improving drug therapy in disabled elderly people. Isr Med Assoc J. 2007;9(6):430–4. Medline:17642388

Hajjar ER, Cafiero AC, Hanlon JT. Polypharmacy in elderly patients. Am J Geriatr Pharmacother. 2007;5(4):345–51. http://dx.doi.org/10.1016/j.amjopharm.2007.12.002. Medline:18179993

Klotz U. Pharmacokinetics and drug metabolism in the elderly. Drug Metab Rev. 2009;41(2):67–76. http:// dx.doi.org/10.1080/03602530902722679. Medline:19514965

Mintzer J, Burns A. Anticholinergic side-effects of drugs in elderly people. J R Soc Med. 2000;93(9):457–62. Medline:11089480

ADDITIONAL E-RESOURCES

Drugs.com: http://www.drugs.com/

Wolters Kluwer clinical drug information: ww.wolterskluwercdi.com

4.5 Psychosocial Aspects of Care in Geriatric Psychiatry

Carole Cohen, MD, FRCPC

DISCLAIMER

This chapter is not meant to provide legal advice or specific recommendations for those acting as legal experts.

INTRODUCTION

In this section, an array of ethical and practical topics pertaining to the psychiatric care of older adults is discussed.

Consent and Capacity Assessments of the Elderly. This book outlines approaches to treatment for many mental disorders, and it is critical that the geriatric psychiatrist understand the options thoroughly, and be able to effectively communicate the pros and cons of the various options to patients. However, many older adults have impairment of cognition and insight that may affect their capacity to understand and appreciate this discussion. The geriatric psychiatrist needs to be able to recognize when the symptoms and impairments of illness bear relevance on the capacity to make treatment decisions. In this chapter, Dr Cohen outlines important principles and approaches to understanding issues of capacity and consent, including treatment and other decisions facing the older adult with mental illness.

Psychiatry in Long-term Care and Community Settings. Principles and practice patterns of geriatric psychiatry that are taught in academic hospital settings form the bulk of evidence-based geriatric mental health. Dr Cohen considers adaptations that are needed in order to provide effective care to our patients in settings outside of hospitals, in long-term care homes and other community settings.

Caregiver Burden, Abuse, and Neglect. Our colleagues in child psychiatry use the term "identified patient," and in geriatric psychiatry, we face daily reminders of just how devastating mental illness can be for the family caregivers. The ideal of an empathic caregiver with endless patience is not always achievable, and abuse can be both the precipitant and consequence of late-life mental illness. In this chapter, Dr Cohen discusses caregiver burden, as well as elder abuse and neglect. The case scenarios provided here highlight some of the challenges associated with these topics.

CASE SCENARIOS

Scenario 1. Mr K. is an 85-year-old married man who is a retired construction worker. He was admitted to a long-term care (LTC) facility from his home where he resided with his wife of 60 years. He has a history of moderate dementia (mixed Alzheimer's disease [AD] and vascular dementia [VaD]), significant vascular risk factors, poor eyesight, chronic kidney disease, and anaemia. He is referred for a psychogeriatric assessment because of resistance to personal care in the LTC home. His wife spends all her days at the LTC home and never seems satisfied with the staff's interactions with her husband. She believes the staff may be poisoning her husband, as he often states, and also seems depressed.

1. How would you approach the psychogeriatric assessment and subsequent treatment of Mr K.?
2. What factors may predispose Mrs K. to depression?

Scenario 2. Mrs C. is a 72-year-old widowed woman living with her 35-year-old unemployed son in a house she owns. She is referred for a psychogeriatric assessment because she is failing to attend scheduled appointments with her family physician as she previously did, does not seem to be taking her thyroid replacement medication consistently, and is using excessive quantities of Tylenol #3. The social worker at the local community agency has visited Mrs C. and found it difficult to interview her alone without her son. She found the house in need of cleaning and minor repairs, and Mrs C. unkempt and unable to give a consistent history.

3. How would you approach the psychogeriatric assessment of Mrs C.?
4. If you were asked to assess Mrs C.'s capacity to manage her finances, how would you proceed?

OVERVIEW

1. Consent and Capacity

1.1 General Principles

- Presumption of capacity
- Right to self-determination
- Use the least restrictive approach

1.2 Additional Principles of Capacity

- Situation specific
- Task specific
- Jurisdiction specific
- Not determined by diagnosis or committal status
- Not the same as agreement with the clinician
- Not determined by a Mini Mental State Examination (MMSE) score

1.3 Substituted Judgment

- Before incapacity – assign a proxy or power of attorney (POA); outline advance directives/living wills
- After incapacity – clinician seeks valid proxy consent from substitute decision maker (SDM), who follows prior expressed wishes or best interest standard
- Finding of incapacity may be challenged
- If clinician disagrees with SDM → ethical or legal process to resolve this potential conflict

1.4 Supported Decision Making

- An alternative process in which the patient may not be formally declared incapable
- Clinician seeks consent from patient who may have support from others to assist in decision making

1.5 Clinical Assessments vs Capacity Assessments

- Clinical assessments are for diagnosis and treatment; they try to "solve problems," enable clinicians to do the best for the patient, and increase the patient's ability to thrive
- Capacity assessments are to make a capacity determination. The "assessor" is making a judgment about decision-making ability and determining if someone's rights may be removed

1.6 Points to Consider in Conducting Capacity Assessments

Trigger
- What domain/what legal jurisdiction
- Why an assessment is needed
- Are other options available?

Information from others

Education and involvement of the client
- Proposed treatment, current finances
- Options: what are the consequences of status quo or potential options/ interventions?

Optimize functioning during the assessment
- Treat reversible conditions
- Pay attention to the time of day
- Optimize vision and hearing
- Use a translator

Clinical considerations
- Diagnosis
- Cognitive functioning
- Functional abilities

Understanding of preferences and values

Knowing when to consult others

Decision-making capacity
- Understanding of information
- Appreciating the relevance for the person
- Rationally manipulate the information (reasoning)
- Expressing a consistent choice

Documentation
- Link (in)ability to understand/appreciate to diagnosis, cognitive, functional impairment
- Link impairment in decision making to actual or predictable inability to manage property or personal care
- Use language in relevant legislation

1.7 Assessing Reasoning and Insight

- Research findings suggest that ability to identify decision options, ability to understand consequences, and ability to implement a decision are necessary but not always sufficient to the assessment of decision-making capacity (Silberfeld, 1994)
- The "gold standard" is a clinical interview
- The interview should consist of decision-specific probing of reasoning and insight using specific examples from the patient's situation
- The interviewer (assessor) should probe and verify

1.8 Regional Geriatric Program Toolkit (4 C's) to Assess Reasoning
(Scott, 2008)

- Context – does the person understand his or her situation (and problems)?
- Choices – does the person understand his or her choices?
- Consequences – does the person understand the ramifications of the choice?
- Consistency – does the person make a consistent choice?

1.9 Informed Consent Dialogue for Treatment
(Sessums, Zembrzuska, & Jackson, 2011; Hall, Prochazka, & Fink, 2012)

- Information
  - Diagnosis
  - Proposed treatment
  - Risks and benefits of treatment
  - Alternate treatment and risks
  - Risks and benefits of declining treatment
- Voluntariness
  - Consider setting and power gradient
- Capacity
  - Focus on issues related to treatment
- Emergency situations
  - Use prior expressed wishes
- Consider using the Aid to Capacity Evaluation (Etchells et al., 1996)

1.10 Financial Issues

(Widera et al. 2011; Marson, 2013)

Physicians' role

- Educate patients, families about the need for advanced planning
- Recognize the signs of possible impaired financial capacity
- Clinician assessment of financial impairment, financial abuse, or both (in certain circumstances)
- Practical interventions to help patients maintain financial independence, e.g., automatic bill paying/deposit of checks
- When to make medical/legal referrals for legal advice or formal financial capacity assessment

POA issues

- Effective when signed unless otherwise stated (delayed effectiveness or triggers)
- Capacity to grant POA often lower "test" than capacity to manage finances
- Issues with banks and activation – what is the role of the physician?

Capacity assessment issues

- What are the procedures in your jurisdiction?
- Consider current situation (size of estate)
- Take into consideration past management of finances
- Assess understanding and appreciation of current finances, options, outcomes

1.11 Capacity Re Admission to a Supervised Setting

- Not easily assessed in office setting
- Need collateral information
- Probe reasoning and insight with attention to cognitive decision making and objective functional abilities
- "How will you know it is time to move?" is a helpful question to pose

1.12 Risk and Capacity Assessment

Definitions of risk

- "Safe" → "At risk of harm": is a continuum
- Risk = degree of harm X probability of harm

Factors to consider in doing capacity assessments involving risk

- Clarify concerns
- Clarify whether this is a decision that is controlled by legislation and whether a formal assessment of capacity will help
- Determine client's ability to participate in decision making (capacity) – risk is factored into discussion regarding capacity but does not determine capacity
- Clarify substitute decision maker concerns (promises made, disagreements)
- Find a balance: decide if interference is justified
- Reassess over time if necessary to determine if capacity has changed

2. Psychiatry in Long-Term Care Settings

2.1 Models of Care

Long-term care
- Regulated by provinces and states
- Based on medical model
- Similarities with hospital – nurses, charts, medication monitoring, medical interventions
- Future directions – environmental design, videoconferencing, academic affiliation

Assisted living
- Regulations vary
- Based on social model
- "Aging in place"
- Variable availability of medical services
- "Specialized" dementia units
- Future directions – monitoring via technology

2.2 Challenges of Diagnosing and Treating Psychiatric Disorders in Long-Term Care

- Lack of long-term care home staff
- Lack of previous history
- Misdiagnosis, underdiagnosis
- Common psychological issues – grief, loss, feelings of abandonment
- Overprescription of medication
- Challenges in collaboration with physicians and allied health team members re treatment plan
- Resident heterogeneity
- Lack of staff training
- Physical environment
- Resident frailty and risk of side effects
- Lack of psychiatric consultants

2.3 Essential Knowledge and Skills Needed to Provide Care in Long-Term Care

- Epidemiology of psychiatric disorders
- Long-term care home culture – structures, policies, community context, partnerships
- Ability to work as part of a team

2.4 Assessments in Long-Term Care

- Review records
- Talk with informants about history, personality, preferences
- Thorough assessment (biopsychosocial); rule out delirium, delusions, depression, pain (Ishii, Streim, & Saliba, 2010)

- Observe resident behaviour over time
- Documentation – ABC (antecedent, behaviour, consequences) behavioural charting or DOS (Dementia Observational System) to record specific behaviours and timing

2.5 Management Principles in Long-Term Care

- Individualized care plans (person centred)
- Set realistic goals (may be care not cure)
- Attention to consistent care (bathing, dressing, meal times)
- Attention to unmet needs (thirst, hunger, need for toileting, communication, activity)
- Utilize residents' remaining abilities
- Attention to safety of residents and staff
- Optimize Rx of medical conditions (rule out delirium)
- ↓ sensory impairment
- ↓ pain
- Behavioural/psychological interventions
- Environmental manipulation
- Appropriate drug treatment
- Promotion of team work
- Involvement of family
- End-of-life care
- Monitor interventions for efficacy and adverse reactions

2.6 Role of Geriatric Psychiatrist in Long-Term Care

- Consultation/liaison – part of a multidisciplinary team, consultant to team, supervision of other team members
- Staff education
- Administrative consultation (re programs and policies)

2.7 What Works in Long-Term Care

- More studies on long-term care populations, but there are many methodological issues
- Use of screening tools: depression (Geriatric Depression Scale [GDS], Cornell); cognition (MMSE, MoCA); behaviour (Neuropsychiatric Inventory [NPI], Cohen Mansfield) (Koopmans et al., 2010)
- Comprehensive, integrated, multidisciplinary assessment interventions helpful in long-term care homes (assessment, education of staff) (Collet et al., 2010)
- Psychosocial interventions – group and individual psychotherapy, behavioural management, cognitive stimulation, physical activity (structured activities, massage, reminiscence, aromatherapy, music therapy) (Vernooij-Dassen et al., 2010; Conn et al., 2006)
- Staff education, training, and coaching results in ↓ use of restraints, inappropriate drugs and ↑quality of life, staff-resident interactions (Moyle et al., 2010)
- P.I.E.C.E.S. (U-First) introduced in many provinces in Canada and provides an organized approach (www.pieceslearning.com)

- Other training – Montessori, Gentle Persuasive Approaches
- Regular reassessment of need for antipsychotic medication and discontinuation
- Good environment design (Fleming & Purandare, 2010)
- Use of quality indicators – organizational structures, environmental, care approaches, relationship with care providers (Gibson et al., 2010)
- See also chapter 1.4.

3. Geriatric Psychiatry in Community Settings

3.1 Challenges of Diagnosing and Treating Psychiatric Disorders in Community Care

- Need to attend to early diagnosis and prevention
- Many caregivers (formal and informal)
- Lack of staff training
- Home setting
- Fragmented system of care
- Difficulty accessing services
- Medical comorbidities
- Functional impairments
- Assessments take time
- Consent and capacity issues

3.2 Factors Affecting Seniors' Mental Health
(Parent, Anderson, & Huestis, 2002)

- Physical factors (exercise, nutrition, sleep, illness/disability)
- Emotional factors (self-esteem, self-knowledge, coping skills, etc.)
- Income
- Transportation and mobility
- Social factors (personal relationships, meaningful activity)
- Services (health, hearing, dental, recreation, vision, food services)
- Spiritual factors (nature and meaning of one's life, balancing what can and cannot be changed, religious beliefs, formal religion)

3.3 Essential Knowledge and Skills Needed to Provide Care in the Community

- Epidemiology, determinants of mental health in late life
- Community resources, policies, culture
- Ability to deal with uncertainty and risk

3.4 Focus of Assessment in Community Care

- Functional skills
- Social supports (formal and informal)
- Capacity to consent to treatment, manage finances, choose a place of residence
- Risk (tolerable and intolerable)

3.5 Management Principles in Community Care

- Collaborative care model – primary care physicians and other service providers
- Integration of medical and social services
- Clearly defined roles and responsibilities of team members – communication
- Medication reconciliation
- Attention to transitions in care
- Ongoing support to caregivers
- Attention to cultural issues
- Attention to ethical/legal issues
- Attention to functional outcomes
- End-of-life care

3.6 Role of the Geriatric Psychiatrist in Community Care

- Consultation/liaison
- Staff education
- System and policy development

3.7 What Works in Community Care

- Integrated care programs for the elderly that target high-needs populations at risk for admission to long-term care with medical and social interventions and case management, for example:
    - On Lok
    - CHOICE (Comprehensive Home Option of Integrated Care for the Elderly)
    - PRISMA (Program of Research to Integrate the Services for the Maintenance of Autonomy)
- Multidisciplinary psychogeriatric outreach teams (Sullivan et al., 2004)
- Depression care manager in primary care (PROSPECT) (Bruce et al., 2004)
- Problem adaptation therapy (PATH) – home delivered intervention to ↓depression and disability in patients with dementia; uses problem-solving therapy (Kiosses et al., 2010)
- Prevention of depression in high-risk groups with cognitive behavioural therapy and problem-solving techniques (Cole, 2008)
- Allied health professionals diagnose dementia in home setting (Page et al., 2012)
- Dementia care managers in primary care (Cherry et al., 2004)
- Primary care dementia clinic (Lee et al., 2010)

4. Caregiver Burden, Abuse, and Neglect

4.1 Caregiver Facts
(Adelman et al., 2014)

- 2 million informal caregivers in Canada; 65.7 million in the United States
- 25% of caregivers are < 65 years of age
- Woman > men likely to be "high intensity" caregivers
- One-third caregivers not immediate family

4.2 Caregiver Themes
(O'Shaughnessy, Lee, & Lintern, 2010)

- Connectedness and separateness
- Tension between meeting own needs and needs of spouse
- Knowing/not knowing future
- Sense of powerlessness – trying to develop strategies and support

4.3 Negative Effects of Caregiving

- ↑ burden
- ↓ self-rated health
- ↑ rates of anxiety, depression
- ↓ health-promoting behaviours (↑morbidity, mortality)
- ↑ sleep problems

4.4 Caregiver-Related Risk Factors for Negative Effects of Caregiving
(Adelman et al., 2014; Sörensen & Conwell, 2011)

- Female
- ↓ socioeconomic status
- # hours providing care
- Duration of caregiving
- Lack of knowledge re dementia
- Social isolation
- Coping style/resources
- Fewer perceived benefits or uplifts

4.5 Risk Factors for Negative Effects: "Patient"
(Adelman et al., 2014; Sörensen & Conwell, 2011)

- Impairment in activities of daily living (ADLs), instrumental activities of daily living (IADLs), communication
- Degree of cognitive impairment
- Behavioural problems (verbal, physical aggression, depression)

4.6 Positive Effects of Caregiving

- Company of patient
- Keeping patient at home
- Sense of duty
- Love
- Fulfilling/rewarding
- Associated with ↓ burden and depression, ↑ self-reported health, and ↓ (-) reaction to patient
- May be associated with current decision not to *seek* long-term care placement, but does not affect *actual* placement in long-term care in the future

4.7 What Caregivers Need

- Information about the disease and problem management/coping skills
- Psychological support and treatment for mental health problems
- Assistance with asking for support

4.8 Unsuccessful Caregiver Interventions

- These interventions do not ↓ placement in long-term care or ↓ caregiver depression
- Education alone
- Support groups alone
- Brief interventions
- Treatment patient alone without involving caregiver

4.9 Successful Caregiver Interventions

- These interventions may ↓ placement in long-term care or ↓ caregiver depression
- Continuing relationship between helper and caregiver
- Variety and flexibility of interventions
- Intensive interventions
- Individualized behavioural/coping strategies
- Involvement of patient and caregiver

5. Elder Abuse

5.1 Types of Elder Abuse (% Seniors)
(Mosqueda & Dong, 2011)

- Neglect (5–17%)
- Financial (5–14%)
- Psychological (5–11%)
- Physical (2–6%)
- Sexual (1%)

5.2 Risk Factors for Abuse

5.2.1 Older Adult Risk Factors

- Cognitive impairment
- Aggressive behaviours and psychological distress
- Poor social network and support
- Low household income
- Need for ADL assistance
- Pre-morbid relationship with abuser
- Shared living arrangements

5.2.2 Perpetrator Risk Factors for Abuse

- Family relation
- Substance abuse
- Mental illness
- Dependency
- Unemployment

5.3 Elder Abuse Awareness Tools and Pocket Guides
(National Initiative for the Care of the Elderly [NICE], n.d.)

- Indicators of abuse
- Elder abuse assessment and intervention reference guide
- Elder abuse suspicion index
- Theft by person(s) holding power of attorney

5.4 Mandatory Reporting of Elder Abuse
Exists in many US states, but is limited in Canada

5.5 Self-Neglect

5.5.1 Definitions

- Hoarding: inability to discard/part with possessions; needs space to save items; distress associated with discarding; living space precluded from intended use; impairment in functioning $2°$ to clutter; not explained by another medical, mental disorder (DSM-5)
- Self-neglect: the behaviour of an elderly person that threatens his/her own health and safety (accommodations may or may not be affected) (Mosqueda & Dong, 2011). This group may most resemble elderly at risk of being victims of consumer fraud.
- Severe domestic squalor: living conditions are filthy and unhygienic (self-care may not be affected; hoarding may not be present) (Snowdon & Halliday, 2007)
- Diogenes syndrome: 4th c. BC Greek philosopher – contentment unrelated to material possessions; lack of shame (Clark et al., 1975)

5.5.2 Past Research Findings

- Syndromes overlap
- Different referral sources/bodies of literature
- Heterogeneous group
- No evidence that people hold the core values of Diogenes

5.5.3 Demographics

- Snowdon & Halliday (2011) estimate 1/1000 > 65 years
- ? Gender
- Most live alone
- Socioeconomic status is low in many studies
- Not restricted to the elderly but some risk factors (physical illness, dementia, loss of family, sensory impairment) more common in the elderly

5.5.4 Physical Morbidity

- High number have chronic illness
- Percentage with acute medical illness depends on referral source
- ? role of sensory impairment

5.5.5 Psychiatric Morbidity

- No formal psychiatric diagnosis in up to 50% (higher rate of diagnosis if limited to severe domestic squalor) (Snowdon & Halliday, 2011 referrals to a geriatric psychiatry service)
- 50% have diagnosis of dementia, paranoid disorders (including schizophrenia), alcohol abuse, other psychiatric disorders
- Frontal lobe pathology common
- ? Pre-morbid personality: aloof, stubborn, intelligent

5.5.6 Prognosis

- Depends on referral source
- Up to 50% die during index admission
- Up to 40% of survivors admitted to long-term care, chronic psychiatry units
- ? positive outcomes

5.5.7 Management

- Diagnosis important
- Understanding local legislation is vital (is there an obligation to report?)
- Knowledge of community resources vital
- Planning ahead vital before undertaking any interventions
- Community Ethics Toolkit may be helpful (Community Ethics Network, 2008)

5.6 Consumer Fraud

5.6.1 Types of Fraud

- Lottery scam/prize scam
- Romance scam
- Charity scam
- Grandson in jail scam
- Phishing – asking to confirm personal information
- Others

5.6.2 Consumer Fraud Statistics

- Financial abuse up to 14% of seniors
- Consumer fraud > 10% of seniors
- Difficult to identify
- Contact lists are sold to others
- "Reload" – contact the victim repeatedly

5.6.3 Risk Factors for Fraud

- May vary for different schemes
- ? ↑ with age

- ? cohort effect for current seniors (wealthy and trusting)
- Social isolation
- Sensory impairment
- Cognitive impairment (executive functioning)
- Personality traits (independent, optimistic, self-reliant)
- Negative life events → dependency
- Being a previous victim

QUESTIONS

Consent and Capacity Questions

1. List the four components of decision-making capacity.
2. List the three components of informed consent.
3. Should physicians be involved in capacity assessments regarding decisions related to management of property or admission to supervised settings?
4. What expertise/information are physicians in the best position to contribute to these capacity assessments?

Psychiatry in Long-Term Care and Community Settings Questions

1. List five factors that contribute to the challenges in diagnosing and treating psychiatric disorders in LTC facilities.
2. List five factors that affect seniors' mental health in community settings.
3. Would geriatric psychiatrists be more likely to improve the mental health of residents in LTC facilities by focusing their efforts on staff education instead of direct patient/resident consultation?

Caregiver Burden, Abuse, and Neglect Questions

1. List five characteristics of caregivers that predispose them to negative outcomes.
2. List the four types of elder abuse.
3. How does one balance the needs of caregivers and patients when you provide care to vulnerable seniors?
4. How can geriatric psychiatrists ensure the development of better systems of support and appropriate interventions for caregivers?
5. Should adult protective legislation (i.e., duty to report elder abuse) be widely introduced?

ANSWERS

Consent and Capacity Answers

1. The four components of decision-making capacity are:
    - Understanding of information
    - Appreciating the relevance for the person
    - Rationally manipulate the information (reasoning)
    - Expressing a consistent choice

2. The three components of informed consent are:
    *   Information about diagnosis, proposed treatment, risks and benefits of treatment, alternate treatment and risks, and risks and benefits of declining treatment
    *   Voluntariness (i.e., free of coercion) – especially important when the patient is at risk of abuse, when the patient is institutionalized, and when discussing admission to a LTC facility or organ donation
    *   Capacity to consent to treatment

3. Many physicians feel uncomfortable doing these types of assessments, particularly if they are uncertain as to their role in their jurisdiction and lack knowledge about the appropriate legislation. Specialists have an important role to play, but will need more information and education to allow them to feel comfortable understanding their obligations, their role, the process, and potential conflicts of interest.

4. Geriatric specialists have expertise in diagnosis and assessment of these patients. Information that may be helpful would include diagnoses that affect function; current and expected future cognitive functioning; presence/absence of psychotic symptoms (e.g., delusions) that may affect capacity; assessment of insight and judgment; exploration of patient's values, preferences, and previous level of functioning; evaluation of risk of harm; and means to potentially improve capacity.

Psychiatry in Long-Term Care and Community Settings Answers

1. Factors contributing to challenges in diagnosing and treating psychiatric disorders in LTC facilities include:
    *   Resident heterogeneity in these settings
    *   Lack of previous patient history
    *   Misdiagnosis/underdiagnosis of common psychiatric disorders (e.g., delirium, depression)
    *   Understaffing in LTC facilities
    *   Lack of staff training in these facilities about psychiatric issues
    *   Physician and non-physician input about diagnosis, treatment, and outcome
    *   Physical environment in many LTC facilities
    *   Overprescription of psychotropic medications leading to polypharmacy
    *   Common psychological issues (e.g., grief, loss, feelings of abandonment) experienced by residents
    *   Resident frailty and risk of side effects from medications
    *   Lack of psychiatric consultants to provide these services
    *   Medical comorbidity
    *   Lack of screening
    *   Atypical presentations

2. Factors affecting seniors' mental health in community settings include:
    *   Physical health (e.g., cognitive disorders, substance use)
    *   Emotional factors (e.g., self-esteem, coping skills)
    *   Social factors (e.g., relationships, meaningful activity, stigma)

- Spiritual factors
- Service availability and structure (e.g., healthcare, community, other)
- Income
- Transportation
- Housing
- Having multiple caregivers
- Functional status
- Consent and capacity issues
- Demographic factors (e.g., age, gender, ethnicity)
- Health behaviours

3. Whether geriatric psychiatrists have more impact via education than direct patient contact depends to a great extent on factors within the system the physician is operating in:
   - What other types of clinicians are working to assist staff and residents in LTC (nurse practitioners, psychiatric registered nurses, primary care physicians with expertise in elder care)?
   - Is there administrative/leadership support at the LTC facility?
   - What is the relationship between the geriatric psychiatrist and the other staff in the facility?
   - What models of care have been adopted for this region?

Caregiver Burden, Abuse, and Neglect Answers

1. Characteristics of caregivers that predispose them to negative outcomes include:
   - Sociodemographic variables (e.g., socioeconomic status, ethnicity/culture, gender, age, rural/urban residence)
   - Lack of knowledge about dementia
   - Intrapersonal resources (e.g., personality/coping styles)
   - Poor physical or mental health
   - Availability, quality of informal support
   - Negative appraisal of caregiving
   - Lack of positive appraisal/uplifts of caregiving
   - Overestimating patient's abilities
   - Dysfunctional family interaction pattern
   - Overinvolvement
   - Caregivers who minimize the patient's deficits
   - Lack of sleep
   - Caregiver's perceived agency in dealing with issues
   - Unmet needs of caregivers

2. Types of elder abuse include:
   - Physical
   - Psychological/emotional
   - Financial
   - Sexual

3. Balancing the needs of caregivers and patients when providing care to vulnerable seniors can be very challenging, particularly if you are working alone without the assistance of an interprofessional team or other supports. It is often challenging to advocate for both patient and caregiver simultaneously. If necessary, one may need to refer the caregiver to his or her own clinician, therapist, or physician.

4. It is helpful to always keep caregiver issues in mind when working with seniors. One may need to advocate for caregiver needs to be met by others who work in a variety of programs (e.g., First Link at the Alzheimer Society, Home Care, primary care, etc.). Caregiver needs can be thought of as falling in three major categories:
   • Information and education
   • Psychological support
   • Assistance mobilizing social support (informal and formal)

It is helpful to think about who in the "system" can provide this type of support to caregivers longitudinally, and identify vulnerable caregivers and target their stress management abilities.

5. The proposal that adult protective legislation (i.e., duty to report elder abuse) be widely introduced is an interesting question, and some elder law lawyers argue that this is not the preferred option because the outcomes may be less than desirable. With too much intervention, seniors' independence may be limited. It may be more helpful to increase awareness of elder abuse among all those who work with seniors and to work collaboratively to assist those individuals affected. For an interesting Canadian commentary on this issue, see the Law Commission of Ontario report: *A Framework for the Law as It Affects Older Adults* (April 2012, available online at http://www.lco-cdo .org/en/content/older-adults).

CASE DISCUSSION

1. The assessment and treatment of Mr K. would involve the following considerations:
   • Assessment should cover medical/physical issues, including ruling out delirium, investigating pain and fatigue, sensory impairment (vision and hearing), cognitive issues (language skills, memory, apraxia, capacity, etc.), other psychiatric symptoms (depression, psychosis), previous personality, habits related to personal care, his relationship with his wife, her role in caregiving prior to admission and the "meaning" of having chosen a LTC facility for this man, and relevant cultural issues related to personal care.
   • It would be very helpful to have some behavioural charting done to clarify when the issues arise in personal care and how the staff is responding to them.
   • It would be helpful to have someone interview Mrs K. to understand her assessment of the situation, how she is intervening on a daily basis, and what she views as a successful outcome; if possible, it would be helpful to include other family members and try to ensure that someone clarifies the goals of care.
   • A treatment plan would try to address all of the above with an emphasis on behavioural interventions, and treatment of any psychiatric (e.g., delusions), medical, or physical factors.

- Psychotropic medications may be needed to treat the delusions or depression, or if behavioural interventions are not successful and there is significant risk of physical aggression.
- Attention to the wife's needs will also be important.
- Must be aware of cultural expectations with regard to interactions with physicians, and expectations and interpretation of care.

2. The following factors may predispose Mrs K. to depression:
   - Previous history of anxiety, depression, other mental health problems, and/or poor coping skills
   - Feelings of guilt about having been unable to continue to care for her husband at home
   - Feeling that only she can provide care to him in an appropriate manner and/or taking great pride in her role as a caregiver; therefore, the loss of the caregiver role may predispose her to depression
   - Lacking the necessary information and education to help her understand her husband's situation
   - Social isolation with few supports or lesser ability to access them
   - South Asian ethnicity
   - Female gender
   - Language/communication barrier
   - Feelings of inadequacy due to cultural expectations of caregivers

3. The psychogeriatric assessment of Mrs C. would include the following considerations:
   - It will be difficult to figure out how to speak to Mrs C. alone without her son; this may take time and it will be important to work with others to figure out how to accomplish this; you may have to work with the other care providers involved (i.e., indirect consultation) to assist them in obtaining relevant information, which may require a preliminary meeting of all those involved.
     - This might help clarify roles, what information is available and lacking, what has been tried to date and why it "failed," and what legislation might be appropriate to use in this situation.
     - A home visit by two individuals trusted by Mrs C. (ideally family physician and social worker) might afford the opportunity to interview this patient alone.
   - The first goal would be to get information about Mrs C.'s safety in the home, risk of different types of abuse, and whether the situation is urgent and requires immediate action.
   - It will also be important to understand what problems the son is experiencing and what resources might be helpful in addressing them.
   - Involvement of the police to accompany clinicians on a home visit might be helpful; many jurisdictions have officers knowledgeable about elder abuse.
   - Attempts to bring the patient back to the family physician with the son might be appropriate.
   - Medical and psychiatric history

- Substance and medication use
- Cognitive assessment (e.g., MMSE or MoCA)
- Functional assessment

4. Regarding Mrs C.'s capacity to manage her finances:
   - One would only want to embark on a capacity assessment regarding finances or admission to a LTC facility if this will help in the current situation.
   - In order to assess her capacity to manage finances, one would want to be familiar with the legislation in one's jurisdiction to understand the definition of capacity and the forms that need to be completed (if any) after the assessment.
   - One would want to know something about her previous involvement in managing finances, how the finances are being managed at this time and any problems that are present (e.g., unpaid bills, etc.).
   - Try to determine her previous preferences and values with respect to money (e.g., was she someone who always gave financial gifts to this son, and if so why?).
   - If she was not involved in managing finances in the past, she may need education about her financial situation (if this information can be obtained) prior to any formal capacity assessment.
   - Think about whether there are any remediable problems that should be addressed or treated first (e.g., pain, UTI).
   - Ensure that she can see and hear you adequately during the interview.
   - Consider what cognitive problems she has that may interfere with capacity such as short-term memory problems and executive dysfunction; this may assist in planning the interview and knowing where there are likely to be more difficulties (understand vs appreciate).
   - Explore her understanding of her current financial situation (e.g., income, expenses, and other obligations such as support of dependents, how much money is going to her son).
   - Explore her understanding and explanation of any current problems with finances (e.g., why are bills not being paid? what other options are there available to insure that bills can be paid?).
   - She should be questioned about her appreciation of what will occur if the problems persist (e.g., loss of power, telephone, debt, etc.), and to determine her understanding and appreciation of the potential financial impact of her son's day-to-day involvement.

RECOMMENDED RESOURCES FOR REVIEW

Although these resources may not be specifically cited in the text, their approach informed the contents of the chapter, and they are recommended as useful further reading.

American Bar Association (ABA) Commission on Law and Aging; American Psychological Association (APA). Assessment of older adults with diminished capacity: a handbook for psychologists. Washington, DC: ABA/APA; 2008. http://www.apa.org/pi/aging/programs/assessment/capacity-psychologist-handbook.pdf

International Psychogeriatric Association (IPA). The IPA complete guides to behavioral and psychological symptoms of dementia (BPSD). Milwaukee, WI: IPA; 2012. https://www.ipa-online.org/publications/guides-to-bpsd

Lai JM, Karlawish J. Assessing the capacity to make everyday decisions: a guide for clinicians and an agenda for future research. Am J Geriatr Psychiatry. 2007;15(2):101–11. http://dx.doi.org/10.1097/01.JGP.0000239246.10056.2e. Medline:17272730

MacCourt P, Wilson K, Tourigny-Rivard M-F; Seniors Advisory Committee, Mental Health Commission of Canada. Guidelines for comprehensive mental health services for older adults in Canada. Calgary, AB: Mental Health Commission of Canada; 2011. http://www.mentalhealthcommission.ca/English/document/279/mental-health-commission-canada-seniors-guidelines-print

Moye J, Butz SW, Marson DC, et al.; ABA-APA Capacity Assessment of Older Adults Working Group. A conceptual model and assessment template for capacity evaluation in adult guardianship. Gerontologist. 2007;47(5):591–603. http://dx.doi.org/10.1093/geront/47.5.591. Medline:17989401

Munson J; Ontario Ministry of the Attorney General, Capacity Assessment Office. Guidelines for conducting assessments of capacity. Toronto: Ontario Ministry of the Attorney General; 2005. https://www.attorneygeneral.jus.gov.on.ca/english/family/pgt/capacity.php

O'Connor D. Incapability assessments: a review of assessment and screen tools – final report. Vancouver, BC: Public Guardian and Trustee of British Columbia; 2009. http://www.trustee.bc.ca/documents/STA/Incapability_Assessments_Review_Assessment_Screening_Tools.pdf

REFERENCES

Adelman RD, Tmanova LL, Delgado D, et al. Caregiver burden: a clinical review. JAMA. 2014;311(10):1052–60. http://dx.doi.org/10.1001/jama.2014.304. PMID:24618967

Bruce ML, Ten Have TR, Reynolds CF III, et al. Reducing suicidal ideation and depressive symptoms in depressed older primary care patients: a randomized controlled trial. JAMA. 2004;291(9):1081–91. http://dx.doi.org/10.1001/jama.291.9.1081. Medline:14996777

Cherry DL, Vickrey BG, Schwankovsky L, et al. Interventions to improve quality of care: the Kaiser Permanente-alzheimer's Association Dementia Care Project. Am J Manag Care. 2004;10(8):553–60. Medline:15352531

Clark AN, Mankikar GD, Gray I. Diogenes syndrome. A clinical study of gross neglect in old age. Lancet. 1975;305(7903):366–8. http://dx.doi.org/10.1016/S0140-6736(75)91280-5http://www.ncbi.nlm.nih.gov/entrez/query.fcgi?cmd=Retrieve&db=PubMed&list_uids=46514&dopt=Abstract

Cole MG. Brief interventions to prevent depression in older subjects: a systematic review of feasibility and effectiveness. Am J Geriatr Psychiatry. 2008;16(6):435–43. http://dx.doi.org/10.1097/JGP.0b013e318162f174. Medline:18515687

Collet J, de Vugt ME, Verhey FRJ, et al. Efficacy of integrated interventions combining psychiatric care and nursing home care for nursing home residents: a review of the literature. Int J Geriatr Psychiatry. 2010;25(1):3–13. Medline:19513988

Community Ethics Network. Ethical decision-making in the community health and support sector: community ethics toolkit. Toronto: Toronto Central Community Care Access Centre; 2008. http://communityethicsnetwork.ca/wordpress/?page_id=531

Conn D, Gibson M, Feldman S, et al.; Canadian Coalition for Seniors' Mental Health (CCSMH). National guidelines for seniors' mental health: the assessment and treatment of mental health issues in long term care homes (focus on mood and behaviour symptoms). Toronto: CCSMH: 2006. www.ccsmh.ca/en/natlGuidelines/ltc.cfm

Etchells E, Darzins P, Silberfeld M, et al. Aid to capacity evaluation. Toronto: Joint Centre for Bioethics; 1996. http://www.jcb.utoronto.ca/tools/ace_download.shtml. http://dx.doi.org/10.1037/t05021-000

Fleming R, Purandare N. Long-term care for people with dementia: environmental design guidelines. Int Psychogeriatr. 2010;22(7):1084–96. http://dx.doi.org/10.1017/S1041610210000438. Medline:20478095

Gibson MC, Carter MW, Helmes E, et al. Principles of good care for long-term care facilities. Int Psychogeriatr. 2010;22(7):1072–83. http://dx.doi.org/10.1017/S1041610210000852. Medline:20598194

Hall DE, Prochazka AV, Fink AS. Informed consent for clinical treatment. CMAJ. 2012;184(5):533–40. http://dx.doi.org/10.1503/cmaj.112120. Medline:22392947

Ishii S, Streim JE, Saliba D. Potentially reversible resident factors associated with rejection of care behaviors. J Am Geriatr Soc. 2010;58(9):1693–700. http://dx.doi.org/10.1111/j.1532-5415.2010.03020.x. Medline:20863329

Kiosses DN, Arean PA, Teri L, et al. Home-delivered problem adaptation therapy (PATH) for depressed, cognitively impaired, disabled elders: a preliminary study. Am J Geriatr Psychiatry. 2010;18(11):988–98. http://dx.doi.org/10.1097/JGP.0b013e3181d6947d. Medline:20808092

Koopmans RT, Zuidema SU, Leontjevas R, et al. Comprehensive assessment of depression and behavioral problems in long-term care. Int Psychogeriatr. 2010;22(7):1054–62. http://dx.doi.org/10.1017/S1041610210000736. Medline:20843390

Lee L, Hillier LM, Stolee P, et al. Enhancing dementia care: a primary care-based memory clinic. J Am Geriatr Soc. 2010;58(11):2197–204. http://dx.doi.org/10.1111/j.1532-5415.2010.03130.x. Medline:20977435

Marson DC. Clinical and ethical aspects of financial capacity in dementia: a commentary. Am J Geriatr Psychiatry. 2013;21(4):382–90. http://dx.doi.org/10.1016/j.jagp.2013.01.033. Medline:23498385

Mosqueda L, Dong X. Elder abuse and self-neglect: "I don't care anything about going to the doctor, to be honest...". JAMA. 2011;306(5):532–40. http://dx.doi.org/10.1001/jama.2011.1085. Medline:21813431

Moyle W, Hsu MC, Lieff S, et al. Recommendations for staff education and training for older people with mental illness in long-term aged care. Int Psychogeriatr. 2010;22(7):1097–106. http://dx.doi.org/10.1017/S1041610210001754. Medline:20843396

National Initiative for the Care of the Elderly (NICE). Elder abuse tools. Toronto: NICE; n.d. http://www.nicenet.ca/tools-elder-abuse

O'Shaughnessy M, Lee K, Lintern T. Changes in the couple relationship in dementia care: spouse carers' experiences. Dementia. 2010;9(2):237–58. http://dx.doi.org/10.1177/1471301209354021

Page S, Hope K, Maj C, et al. 'Doing things differently'–working towards distributed responsibility within memory assessment services. Int J Geriatr Psychiatry. 2012;27(3):280–5. http://dx.doi.org/10.1002/gps.2716. PMID:21472781

Parent K, Anderson M, Huestis L. Supporting seniors' mental health through home care policy: a policy guide. Toronto: Canadian Mental Health Association; 2002. http://www.cmha.ca/public_policy/supporting-seniors-mental-health-through-home-care-a-policy-guide/#.VykU9fkguUk

P.I.E.C.E.S.™ learning & development model: supporting relationships for changing health and health care [Internet]. www.pieceslearning.com

Scott D. Toolkit for primary care: capacity assessment. Toronto: Geriatrics Interprofessional Interorganizational Collaboration (GiiC); 2008. http://giic.rgps.on.ca/capacity-assessment

Sessums LL, Zembrzuska H, Jackson JL. Does this patient have medical decision-making capacity? JAMA. 2011;306(4):420–7. http://dx.doi.org/10.1001/jama.2011.1023. Medline:21791691

Silberfeld M. Evaluating decisions in mental capacity assessments. Int J Geriatr Psychiatry. 1994;9(5):365–71. http://dx.doi.org/10.1002/gps.930090504

Snowdon J, Halliday G. A study of severe domestic squalor: 173 cases referred to an old age psychiatry service. Int Psychogeriatr. 2011;23(2):308–14. http://dx.doi.org/10.1017/S1041610210000906. Medline:20678298

Snowdon J, Shah A, Halliday G. Severe domestic squalor: a review. Int Psychogeriatr. 2007;19(1):37–51. http://dx.doi.org/10.1017/S1041610206004236. Medline:16973099

Sörensen S, Conwell Y. Issues in dementia caregiving: effects on mental and physical health, intervention strategies, and research needs. Am J Geriatr Psychiatry. 2011;19(6):491–6. http://dx.doi.org/10.1097/JGP.0b013e31821c0e6e. Medline:21502853

Sullivan MP, Kessler L, Le Clair JK, et al. Defining best practices for specialty geriatric mental health outreach services: lessons for implementing mental health reform. Can J Psychiatry. 2004;49(7):458–66. Medline:15362250

Vernooij-Dassen M, Vasse E, Zuidema S, et al. Psychosocial interventions for dementia patients in long-term care. Int Psychogeriatr. 2010;22(7):1121–8. http://dx.doi.org/10.1017/S1041610210001365. Medline:20813074

Widera E, Steenpass V, Marson D, et al. Finances in the older patient with cognitive impairment: "He didn't want me to take over". JAMA. 2011;305(7):698–706. http://dx.doi.org/10.1001/jama.2011.164. Medline:21325186

ADDITIONAL E-RESOURCES ON ELDER ABUSE

Canadian Anti-Fraud Centre. http://www.antifraudcentre-centreantifraude.ca/index-eng.htm.

Competition Bureau Canada. The little black book of scams" your guide to protection against fraud. Canadian edition. Reproduced with permission from the Australian Competition and Consumer Commission. Ottawa: Competition Bureau Canada; 2012. http://www.competitionbureau.gc.ca/eic/site/cb-bc.nsf/eng/03074.html.

Law Commission of Ontario. A framework for the law as it affects older adults: advancing substantive equality for older persons through law, policy and practice. Toronto: Law Commission of Ontario; April 2012. http://www .lco-cdo.org/en/content/older-adults

Texas Consortium Geriatric Education Center, Baylor College of Medicine; Investor Protection Trust. Pocket guide on elder investment fraud and financial exploitation. www.investorprotection.org/downloads/ EIFFE_Clinicians_Pocket_Guide_National.pdf.

4.6 Palliative Care in Geriatric Psychiatry

Daphna Grossman, MD, CCFP(PC), FCFP
Jeffrey Myers, MD, MSEd, CCFP(PC)

INTRODUCTION

The bulk of this book has focused on the assessment and active treatment of mental disorders in later life. However, when the older patient is close to death, the processes involved with diagnoses and management need to be adapted. The goals of care are reassessed, the balance of risks and benefits shifts, and an understanding of the desire for and fear of death becomes more immediately salient. The palliative approach to care provides a helpful alternative way of thinking about psychiatric illness among dying older adults and those with end-stage incurable disease. Our colleagues in palliative medicine highlight the team-based approach to care using several complex cases as the springboards to explore the relevant medical and psychosocial issues. As such, the overview section in this chapter is very brief in favour of an expanded question and answer format.

CASE SCENARIOS

Scenario 1. Mr K.L. is a 76-year-old male with a long-standing history of coronary artery disease (CAD), type I diabetes mellitus, hypertension, and hypercholesterolemia. His first myocardial infarction (MI) was at age 50, and he underwent a triple bypass at age 56. He has always been vigilant regarding control of his blood sugars and ensured adequate exercise. Four years ago, he developed congestive heart failure (CHF) following a second MI, after which a number of medical issues surfaced, including chronic kidney disease (CKD) and peripheral vascular disease (PVD). At that time, he had a pacemaker and implantable defibrillator inserted.

Over the past year, he has experienced a substantial progression of his symptoms, including breathlessness, fatigue, and leg pain. These have greatly impacted the level of enjoyment he experiences in daily life. Historically, his routine included going out with friends to plays, movies, and for long walks. He now finds walking from house to car causes significant breathlessness and pain. He recently learned surgery is not an option for managing his leg claudication. You met him briefly during his last hospitalization a year ago: consulted for transient agitation.

Past medical history is remarkable for CAD, CHF, CKD, hypercholesterolemia, hypertension, type I diabetes mellitus, PVD.

Medications include bisoprolol 5 mg bid; furosemide 80 mg od; nitroglycerin patch 0.4 mg; ASA 81 mg od; ramipril 2.5 mg od; atorvastatin 20 mg od; Novolin®30/70 20U ACB and 15U ACD.

A few days ago you received a call from his concerned wife who requested guidance because he has stated several times over the past week that he wants to have his pacemaker and implantable defibrillator turned off. She is very concerned about this request, as turning this device off would result in his dying, likely imminently. She wonders if he might be depressed and this is in fact an attempt to hasten his own death. Furthermore, she knows that a medical professional must turn off the pacemaker and wouldn't that be the same as physician-hastened death?

1. How would you assess Mr K.L. to determine whether his request to turn off his pacemaker/defibrillator is secondary to depression and suicidal ideation?
2. Is having a physician turn off the pacemaker an example of physician-assisted suicide?

Later, you receive a request for consultation from the coronary care unit (CCU) attending team as Mr K.L. had been admitted again to their unit five days earlier following another MI. The reason for referral is stated to be "severe agitation." Upon reviewing his chart, you note that the patient's performance (functional) status has progressively deteriorated over the past three days; he has repeatedly pulled out both his IV and urinary catheters and persistently pulls off his oxygen mask. These behaviours occur more often at night. The CCU attending team indicates the family has clarified the goals for his care to be comfort, and because of his exceptionally poor heart function, they believe his prognosis to be in the order of days. When you arrive at Mr K.L.'s room, you find he is mumbling, occasionally opens his eyes, and in general appears uncomfortable. With family members sitting around his bed, Mrs K.L. looks up at you and says, "You have to do something. He's suffering so much and would not want to have lived like this."

3. How will you respond to Mrs K.L. in the moment, and how will you approach management?

Scenario 2. You have been caring for an elderly patient with behavioural and psychological symptoms of dementia (BPSD) who has been managed at home with an atypical antipsychotic. He has now been admitted to a palliative care unit with end-stage lung cancer. He is becoming increasingly agitated, continuously falling out of bed, and striking out at both his family and the medical staff. Because these behaviours are "very distressing," his wife asks if a more sedating medication could be used and "allow him to sleep until he dies."

4. In scenario 2, how would you respond to the request?

OVERVIEW

- "Palliative care is an approach that improves the quality of life of patients and their families facing the problem associated with life-threatening illness, through the prevention and relief of suffering by means of early identification and impeccable assessment and treatment of pain and other problems, physical, psychosocial and spiritual" (World Health Organization, 2016).
  - Palliative care is provided by a team of physicians, nurses, social workers, spiritual care providers, and other professions, all of whom work with a patient's other healthcare teams to provide an additional layer of care.
  - Palliative care is appropriate at any age and any stage of a serious illness, and it may be provided concurrently with curative treatment.

- If curative treatment is no longer an option, palliative care may become the sole focus of care.
- A number of clinical areas of focus are shared between palliative care and geriatric psychiatry, particularly the general elements of preserving function and quality of life, managing symptoms, focus on psychosocial aspects of care, and the coordination of multiple care teams.
- The following are the specific areas of focus warranting the detailed attention for this chapter in the case scenarios above and the questions below.
  - Approach to psychosocial, spiritual, and existential distress
  - Depression among older persons with serious illness
  - Screening
  - Varied management approach based on survival estimation
  - Delirium among older persons with serious illness
  - Varied work-up and management based on survival estimation
  - Palliative care use of medications common for the psychiatry setting
  - Special considerations for the palliative care of a nonverbal patient
  - Palliative sedation therapy
  - Request for hastened death
  - Physician-hastened death ("medical assistance in dying")

QUESTIONS

1. Many of the psychomotor features associated with the diagnosis of depression are also symptoms commonly experienced by patients with advanced incurable disease. Identify tools for screening for depression among older persons in the palliative care setting.
2. List the antidepressant medications thought to be appropriate for use among older persons with a survival estimate of less than two months.
3. Outline your approach to the work-up of the older person with delirium for each of the following estimated survival durations: four months, one month, and one week.
4. Antipsychotic and antidepressant medications have adjuvant benefits in the palliative care setting, which are different from their conventional use in psychiatry. Identify three such medications, how and why each is used "off label" in the palliative care setting, and address route of administration when the patient is very near the end of life and no longer able to swallow.
5. Describe an approach for assessing the psychosocial, spiritual, or existential components of distress in a patient in the palliative care setting, and outline in detail one clinical intervention aimed to address this distress.
6. Pain and delirium are very common symptoms in the palliative care setting. A non-verbal elderly person with dementia suffering pain may show agitated, aggressive behaviour, which is similar to the behaviour seen in delirium. Given the management of each is significantly different, how might pain and delirium be differentiated in this setting?

ANSWERS

1. Options for screening for depression among older persons in the palliative care setting include (Rayner et al., 2011):
   - Hospital Anxiety and Depression Scale (HADS): score above 8
   - Clinical interview:
     - Single item: in patients not cognitively impaired, asking directly "Are you depressed?" has a high yield for depression screening.
     - Two items: in addition to mood, assessing a patient's level of interest in activities increases the yield for diagnosing depression.
   - Edmonton Symptom Assessment Scale (ESAS): numeric rating scale (0–10) that assesses the severity of nine different symptoms; depression and anxiety are two of the nine
   - Brief Edinburgh Depression Scale (BEDS): Edincott criteria
     - Edincott substitution criteria: substitution of cognitive symptoms for the somatic symptoms that commonly manifest in older patients in the palliative care setting (Noorani & Montagnini, 2007)
   - Patient Dignity Index (limited evidence, but increasing interest in its use in geriatric palliative care settings)

2. For a depressed patient in the palliative care setting, the patient's likely survival duration may influence treatment choice. One must be aware of the data showing that clinicians are notoriously inaccurate with survival estimates, with a substantial tendency to overestimate. Therefore prognosis is often described as hours to days, days to weeks, weeks to months, and months to years.

   There is no evidence of superior efficacy for any one medication; however clinical practice guidelines most frequently identify medications in the selective serotonin reuptake inhibitor (SSRI) class, in particular citalopram, sertraline, and escitalopram. Less common medication choices are amitriptyline, nortriptyline, fluoxetine, and paroxetine. The anticholinergic effects of tricyclic antidepressants (TCAs) increase the risk of delirium. Fluoxetine and paroxetine may affect the metabolism of opioids. These medications (except escitalopram) have a delayed onset of action, which affect their usefulness in a person with a short prognosis.

   Other medications commonly included within clinical practice guidelines are venlafaxine, duloxetine, and mirtazapine.

   - The side effects of mirtazapine include increased appetite, and sedation may be considered favourable or beneficial for certain patients in the palliative care setting.
   - Venlafaxine and duloxetine may have adjuvant properties in the treatment of neuropathic pain.

   There is some evidence for efficacy of mirtazapine and escitalopram within 2 weeks of initiation (important for a patient with expected survival duration in the order of months).

   Psychostimulants such as methylphenidate, modafinil, and dexamethasone may be useful for patients with a prognosis of weeks.

It is also acceptable to temporarily combine an antidepressant with a psychostimulant to allow for a rapid onset of action while awaiting the onset of the antidepressant's effect.

- Psychostimulants are often used in the management of other common symptoms in the palliative care setting:
    - Methylphenidate and modafinil may increase appetite.
    - Dexamethasone is used in the management of pain, fatigue, drowsiness, and poor appetite; benefits must be balanced with side effects (less important for patients with very short life prognosis).
- Psychostimulants should be used with caution in patients with heart disease.

For each patient, consider nonpharmacological interventions such as spiritual care, psychological support/counselling, and music/art/recreational/massage/touch therapy.

3. The approach to work-up and treatment will be guided by the patient's goals of care (Zimmerman et al., 2011). The goal of treating the delirium at any stage is to promote comfort and relieve suffering. The following table outlines work-up and treatment for three estimated survival durations.

4 months ("weeks to months")	1 month ("days to weeks")	1 week ("hours to days")
• More thorough work-up to rule out infection, metabolic imbalance, medication side effect, cardiac etiology, anaemia, hypoxia, space-occupying central nervous system (CNS) lesion, pain, urinary retention, and constipation • Focus of care is the treatment and reversal of the underlying cause	• Must discuss range of investigation options with patient and/or SDM • Can treat pain, urinary retention, constipation, and medication side effects* while being minimally invasive • If aligned with patient's goals of care, treatment of infection and metabolic disturbance may be appropriate • For suspected underlying cardiac etiologies, it is often most appropriate to manage the symptom and not pursue reversal of underlying cause • Anticoagulation to treat an underlying etiology is rarely appropriate • For suspected CNS lesions or other etiologies, imaging is appropriate if managing findings aligns with goals of care	• All investigations often considered inappropriate • Sole focus of care is most commonly symptomatic support (includes assessment for pain, urinary retention, and constipation, as well as review of current medications) • Opioids should be considered if it is felt pain or dyspnea might be contributing to delirium

* Exercise caution if medication side effect is felt to be a contributing factor, as adjustments may worsen other, more distressing symptoms.

4. Regarding "off label" use of antipsychotics and antidepressants in the palliative care setting at the end of life:
   - Haloperidol: anti-dopaminergic properties make it highly effective for nausea
   - Olanzapine: may decrease nausea, improve appetite, decrease secretions, or improve insomnia
   - Mirtazapine: may decrease pruritus in the setting of end-stage liver failure, improve appetite, decrease nausea, or improve insomnia; risk of worsening constipation
   - Citalopram (and other SSRIs): may decrease hot flushes
   - Chlorpromazine: may improve hiccoughs
   - Methotrimeprazine: may improve nausea; anticholinergic side effect of sedation may be desirable; may improve secretions; may decrease colic pain (e.g., in setting of malignant bowel obstruction)
   - Quetiapine: may improve insomnia
   - Acetylcholinesterases: decrease opioid-induced sedation and myoclonus
   - TCA and serotonin norepinephrine reuptake inhibitor (SNRI): adjuvant analgesics and may augment impact of opioids
   - Trazadone: sedation may be desirable

Route of administration at the end of life:
   - Haloperidol – subcutaneous (SC)
   - Methotrimeprazine – SC
   - Olanzapine – sublingually (SL)
   - Midazolam – SL/SC (preferred benzodiazepine)
   - Lorazepam – SL/SC (consider possible paradoxical effect; however, rarely seen in practice and is an important option for this setting)
   - Risperidone – SL
   - General considerations: SC administration is preferred over intramuscular (IM) and intravenous (IV) for the following reasons:
     - With SC administration, a butterfly can be inserted under the skin on the leg, arm, back, or abdomen; given syringe connects directly with port, and needle is not required.
     - Patients in this setting have typically lost muscle mass, thus absorption of medications given IM can be highly variable.
     - Frequent IM injections can be painful and lead to tissue trauma.
     - IV administration may be less comfortable for patients and no more effective than SC (considering goal of care being comfort).

5. The interdisciplinary team should include professionals with skill in assessment of and response to the spiritual and existential issues common to patients with life-threatening illnesses and conditions and their families. In addition, considerations include the following:
   - Regular assessment of spiritual and existential concerns should be documented. This includes, but is not limited to, life review, assessment of hopes and fears, meaning, purpose, beliefs about afterlife, guilt, forgiveness, and life completion tasks.

- Whenever possible a standardized instrument should be used to assess and identify religious or spiritual/existential background, preferences, and related beliefs, rituals, and practices of the patient and family.
- Periodic re-evaluation of the impact of spiritual/existential interventions and patient-family preferences should occur with regularity and be documented.
- Spiritual/existential care needs, goals, and concerns should addressed and documented, and support is offered for issues of life completion in a manner consistent with the individual's and family's cultural and religious values.
- Pastoral care and other palliative care professionals facilitate contacts with spiritual/religious communities, groups, or individuals, as desired by the patient and/or family. Primary importance is that patients have access to clergy in their religious traditions.
- Examples of interventions: dignity therapy, life review interview, mindfulness meditation
  - *Dignity therapy*: brief individualized psychotherapeutic intervention for those experiencing existential distress (a loss of meaning). The goal of the intervention is to engender a sense of meaning and purpose in order to reduce suffering in the time.
  - *Life review interview*: 30 to 60 minute interview that occurs at the bedside with the clinician taking notes, which the clinician then reshapes into a narrative. The narrative is then read to the patient, and in the follow-up session the patient is allowed to edit. It can serve as a potential legacy for loved ones.
  - *Mindfulness meditation*: evidence of improvement in symptom severity and decreased levels of stress, anxiety, and depression.

6. The following suggestions may help differentiate pain from delirium:
   - Exclude common causes of delirium (e.g., constipation, infections, urinary retention).
   - Observe for nonverbal signs of pain; the American Geriatric Society's list of behaviours that may indicate pain include facial expression, verbalizations, body movements, and change in interpersonal interactions, activity pattern, and/or mental status (American Geriatric Society [AGS] Panel on Persistent Pain in Older Adults, 2002).
   - Use one or more of the tools that help identify pain in the nonverbal patient, such as the Pain Assessment in Advanced Dementia (PAINAD), the Adult Faces Scale, MOBID-2 (Mobilization Observation Behaviour Intensity Dementia), Pain Assessment Checklist for Seniors with Limited Ability to Communicate (PACSLAC), the PACSLAC-D for patients with severe dementia (see RQ-1) (AGS Panel, 2002).
   - Consider a trial of analgesics.

CASE DISCUSSION

1. Important elements for assessing the patient Mr K.L. include screening for comorbid psychiatric issues (depression, anxiety, and suicidality), assessing other medical comorbidities that may be producing distress, assessing for and discussing symptom control strategies with the patient and his wife, and selecting those that optimize

symptom control as well as patient dignity. Please refer to review paper by Monica Branigan (2015) in the recommended resources section, which addresses the topic of the "wish to hasten death."

2. This question about turning off the pacemaker aims to address the differences between withdrawal or withholding of life-sustaining treatments and physician-hastened death (Gordon & Grossman, 2015).

- Withholding = not starting treatment that has the potential to sustain life
- Withdrawing = stopping treatment that has the potential to sustain life
- A life-sustaining treatment would include any medical intervention, technology, procedure, or medication that is administered to a patient in order to prolong the patient's life; treatment may or may not relate specifically to the underlying condition or disease of the patient.
  - Examples: respirators, blood transfusions, kidney dialysis, antibiotics, CPR, artificial nutrition, and hydration
- Physician-hastened death is the act of helping someone hasten their own death by providing the means or the information on how to proceed, or both.
- Competent patients may refuse life-sustaining treatment.
- There is no ethical, medical, moral, or clinical difference between withholding or withdrawing life-sustaining treatment.
- Although patients have a clear right to refuse treatment, withdrawal of life-sustaining treatment with the knowledge the patient will subsequently die can be problematic.
- For some, a commitment to preserving life would not allow them to perform this action.
- Others fear acts will be interpreted in a way there is risk for prosecution for a criminal act.

3. In responding to Mrs K.L.'s request concerning her husband's suffering:

- This scenario raises the issue of "hastening death"; there are definite clinical circumstances whereby it is very important to inform patients/family members regarding the legalities surrounding this issue, but it is unlikely necessary for a scenario such as this.
- The "in the moment" response to the wife may simply be seeking to better understand her perspective.
- The best approach to management is likely to involve effectively addressing symptoms associated with delirium (see question 3 above in the question and answer section).
- Although delirium may never be normal, even at the end of life, it is important to remember agitation secondary to delirium is an anticipated symptom associated with dying; the degree to which physicians search for the cause of the underlying delirium may be different depending on the patient's location in the trajectory of his or her illness.
- In this example, it is felt that there is no further treatment that can be offered to improve the patient's cardiac status and that he is dying of terminal CAD; therefore, it is imperative the symptoms of delirium be treated with the appropriate antipsychotic medication, opioids (to treat pain or dyspnea), and benzodiazepines if necessary in order to control agitation.

- Effective symptom management is essential not only for the patient but for the wife who wants to ensure her husband is not suffering in his final hours.

4. Concerning the patient in scenario 2, it will be prudent to evaluate the BPSD, do a delirium work-up, and discuss palliative sedation therapy. (Kapo, Morrison, & Liao, 2007)

- For the evaluation of BPSD and work-up of delirium:
  - The degree of investigation will be somewhat dependent on the survival estimate; underlying etiologies that can be immediately treated include pain, urinary retention, and constipation (see question 3 above).
  - Providing support to the family while addressing the patient's symptoms is very important; speak to the patient's wife about prior expressed wishes and try to reach consensus on a treatment approach with her.
  - Communicate both hope and optimism; the patient will likely be aware and able to understand at the end of life.
  - Pain should be excluded at this stage and treated appropriately if present; assessing pain in this patient may require careful attention to nonverbal cues and/or subjective reports from the caregiver.
  - If the atypical antipsychotic is not helpful, a trial of haloperidol for agitation can be initiated while awaiting results of investigation.
  - Differentiating pain from agitation in this context can be difficult; however, some tools are available including the PAINAD, Adult Faces Scale, MOBID-2, and PACSLAC.
    - Example: PAINAD: assign 0, 1, or 2 for (I) severity of breathing, (II) vocalization, (III) facial expression, (IV) body language, and (V) consolability; total score out of 10 provides the pain rating (Zwakhalen, van der Steen, & Najim, 2012).
  - Identifying causes of delirium may be inconsistent with the patient's goals of care, and may be inappropriate for patients with a likely survival duration of hours to days or, in some cases, days to weeks; in these cases, treating the agitation rather than the underlying cause would be most appropriate.
  - "Terminal delirium" is a diagnosis made in the hours to days prior to death, with the most common symptoms being somnolence, communication difficulty, memory disturbance, thinking difficulty, and disorientation; in general, the level of distress present determines the management approach.
- Palliative sedation therapy:
  - Given the attention palliative sedation therapy has recently received in the media (often accompanying discussions addressing euthanasia and physician-hastened death), be sure to be clear on definitions (Dean et al., 2012).
  - Palliative sedation therapy is the use of controlled sedation for the management of symptoms that are both intolerable and refractory to all other interventions. It is important to distinguish between a difficult/complex and a refractory symptom.
    - A refractory symptom is one for which there has been insufficient relief despite aggressive efforts short of sedation, and any additional treatments are not thought to be capable of providing relief.
    - As an example, if a patient has severe intractable pain and all treatment including opioids and adjuvant therapies have been used, it may be decided that the only way to relieve this intractable symptom is

to decrease the patient's awareness of the symptom, i.e., sedate the patient. This would be considered palliative sedation. In contrast, when managing delirium, "sedation" may be an outcome of the delirium management, but not necessarily the intent. This treatment would not be considered palliative sedation.

- Palliative sedation therapy is most often used very near the end of life (i.e., likely survival of a small number of weeks).
  - A key element often overlooked is the requirement of patient/SDM consent.
  - Many protocols have psychological and spiritual assessments by skilled clinicians/clergy as elements.
  - The historical ethical debate has centred on the possibility that palliative sedation therapy hastens death. However, the ethical principle of double effect is of greatest significance, as the intent of palliative sedation therapy is relief from the associated intractable suffering.

Note to readers: At the time of publication, medical assistance in dying (MAID) had been decriminalized in Canada. However, federal and provincial legislation had not yet been passed. As a result this section has limited content on this topic.

RECOMMENDED RESOURCES FOR REVIEW

Although these resources may not be specifically cited in the text, their approach informed the contents of the chapter, and they are recommended as useful further reading.

Branigan M. Desire for hastened death: exploring the emotions and the ethics. Curr Opin Support Palliat Care. 2015;9(1) 64–71. http://dx.doi.org/10.1097/SPC.0000000000000109. Medline:25581449

Kapo J, Morrison LJ, Liao S. Palliative care for the older adult. J Palliat Med. 2007;10(1):185–209. http://dx.doi.org/10.1089/jpm.2006.9989. Medline:17298269

Zimmerman K, Rudolph J, Salow M, et al. Delirium in palliative care patients: focus on pharmacotherapy. Am J Hosp Palliat Care. 2011;28(7):501–10. http://dx.doi.org/10.1177/1049909111403732. Medline:21454319

REFERENCES

American Geriatrics Society (AGS) Panel on Persistent Pain in Older Adults. The management of persistent pain in older adults. J Am Geriatr Soc. 2002;50(S6):S205–24. http://dx.doi.org/10.1046/j.1532-5415.50.6s.1.x. Medline:12067390

Dean MM, Cellarius V, Henry B, et al.; Canadian Society of Palliative Care Physicians Taskforce. Framework for continuous palliative sedation therapy in Canada. J Palliat Med. 2012;15(8):870–9. http://dx.doi.org/10.1089/jpm.2011.0498. Medline:22747192

Gordon M, Grossman D. Ethical and legal implications of pacemaker withdrawal toward the end of life. Ann Longterm Care. 2015;23(10):35–9.

Noorani NH, Montagnini M. Recognizing depression in palliative care patients. J Palliat Med. 2007;10(2):458–64. http://dx.doi.org/10.1089/jpm.2006.0099. Medline:17472517

Rayner L, Price A, Hotopf M, et al. Expert opinion on detecting and treating depression in palliative care: a Delphi study. BMC Palliat Care. 2011;10(1):10. http://dx.doi.org/10.1186/1472-684X-10-10. http://www.ncbi.nlm.nih.gov/pubmed/21619580Medline:21619580

World Health Organization. WHO definition of palliative care. World Health Organization [website], 2016. http://www.who.int/cancer/palliative/definition/en/

Zwakhalen SM, van der Steen JT, Najim MD. Which score most likely represents pain on the observational PAINAD pain scale for patients with dementia? J Am Med Dir Assoc. 2012;13(4):384–9. http://dx.doi.org/10.1016/j.jamda.2011.04.002. Medline:21640656

4.7 What Else?

Although this book covers a huge array of topics in geriatric psychiatry, it has been impossible to assemble a comprehensive brief review of all topics. In recognition of this, we are providing a list of up-to-date reference articles that give a helpful review of topics that we have left out or covered only in a cursory fashion in this book.

Topic	References
Successful aging	Depp C, Vahia IV, Jeste D. Successful aging: focus on cognitive and emotional health. Annu Rev Clin Psychol. 2010;6:527–50. PMID:20192798
Psychosocial factors in aging	Larzelere MM, Campbell J, Adu-Aarkodie NY. Psychosocial factors in aging. Clin Geriatr Med. 2011;27(4):645–60. PMID:22062446
Pharmacological treatment of behavioural disturbances of dementia (other than antipsychotics covered in chapter 4.3)	Sink KM, Holden KF, Yaffe K. Pharmacological treatment of neuropsychiatric symptoms of dementia: a review of the evidence. JAMA. 2005;293(5):596–608. PMID:15687315
• Antidepressants in dementia	Nelson JC, Devanand DP. A systematic review and meta-analysis of placebo-controlled antidepressant studies in people with depression and dementia. J Am Geriatr Soc. 2011;59(4):577–85. PMID:21453380
	Porsteinsson AP, Drye LT, Pollock BG, et al. Effect of citalopram on agitation in Alzheimer disease: the CitAD randomized clinical trial. JAMA. 2014;311(7):682–91. PMID:24549548
	Seitz DP, Adunuri N, Gill SS, et al. Antidepressants for agitation and psychosis in dementia. Cochrane Database Syst Rev. 2011;16;(2): CD008191. PMID:21328305
• Anticonvulsants in dementia	Gallagher D, Herrmann N. Antiepileptic drugs for the treatment of agitation and aggression in dementia: do they have a place in therapy? Drugs. 2014;74(15):1747–55. PMID:25239267
• Psychostimulants in dementia	Mitchell RA, Herrmann N, Lanctôt KL. The role of dopamine in symptoms and treatment of apathy in Alzheimer's disease. CNS Neurosci Ther. 2011; 17(5):411–27. PMID:20560994
	Rosenberg PB, Lanctôt KL, Drye LT, et al. Safety and efficacy of methylphenidate for apathy in Alzheimer's disease: a randomized, placebo-controlled trial. J Clin Psychiatry. 2013;74(8):810–6. PMID:24021498
Neuroimaging in dementia	Tang-Wai DF. A quick guide for neuroimaging of common dementias seen in clinical practice. Canadian Geriatrics Society Journal of CME. 2012;2(1):18–25.

Topic	References
Dysthymia and subsyndromal depression in the elderly	Meeks TW, Vahia IV, Lavretsky H, et al. A tune in "a minor" can "b major": a review of epidemiology, illness course, and public health implications of subthreshold depression in older adults. J Affect Disord. 2011;129(1–3):126–42. PMID:20926139
Cognitive dysfunction in major depression in the elderly	Wilkins CH, Mathews J, Sheline YI. Late life depression with cognitive impairment: evaluation and treatment. Clin Interv Aging. 2009;4:51–7. PMID:19503765
Screening tools for depression	Dennis M, Kadri A, Coffey J. Depression in older people in the general hospital: a systematic review of screening instruments. Age Ageing. 2012; 41(2):148–54. PMID:22236655
Neurological examination in geriatric psychiatry	Gladstone DJ, Black SE. The neurological examination in aging, dementia and cerebrovascular disease. Geriatr & Aging. 2002;5(7):36–57.
Alcohol and substance disorders in older adults	Han B, Gfroerer JC, Colliver JD, et al. Substance use disorder among older adults in the United States in 2020. Addiction. 2009:104(1):88–96. PMID:19133892
	Oslin DW. Late-life alcoholism: issues relevant to the geriatric psychiatrist. Am J Geriatr Psychiatry. 2004;12(6):571–83. PMID:15545325
Depression and macular degeneration in older adults	Casten RJ, Rovner BW. Update on depression and age-related macular degeneration. Curr Opin Ophthalmol. 2013;24(3):239–43. PMID:23429599
Seizure disorders in older adults	McLaughlin DP, Pachana NA, McFarland K. The impact of depression, seizure variables and locus of control on healthv related quality of life in a community dwelling sample of older adults. Seizure. 2010;19(4):232–6. PMID:20338790
Chronic pain management in older adults	Fine PG. Treatment guidelines for the pharmacological management of pain in older persons. Pain Med. 2012;13(Suppl 2):S57–66. PMID:22497749
	McGuire BE, Nicholas MK, Asghari A, et al. The effectiveness of psychological treatments for chronic pain in older adults: cautious optimism and an agenda for research. Curr Opin Psychiatry. 2014;27(5):380–4. PMID:25010990
Diabetes and psychiatric disorders in older adults	Alagiakrishnan K, Sclater A. Psychiatric disorders presenting in the elderly with type 2 diabetes mellitus. Am J Geriatr Psychiatry. 2012;20(8):645–52. PMID:21989315
Frailty in older adults	Andrew MK, Rockwood K. Psychiatric illness in relation to frailty in community-dwelling elderly people without dementia: a report from the Canadian Study of Health and Aging. Can J Aging. 2007;26(1):33–8.
	Clegg A, Young J, Iliffe S, et al. Frailty in elderly people. Lancet. 2013;381(9868):752–62. PMID:23395245
Falls and incontinence in older adults	Carlson C, Merel SE, Yukawa M. Geriatric syndromes and geriatric assessment for the generalist. Med Clin North Am. 2015;99(2):263–79. PMID:25700583
	Denkinger MD, Lukas A, Nikolaus T, et al. Factors associated with fear of falling and associated activity restriction in community-dwelling older adults: a systematic review. Am J Geriatr Psychiatry. 2015;23(1):72–86. PMID:24745560
	Vaughan CP, Goode PS, Burgio KL, et al. Urinary incontinence in older adults. Mt Sinai J Med. 2011;78(4):558–70. PMID:21748744

Abbreviations

3MSE	Modified Mini Mental State Examination
5-HT	serotonin (5-hydroxytryptamine)
AA	anticholinergic activity
AAN	American Academy of Neurology
ACE	angiotensin-converting enzyme
ACEI	angiotensin-converting enzyme inhibitor
Ach	acetylcholine
AChE	acetylcholinesterase
AChEI	acetylcholinesterase inhibitor
AD	Alzheimer's disease
ADAMS	Aging, Demographics, and Memory Study
ADL	activity of daily living
ADS	Anticholinergic Drug Scale
AE	adverse event
AGS	American Geriatrics Society
APOE	apolipoprotein E
ASA	acetylsalicylic acid
BAI	Beck Anxiety Inventory
BBB	blood-brain barrier
BDI	Beck Depression Inventory
BDNF	brain-derived neurotrophic factor
BEDS	Brief Edinburgh Depression Scale
BEHAVE-AD	behavioural pathology in Alzheimer's disease
BF	bifrontal
BMI	body mass index
BMT	behavioural management therapy
BNA	behavioural neurology assessment
BP	blood pressure
BPSD	behavioural and psychological symptoms of dementia
BRD	bereavement-related depression
BT	bitemporal
BuChE	butyrylcholinesterase
bvFTD	behavioural variant frontotemporal dementia
CAA	cerebral amyloid angiopathy
CABG	coronary artery bypass graft
CAC	Clinical Assessment of Confusion
CAD	coronary artery disease

CADRES	Caring for Aged in Dementia Care Resident Study
CAGP	Canadian Academy of Geriatric Psychiatry
CAM	Confusion Assessment Method
CAMI-SF	Columbia Autobiographical Memory Interview – Short Form
CANECTS	Canadian Electroconvulsive Therapy Survey
CANMAT	Canadian Network for Mood and Anxiety Treatments
CAT	choline acetyltransferase
CATIE-AD	Clinical Antipsychotic Trials of Intervention Effectiveness – Alzheimer's Disease
CBC	complete blood count
CBS	corticobasilar degeneration syndrome
CBT	cognitive behavioural therapy
CBT-I	cognitive behavioural therapy of insomnia
CCCDTD3	3rd Canadian Consensus Conference on the Diagnosis and Treatment of Dementia
CCCDTD4	4th Canadian Consensus Conference on the Diagnosis and Treatment of Dementia
CCHS	Canadian Community Health Survey
CCSMH	Canadian Coalition for Seniors' Mental Health
CCU	coronary care unit
CDT	clock drawing test
CG	complicated grief
CGI	Clinical Global Improvement
CGT	complicated grief treatment
ChAT	choline acetyltransferase
ChEI	cholinesterase inhibitor
CHF	congestive heart failure
CI	confidence interval
CIHR	Canadian Institutes of Health Research
CIND	cognitive impairment no dementia
CIWA-Ar	Clinical Institute Withdrawal Assessment of Alcohol Scale, Revised
CKD	chronic kidney disease
CMAI	Cohen-Mansfield Agitation Inventory
CNS	central nervous system
COPD	chronic obstructive pulmonary disease
CORE	Consortium of Researchers for ECT
CPAP	continuous positive airway pressure
CPG	clinical practice guideline
CrCl	creatinine clearance
CRF	corticotropin-releasing factor
CSA	central sleep apnea
CSDD	Cornell Scale for Depression in Dementia
CSF	cerebrospinal fluid
CSHA	Canadian Study of Health and Aging
CT	computerized tomography
CVA	cerebrovascular accident
CVAE	cerebrovascular adverse event
CYP450	cytochrome P450
DA	dopamine
DART-AD	Dementia Antipsychotic Withdrawal Trial

DDI	drug-drug interaction
DIMS-R	drugs, infection, metabolic, structural, retention
DLB	dementia with Lewy bodies
DLPFC	dorsolateral prefrontal cortex
DM	diabetes mellitus
DOPA	dihydroxyphenylalanine
DOS	Dementia Observation System
DOSS	Delirium Observation Screening Scale
DRS-R-98	Delirium Rating Scale Revised-98
DSM	Diagnostic and Statistical Manual of Mental Disorders
DWMH	deep white matter hyperintensities
ECA	Epidemiologic Catchment Area Study
ECG	electrocardiogram
ECT	electroconvulsive therapy
EEG	electroencephalogram
eGFR	estimated glomerular filtration rate
EMDR	eye-movement desensitization reprocessing
EPS	extrapyramidal symptoms
ESA	Enquête sur la Santé des Aînés Study
ESAS	Edmonton Symptom Assessment Scale
ESL	English as a second language
FAB	Frontal Assessment Battery
FBG	fasting blood glucose
FDA	Food and Drug Administration (US)
FDG	fluorodeoxyglucose
FFT	family-focused therapy
FTD	frontotemporal dementia
FTD-MND	frontotemporal dementia with motor neuron disease
FTLD	frontotemporal lobar degeneration
GABA	γ-aminobutyric acid
GAD	generalized anxiety disorder
GAR	Global Attentiveness Rating
GCS	Glasgow Coma Scale
GDS	Geriatric Depression Scale
GFR	glomerular filtration rate
GHB	gammahydroxybutyrate
GI	gastrointestinal
GMC	general medical condition
GPCOG	General Practitioner Assessment of Cognition
GPS	Gerontological Personality Disorder Scale
GSIS	Geriatric Suicide Ideation Scale
GSK	glycogen synthase kinase
HADS	Hospital Anxiety and Depression Scale
HAM-A	Hamilton Rating Scale for Anxiety
HAM-D	Hamilton Rating Scale for Depression
HBS	Harmful Behaviours Scale
HELP	Hospital Elder Life Program
HIV	human immunodeficiency virus
HPA	hypothalamic-pituitary-adrenal
HR	hazard ratio

HVA	homovanillic acid
IADLs	instrumental activities of daily living
ICD	impulse control disorder
ICG	Inventory of Complicated Grief
IM	intramuscular
IMPACT	Improving Mood-Promoting Access to Collaborative Treatment
IPA	International Psychogeriatric Association
IPT	interpersonal psychotherapy
ISDB	indirect self-destructive behaviours
ISEN	International Society of ECT and Neurostimulation
IV	intravenous
KT	knowledge translation
LASA	Longitudinal Aging Study Amsterdam
LBBB	left bundle branch block
LTC	long-term care
lvPPA	logopenic variant primary progressive aphasia
MADRS	Montgomery-Åsberg Depression Rating Scale
MAID	medical assistance in dying
MAO	monoamine oxidase
MAOI	monoamine oxidase inhibitor
MB	microbleed
MCI	mild cognitive impairment
MCV	mean corpuscular volume
MDAS	Memorial Delirium Assessment Scale
MDD	major depressive disorder
MDE	major depressive episode
MI	myocardial infarction
MMSE	Mini Mental State Examination
MoCA	Montreal Cognitive Assessment
MRI	magnetic resonance imaging
MTA	medial temporal lobe atrophy
MTL	medial temporal lobe
NAMCS	National Ambulatory Medical Care Surveys (US)
NbM	nucleus basalis of Meynert
NCD	neurocognitive disorder
NCS-R	National Comorbidity Study – Replication Study
NDI	nephrogenic diabetes insipidus
NE	norepinephrine
nfPPA	non-fluent primary progressive aphasia
NICE	National Institute for Health and Clinical Excellence (UK)
NMDA	N-methyl-D-aspartate
NMS	neuroleptic malignant syndrome
NNH	number needed to harm
NNT	number needed to treat
NPH	normal pressure hydrocephalus
NPI	Neuropsychiatric Inventory
NPS	neuropsychiatric symptoms
NPV	negative predictive value
NREM	non-rapid eye movement
NSAID	non-steroidal anti-inflammatory drug

OA	osteoarthritis
OCD	obsessive-compulsive disorder
OR	odds ratio
OSA	obstructive sleep apnea
OSAH	obstructive sleep apnea/hypopnea
PACSLAC	Pain Assessment Checklist for Seniors with Limited Ability to Communicate
PAINAD	Pain Assessment in Advanced Dementia
PANSS	Positive and Negative Syndrome Scale
PATH	problem adaptation therapy
PCBD	persistent complex bereavement disorder
PCC	person-centred care
PD	Parkinson's disease
PDD	Parkinson's disease dementia
PET	positron emission tomography
PGD	prolonged grief disorder
PHQ-2	Patient Health Questionnaire-2
PIM	potentially inappropriate medication
PLM	periodic limb movement
PO	by mouth
POA	power of attorney
PP	psychodynamic psychotherapy
PPA	primary progressive aphasia
PPI	proton pump inhibitor
PPV	positive predictive value
PQoL	perceived quality of life
PRIDE	Prolonged Remission in Depressed Elderly Trial
PROSPECT	Prevention of Suicide in Primary Care Elderly: Collaborative Trial
PSD	post-stroke depression
PSP	progressive supranuclear palsy
PST	problem-solving therapy
PTH	parathyroid hormone
PTSD	post-traumatic stress disorder
PVD	peripheral vascular disease
QOL	quality of life
RAVLT	Rey Auditory Verbal Learning Test
RBD	REM sleep behaviour disorder
RCT	randomized controlled trial
REM	rapid eye movement
RFL-OA	Reasons for Living Scale – Older Adults
RLS	restless legs syndrome
ROC	receiver operating characteristics
RP	reminiscence psychotherapy
RR	relative risk
rTMS	repetitive transcranial magnetic stimulation
RUDAS	Rowland Universal Dementia Assessment Scale
RUL	right unilateral
SAMHSA	Substance Abuse and Mental Health Services Administration
SBPW	standard/brief pulse width
SC	subcutaneous

SCIE	Social Care Institute for Excellence
SD	standard deviation
SDH	subdural hemorrhage
SDM	substitute decision maker
SES	socioeconomic status
SH	sleep hygiene
SHAFT	shopping, housework/hobbies, accounting, food preparation, transportation (ADLs)
SIADH	syndrome of inappropriate antidiuretic hormone secretion
SIB	Severe Impairment Battery
SIS	Suicidal Ideation Scale
SL	sublingually
SMILE	Sydney Multisite Intervention for LaughterBosses and ElderClowns
sMMSE	standardized MMSE scoring
SNRI	serotonin norepinephrine reuptake inhibitor
SOAP	Suicidal Older Adults Protocol
SPECT	single-photon emission computerized tomography
SSRI	selective serotonin reuptake inhibitor
ST	seizure threshold
STI	Serial Trial Intervention
SUDS	Subjective Units of Distress Scale
svPPA	semantic variant primary progressive aphasia
TBI	traumatic brain injury
TCA	tricyclic antidepressant
TD	tardive dyskinesia
TIA	transient ischemic attack
TIP	treatment initiation and participation
TREA	Treatment Routes for Exploring Agitation
TSH	thyroid stimulating hormone
TURP	transurethral resection of prostate
UBPW	ultrabrief pulse width
USPSTF	United States Preventive Services Task Force
UTI	urinary tract infection
VaD	vascular dementia
VCI	vascular cognitive impairment
Vd	volume of distribution
VDRL	venereal disease research laboratory (test)
WBC	white blood count
WHO	World Health Organization
WMD	weighted mean difference
XR	extended release

Authors and Affiliations

Daniel M. Blumberger, *MD, MSc, FRCPC*, Medical Head, Temerty Centre for Therapeutic Brain Intervention, Centre for Addiction and Mental Health; Associate Professor, Department of Psychiatry, University of Toronto, Toronto, Ontario.

Keri-Leigh Cassidy, *MD, FRCPC*, Professor, Department of Psychiatry, Dalhousie University, Halifax, Nova Scotia.

Peter Chan, *MD, FRCPC*, Geriatric and Consultation-Liaison Psychiatrist, Neurostimulation Program Medical Head, Vancouver General and UBC Health Science Hospitals; Clinical Professor, Department of Psychiatry, University of British Columbia, Vancouver, British Columbia.

Carole Cohen, *MD, FRCPC*, Professor, Psychiatry, University of Toronto, Sunnybrook Health Sciences Centre, Toronto, Ontario.

Jonathan Fleming, *MB, FRCPC*, Associate Professor Emeritus, Associate Head, Education Department of Psychiatry, University of British Columbia, Vancouver, British Columbia.

Janya Freer, *MD, FRCPC*, Assistant Professor, Department of Psychiatry, Dalhousie University, Halifax, Nova Scotia.

Laura Gage, *MD, FRCPC*, Assistant Professor, Psychiatry, University of Toronto, Toronto East General Hospital, Toronto, Ontario.

Sudeep S. Gill, *MD, MSc, FRCPC*, Associate Professor, Department of Medicine (Division of Geriatric Medicine), Queen's University, Kingston, Ontario.

Cindy Grief, *MD, MSc, FRCPC*, Assistant Professor, Psychiatry, University of Toronto; Medical Director for Mental Health, Baycrest Health Sciences, Toronto, Ontario.

Daphna Grossman, *MD, CCFP(PC), FCFP*, Assistant Professor, Division of Palliative Care, Department of Family and Community Medicine, University of Toronto, North York General Hospital, Toronto, Ontario.

Marnin J. Heisel, *PhD*, *CPsych*, Associate Professor, Departments of Psychiatry and Epidemiology & Biostatistics, The University of Western Ontario; Director of Research, Department of Psychiatry, The University of Western Ontario; Scientist, Lawson Health Research Institute , London, Ontario; Adjunct Faculty, Center for the Study and Prevention of Suicide, University of Rochester Medical Center, Rochester , New York.

Nathan Herrmann, *MD*, *FRCPC*, Head, Division of Geriatric Psychiatry, Sunnybrook Health Sciences Centre; Professor, Faculty of Medicine, University of Toronto, Toronto, Ontario.

Maria Hussain, *MD*, *FRCPC*, Assistant Professor, Department of Psychiatry, Queen's University, Kingston, Ontario.

Benoit H. Mulsant, *MD*, *MS*, *FRCPC*, Professor and Chair, Department of Psychiatry, University of Toronto; Senior Scientist, Centre for Addiction and Mental Health, Toronto, Ontario.

Jeff Myers, *MD*, *MSEd*, *CCFP(PC)*, W. Gifford-Jones Professor in Pain and Palliative Care, Head and Associate Professor – Division of Palliative Care, Department of Family and Community Medicine, Faculty of Medicine, University of Toronto; Head – Palliative Care Consult Team, Sunnybrook Health Sciences Centre, Toronto, Ontario.

Tarek K. Rajji, *MD*, *FRCPC*, Canada Research Chair in Neurostimulation for Cognitive Disorders; Chief, Geriatric Psychiatry Division, Centre for Addiction and Mental Health; Associate Professor of Psychiatry, University of Toronto, Toronto, Ontario.

Mark J. Rapoport, *MD*, *FRCPC*, Associate Professor of Psychiatry, University of Toronto; Staff Psychiatrist, Sunnybrook Health Sciences Centre, Toronto, Ontario.

Suzane Renaud, *MD*, *CRCP(P)*, *CSMQ*, *LDFAPA*, *FCPA-APC*, Associate Professor of Psychiatry, McGill University, Montreal, Quebec.

Dallas Seitz, *MD*, *PhD*, *FRCPC*, Associate Professor, Division of Geriatric Psychiatry, Queen's University, Kingston, Ontario.

Kenneth Shulman, *MD*, *FRCPC*, Professor, Department of Psychiatry, University of Toronto; Staff Psychiatrist, Sunnybrook Health Sciences Centre, Toronto, Ontario.

Andrew Wiens, *MD*, *FRCPC*, Associate Professor and Head, Division of Geriatric Psychiatry, Department of Psychiatry, University of Ottawa, Ottawa, Ontario.

Lesley Wiesenfeld, *MD*, *FRCPC*, Associate Professor, Department of Psychiatry, Mount Sinai Hospital, University of Toronto, Toronto, Ontario.

Disclosures

The authors were asked to disclose any relationships from industry, peer-reviewed funding, or other sources that may impact the content of their chapter.

Daniel M. Blumberger, *MD, MSc, FRCPC*: Received research support from the Canadian Institutes of Health Research (CIHR), National Institute of Health (NIH), Brain Canada and the Temerty family through the Centre for Addiction and Mental Health (CAMH) Foundation, and the Campbell Research Institute. He received research operating fund support and in-kind equipment support for an investigator-initiated study from Brainsway Ltd., and is the site principal investigator for three sponsor-initiated studies for Brainsway Ltd. He has received in-kind equipment support from Magventure for an investigator-initiated study. He has received medication supplies for an investigator-initiated trial from Invidior.

Keri-Leigh Cassidy, *MD, FRCPC*: None.

Peter Chan, *MD, FRCPC*: None.

Carole Cohen, *MD, FRCPC*: Consulting fees, Capacity Assessment Office, Ministry of the Attorney General of Ontario.

Jonathan Fleming, *MB, FRCPC*: None.

Janya Freer, *MD, FRCPC*: None.

Laura Gage, *MD, FRCPC*: None.

Sudeep S. Gill, *MD, MSc, FRCPC*: None.

Cindy Grief, *MD, MSc, FRCPC*: None.

Daphna Grossman, *MD, CCFP(PC), FCFP*: None.

Marnin J. Heisel, *PhD*, *CPsych*: No financial or in-kind support from outside organizations. Co-developed the Geriatric Suicide Ideation Scale (GSIS), co-led the development of the Canadian Coalition for Seniors' Mental Health (CCSMH) late-life suicide prevention knowledge translation toolkit, paid expert witness for the Canadian Federal Department of Justice in 2011–2012 litigation on assisted suicide. Received research funds from CIHR, SSHRC, the Ontario Ministry of Research, Innovation and Science, the Ontario Mental Health Foundation, the American Foundation for Suicide Prevention, Movember Canada, the Lawson Health Research Institute, and the Departments of Psychiatry at the University of Western Ontario and the University of Rochester. 2008 American Foundation for Suicide Prevention/Pfizer travel award to present AFSP-funded research at the American Association of Suicidology annual conference. Co–principal investigator on a grant funded by OSSU (the Ontario SPOR Support Unit).

Nathan Herrmann, *MD*, *FRCPC*: Research support from Lundbeck, Sanofi-Aventis, Roche, and Elan, and Honoraria from Pfizer and Lundbeck.

Maria Hussain, *MD*, *FRCPC*: None.

Benoit H. Mulsant, *MD*, *MS*, *FRCPC*: Grants/Research support from Brain Canada, Canadian Institute of Health Research, National Institute of Health, and several foundations; Bristol-Myers Squibb (current), Eli Lilly (2008), and Pfizer (current) have provided medications (or matched placebo pills) for NIMH-funded clinical trials; travel support from Roche in 2011.

Jeff Myers, *MD*, *MSEd*, *CCFP(PC)*: None.

Mark J. Rapoport, *MD*, *FRCPC*: Research funding from Alzheimer Society of Canada and Transport Canada. Canadian Institute of Health Research.

Tarek K. Rajji, *MD*, *FRCPC*: During the past five years received research support from Brain Canada, Brain and Behavior Research Foundation, Canada Foundation for Innovation, Canada Research Chair, Canadian Institutes of Health Research, Ontario Ministry of Health and Long-Term Care, Ontario Ministry of Research and Innovation, the US National Institute of Health, and the W. Garfield Weston Foundation. Dr Rajji reports no competing interests.

Suzane Renaud, *MD*, *CRCP(P)*, *CSMQ*, *LDFAPA*, *FCPA-APC*: None.

Dallas Seitz, *MD*, *PhD*, *FRCPC*: Eli Lilly Advisory Board.

Kenneth Shulman, *MD*, *FRCPC*: None.

Andrew Wiens, *MD*, *FRCPC*: None.

Lesley Wiesenfeld, *MD*, *FRCPC*: None.

9 781442 628274